POCKET CONSULTANT

Gastroenterology

S.P.L. Travis MB MRCP
Lecturer in Gastroenterology
Radcliffe Infirmary and Linacre College, Oxford

R.H. Taylor BSc MD FRCP
Professor of Medicine and Consultant Gastroenterologist
Royal Naval Hospital
Haslar, Gosport

J.J. Misiewicz BSc FRCP
Joint Director
Department of Gastroenterology and Nutrition
Central Middlesex Hospital
London

PRESENTED WITH

THE COMPLIMENTS OF

Glaxo Laboratories

OXFORD

Blackwell Scientific Publications

LONDON EDINBURGH BOSTON

MELBOURNE PARIS BERLIN VIENNA

© 1991 by
Blackwell Scientific Publications
Editorial Offices:
Osney Mead, Oxford OX2 0EL
25 John Street, London WC1N 2BL
23 Ainslie Place, Edinburgh EH3 6AJ
238 Main Street, Cambridge,
  Massachusetts 02142, USA
54 University Street, Carlton,
  Victoria 3053, Australia

Other Editorial Offices:

Librairie Arnette SA
2 rue Casimir-Delavigne
75006 Paris
France

Blackwell Wissenschafts-Verlag
Meinekestrasse 4
D-1000 Berlin 15
Germany

Blackwell MZV
Feldgasse 13
A-1238 Wien
Austria

First published 1991
Reprinted 1993

Set by Semantic Graphics, Singapore
Printed and bound in Great Britain
by The Alden Press, Oxford

DISTRIBUTORS

Marston Book Services Ltd
PO Box 87
Oxford OX2 0DT
(*Orders*: Tel: 0865 791155
    Fax: 0865 791927
    Telex: 837515)

USA
Blackwell Scientific Publications, Inc.
238 Main Street
Cambridge, MA 02142
(*Orders*: Tel: 800 759-6102
    617 876-7000)

Canada
Times Mirror Professional Publishing, Ltd
130 Flaska Drive
Markham, Ontario L6G 1B8
(*Orders*: Tel: 800 268-4178
    416 470-6739)

Australia
Blackwell Scientific Publications Pty Ltd
54 University Street
Carlton, Victoria 3053
(*Orders*: Tel: 03 347-5552)

British Library
Cataloguing in Publication Data

Travis, S. P. L.
    Pocket consultant in gastroenterology.
    I. Title II. Taylor, R. H.
    III. Misiewicz, J. J.
    616.33

    ISBN 0-632-01098-3

Contents

Preface

This book is for House Officers on the wards, Senior House Officers or Registrars involved in outpatient clinics, and General Practitioners in their surgeries. The purpose is to provide a practical, concise text on gastroenterology. It will, we hope, be a useful guide and checklist when dealing with unfamiliar situations, and an *aide mémoire* before follow-up consultations, ward rounds, or discussion with senior colleagues. It should also help junior doctors in the management of emergency and elective admissions of patients with alimentary diseases. The style is terse and somewhat dogmatic by necessity, but we have attempted to address common clinical dilemmas.

We are most grateful to our colleagues, listed below, who have helped by reading drafts of the text or by making suggestions; we are, however, solely responsible for any errors. Above all, our thanks go to our families for their forbearance, patience and support.

Acknowledgements
Mrs E.M. Bardolph SRN SEN, Dr G.C. Cook DSc MD FRCP,
Mr C.W. Imrie BSc FRCS, Miss R. James BSc,
Dr D.P. Jewell DPhil FRCP, Dr D. Loft MD MRCP,
Dr A.R.O. Miller MA MRCP DTM & H, Dr D.J. Nolan MD FRCR,
Dr R.P.H. Thompson DM FRCP, Dr C.B. Williams MD FRCP.

The following illustrations are published with the kind permission of Gower Medical Publishing: Figs 1.1, 1.3, 2.1, 2.3–2.5, 3.1, 3.3, 4.2, 6.5, 7.4, 7.5, 8.2, 9.1, 9.3, 9.5.

1 Alimentary Emergencies

1.1 Swallowed foreign body

Children, the mentally handicapped and the elderly most commonly swallow foreign bodies. If no history is available, look for excessive salivation, regurgitation, or chest pain. Objects impact in the pharynx, lower end of the oesophagus, or pylorus. Once through the pylorus, spontaneous passage is the rule.

All patients
• Look in the mouth
• If the object is impacted in the fauces, call the ENT surgeons
• X-ray the chest and abdomen
• Look for surgical emphysema, mediastinal and sub-diaphragmatic gas on X-ray
• Arrange an urgent Gastrografin swallow if the object cannot be seen on plain films

Bones, pins and glass
• Sharp objects should be removed by an experienced endoscopist, unless they have passed the pylorus
• A plastic sleeve over the endoscope helps prevent trauma during withdrawal

Coins and beads
• Almost always pass spontaneously
• Reassure the patient or parents and advise them to check stools for 3 days
• Repeat abdominal X-ray after 36 hours if there is doubt about progress

Body-packing (ingested packets of drugs)
• Smuggled packets of drugs may be swallowed, or secreted per rectum, or per vaginam
• Intact packets can cause intestinal obstruction
• Burst packets cause life-threatening overdose
• Heroin overdose causes constricted pupils, bradypnoea, or coma. Hypoglycaemia or non-cardiogenic pulmonary oedema may occur later. Give intravenous naloxone 0.8 mg rapidly, to a maximum 2.4 mg if necessary
• Cocaine causes dilated pupils, tachycardia and agitation. Convulsions, metabolic acidosis, or coma may occur. Sedate with

intravenous diazepam 5–10 mg and give oral propranolol 40 mg three times daily for a few days
• Severe overdose of any narcotic is an indication for ventilation and surgical removal of the packets, to stop drug absorption
• The doctor's immediate duty is the treatment of the patient if body-packing is discovered. Once treatment has been initiated, the local police and hospital administrator should be informed. The police will inform other authorities (such as Customs and Excise, Drug Squad)
• Questioning of the patient must wait until the patient is fit, and be sanctioned by a senior doctor. Doctors have a moral duty to ensure that the patient understands his/her legal right to consult a Crown-appointed solicitor, through an interpreter if necessary

1.2 Complete oesophageal obstruction
Bolus obstruction causes sudden, complete dysphagia for solids and liquids, with inability to swallow saliva. Food impacted against a benign or malignant stricture is the usual cause. Occasionally the presentation is delayed for a few days in the mentally handicapped or severely debilitated. The obstruction has to be relieved urgently.

Clinical features
Ask about and look for:
• Duration of symptoms preceding obstruction
• Predisposing disease (stricture, carcinoma, Schatzki ring)
• Triggering factors (steak, toast, fibrous foods, tablets)
• Dehydration
• Weight loss (suggests malignant obstruction)
• Supraclavicular nodes (from a carcinoma of the cardia)
• Complications (aspiration pneumonia, perforation)

Investigations
The endoscopist should be contacted as a priority.
• Full blood count—anaemia suggests carcinoma
• Serum electrolytes—high urea indicates dehydration
• Chest X-ray—look for a mediastinal fluid level (obstruction), absent gastric air bubble (obstruction), or right lower lobe consolidation (aspiration)
• Urgent endoscopy—must be done by an experienced endoscopist
• A barium swallow risks aspiration and is not necessary, unless

the diagnosis is in doubt. This is not the same as in dysphagia without obstruction (Section 2.1, p. 48)

Management
- Intravenous fluids
- Endoscopic removal of the obstructing bolus
- Endoscopic dilatation can be done immediately after disimpaction
- Fizzy drinks occasionally disimpact fibrous debris, but endoscopy is needed when a food bolus has been stuck for a few hours
- Fine-bore nasogastric feeding, or nutritional supplements are needed (Section 13.2, p. 376) if dilatation is delayed. Endoscopic placement of the tube is difficult, but indicated if it cannot be inserted in the normal way (p. 377)
- Intravenous metronidazole 500 mg and cefuroxime 750 mg three times daily for 5 days, if aspiration pneumonia is present

Prevention
Simple measures decrease the risk of acute obstruction in patients with oesophageal strictures or prosthetic oesophageal tubes (pp. 55 and 60)
- Avoid fibrous food (apples, oranges), steak and toast
- Wear dentures if edentulous
- Chew all solids well
- Fizzy drinks with meals
- Avoid oral potassium supplements, salicylates and large tablets
- Omeprazole 20 mg daily has not yet been shown to prevent restricturing, but will heal associated oesophagitis

1.3 Oesophageal rupture
Sudden chest pain after vomiting is the cardinal symptom when the distal posterior oesophageal wall tears longitudinally in spontaneous perforation (Boorhaeve's syndrome). Traumatic perforation after instrumentation or chest injury is more common than spontaneous rupture.

Differential diagnosis
Early diagnosis is crucial to survival. Failure to consider the possibility is the commonest reason for misdiagnosis.
- Myocardial infarction (ECG, cardiac enzymes)
- Dissecting aneurysm (pulses, chest X-ray, urgent echocardiogram)

1.3 Oesophageal rupture

- Perforated peptic ulcer (rigid, silent abdomen, erect chest X-ray)
- Acute pancreatitis (amylase >4-fold elevated)
- Spontaneous pneumothorax (chest X-ray in expiration)

Investigations
Confirm the diagnosis.
- Chest X-ray—look for mediastinal or sub-diaphragmatic gas, or a hydro/pneumothorax (Fig. 1.1)
- Gastrografin swallow—in spontaneous rupture, tears are usually large and leak contrast; after instrumental rupture, tears are often small and do not leak contrast

Management

Resuscitation
- Intravenous fluids
- Analgesia—intravenous diamorphine 2.5 mg every hour until pain relieved, then every 4 h
- Involve surgical colleagues at an early stage

Spontaneous rupture
- Nil by mouth
- Surgical repair and drainage is needed within 24 h
- Antibiotics—intravenous metronidazole 500 mg and cefuroxime 750 mg three times daily for 5 days
- Enteral nutrition through a fine-bore tube, if feeding has not restarted within 72 h. Parenteral nutrition is indicated if complications (such as mediastinitis) develop

Instrumental rupture
- Small tears (with minor symptoms and no leakage of contrast) may be managed conservatively in conjunction with the surgeons. Large tears that leak contrast are managed as for spontaneous rupture
- Nil by mouth
- Nasogastric aspiration for 3 days
- Intravenous fluids
- Antibiotics as above
- Indications for surgery are a persistent pyrexia, or pneumothorax after 48 h

1 Alimentary Emergencies

1.3 Oesophageal rupture

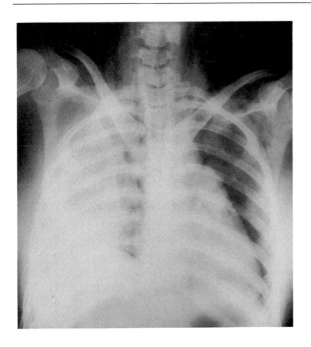

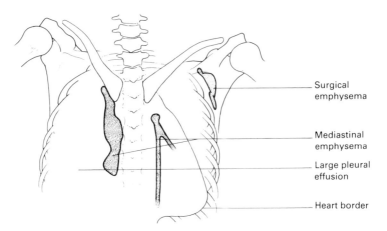

Surgical emphysema

Mediastinal emphysema

Large pleural effusion

Heart border

Fig. 1.1 Chest X-ray in oesophageal rupture showing consequences of oesophageal perforation. There is a large right pleural effusion, mediastinal emphysema and gross surgical emphysema in the neck and upper chest wall.

1.4   Acute bleeding: upper gastrointestinal tract

Most upper gastrointestinal bleeds are from chronic gastric or duodenal ulcers. An increasing proportion in the elderly are from non-steroidal anti-inflammatory drug (NSAID)-associated ulcers. Varices, Mallory–Weiss syndrome, acute haemorrhagic gastritis and some very rare causes (see Table 1.1, p. 9) cause a minority. Most bleeds from peptic ulcers stop spontaneously, but about 20% rebleed in hospital and many of these will need surgical intervention. A standard clinical approach, outlined below, is recommended for every patient, so that the patients at highest risk of rebleeding and death are identified early.

Clinical approach
- Assess severity
- Resuscitate
- Establish the site of bleeding
- Liaise with the surgical and intensive care teams on call
- Medical intervention
- Surgery when appropriate

Assessment
The aim is to identify patients at high risk of rebleeding and death, by clinical and endoscopic examination. All patients with haematemesis or melaena must be treated actively until a stable baseline has been established. There is no room for complacency.
High-risk patients are those with:
- Haematemesis with malaena—twice the mortality of either alone
- Fresh melaena
- Continued bleeding, or a rebleed in hospital
- Age >60 years, or cardiorespiratory disease—adversely affect prognosis
- Elderly female on NSAIDs
- Pulse >100 bpm—suggests the need for transfusion
- Jugular venous pressure (JVP) <1 cm with reference to the sternal angle (normal = 1–5 cm H_2O)—lie the patient flat until visible
- Poor peripheral perfusion—cool, clammy extremities
- Systolic blood pressure <100 mmHg—but it may be preserved until very late in young patients
- Endoscopic stigmata present. These are:
  active arterial bleeding (90% risk of rebleed)
  visible vessel in the ulcer base (70% risk of rebleed)

adherent clot (black dots on the ulcer base; 30% risk of rebleed)
• Oesophageal varices
Lower risk patients:
• Age <60 years
• Coffee-ground vomitus without melaena
• Alcohol induced
• Haemodynamically normal (pulse <100 bpm, JVP 1–5 cm H$_2$O, systolic BP >100 mmHg, warm peripheries)
• Endoscopic stigmata absent
In addition to a record of the assessment of the patient (pp. 8 and 9), *document the following*:
• Preceding symptoms (dyspepsia, vomiting, weight loss)
• Drug and alcohol ingestion
• Presence or absence of melaena on rectal examination
• Signs of chronic liver disease (Table 5.2, p. 139)

Causes
See Table 1.1

Table 1.1 Differential diagnosis of haematemesis or melaena

Common	Less common (<5%)	Rare (1%)
Duodenal ulcer (35%)	Duodenitis	Hereditary telangiectasia
Gastric ulcer (20%)	Oesophageal varices	Aorto-duodenal fistula
Gastric erosions (6%)	Oesophagitis	Haemostatic defect
Mallory–Weiss tear (6%)	Tumours	Pseudoxanthoma elasticum
No lesion found (20%)		Haemobilia
		Pancreatitis
		Angiodysplasia
		Portal hypertensive gastropathy

Investigations and management

Resuscitation on arrival
• Ensure a patent airway and remove false teeth
• Insert a 14 or 16 gauge intravenous cannula (grey or yellow Venflon)
• If pulse >100 bpm, give 500 ml colloid (such as Haemaccel) over 30–60 min and repeat if necessary whilst waiting for blood
• Transfuse blood until haemodynamically stable in the first few hours, because initial haemoglobin is a poor indicator of the

severity of the bleed. Subsequently transfuse up to haemoglobin of 10 g/dl. Synthetic colloid or crystalloid will cause haemodilution: 1000 ml decreases the pre-transfusion haemoglobin by about 10%
• Reserve group O rhesus negative blood for dire emergencies (such as continuing massive bleeding and systolic BP <80 mmHg despite intravenous colloid), when the risk from hypotension exceeds that from uncrossmatched blood
• Insert a urinary catheter in patients who need a central venous line (see below), to monitor urine output for haemodynamic information
• Do not insert a nasogastric tube, because this increases the risk of haemorrhage from gastric lesions
• Consider admission to intensive care unit unless *absolutely* confident that the bleed is trivial and contact surgical colleagues as soon as the patient is resuscitated

Initial investigations
• Full blood count, crossmatch, coagulation studies (when liver disease is present, or suspected) and electrolytes
• Crossmatch 1 unit for every g/dl of haemoglobin less than 14 g/dl. This is usually sufficient to replace blood already lost and allows 2 units in hand should a rebleed occur, but haemodynamic status is a better guide to transfusion requirements than measured haemoglobin
• Arterial gases in those with cardiorespiratory disease
• ECG in high-risk patients
• Chest X-ray in high-risk patients (abdominal films rarely help)

Indications for a central venous line
• Signs of a major haemorrhage (pulse >100 bpm, cool peripheries, systolic BP <100 mmHg), especially in high-risk patients (p. 8)
• Rebleed during the same admission
• Inadequate peripheral venous access
• If a central venous line is needed, monitoring in an intensive care unit is advisable because these patients have a very high risk of further bleeding. Transfer to intensive care should not delay insertion of a central venous line

Establish site of bleeding
• Arrange endoscopy after resuscitation, ideally on the next endoscopy list, within 12–24 h. Mucosal lesions and stigmata for

rebleeding are otherwise missed. Ensure that the presence or absence of stigmata (pp. 8 and 9) is recorded
• Endoscope within 4 h if oesophageal varices are strongly suspected, or if a surgical decision depends on the result
• Profuse haemorrhage may obscure the bleeding site. Gastric lavage to remove clots rarely alters management and can be hazardous. Repeat endoscopy after a further 12 h resuscitation is recommended. Immediate surgery should be a joint decision between surgeons and physicians
• Table 1.1 (p. 9) shows the differential diagnosis

Monitoring
• Pulse, blood pressure, central venous pressure and urine output hourly, until stable
• Re-examine after 4 h
• Coagulation studies if >4 units transfused
• Daily full blood count, urea and electrolytes in high-risk patients
• Keep 2 units in the blood bank for 48 h after bleeding has stopped
• Keep in hospital for 48 h after bleeding has stopped

Medical intervention
These measures are not an alternative to surgery if an operation is indicated, but may help stop bleeding or reduce the risk of rebleeding.
• Ranitidine: 50 mg, in 20 ml saline, intravenously over 2 min three times daily, in all patients. The risk of stress ulcers is decreased, but rebleeding from an existing ulcer is not affected
• Endoscopic therapy—all techniques depend on local expertise and may not be available
  sclerotherapy of varices (p. 14)
  injection of adrenaline (up to 10 ml 1:10 000) or sclerosant (up to 5 ml ethanol), around peptic ulcers
  laser photocoagulation
  thermocoagulation of peptic ulcers
• Other drugs (vasopressin or glypressin for varices, omeprazole or tranexamic acid for haemorrhagic gastritis) are occasionally indicated (p. 15). Somatostatin does not stop acute bleeding from gastroduodenal lesions, but may reduce bleeding from oesophageal varices (p. 13). Oestrogen (ethinyloestradiol 50 mg/day) may

decrease episodes of recurrent acute bleeding from angiodysplasia (such as hereditary telangiectasia)

Rebleeding
Rebleeding greatly increases mortality. Patients at high risk of rebleeding (p. 8) need to be identified and the surgeons told of their admission. Patients (especially those with more than one risk factor) are best admitted to an intensive care unit, where signs of rebleeding should be detected early. Signs of rebleeding are:
• Rise in pulse rate (a sensitive and early sign)
• Fall in central venous pressure
• Decrease in hourly urine output
• Haematemesis or melaena
• Fall in blood pressure (a late and sinister sign)
• Looking at the patient (pallor, pulse, jugular venous and arterial pressures, peripheries) is as important as looking at the charts

Indications for surgery
Contact surgical colleagues at the outset rather than when it is inevitable. The timing of operation depends on the cause of bleeding (late for erosions, earlier for ulcers) and coexisting disease. The severity of bleeding is the most important single factor.
• Severity of the bleed
• Continued bleeding after transfusing:
   6 units, age >60 years
   8 units, age <60 years
• Rebleed during the same admission
• Active bleeding at endoscopy
• A visible vessel in the ulcer base, or adherent clot, are indications for close observation rather than surgery, unless rebleeding occurs

The differential diagnosis of upper gastrointestinal bleeding is shown in Table 1.1 (p. 9). Individual topics are discussed below.

Oesophageal varices

Acute bleeding
• Resuscitate and monitor as above, but do not use intravenous saline. Dextrose, or colloid (synthetic, albumin, or blood) are indicated

1 Alimentary Emergencies

1.4 Acute bleeding: upper gastrointestinal tract

- 30% with known varices have another source of haemorrhage
- Correct disordered coagulation to International Normalized Ratio (INR) <1.5 or prothrombin time <22 sec with fresh frozen plasma
- Sclerotherapy, performed by an experienced endoscopist, at the first endoscopy is ideal
  If sclerotherapy is not available, or bleeding continues:
- Infuse vasopressin 10–20 U/h, or intravenous glypressin 2 mg bolus, then 2 mg every 4 h, for up to 72 h if necessary. Somatostatin (250 μg over 5 min, then infused at 250 μg/h for up to 72 h) has also been shown to decrease bleeding, but is not routinely used
- Use transdermal or buccal nitrate 5–10 mg every 12 h, for patients with cardiac ischaemia

Sengstaken tube
- Indicated for uncontrolled variceal bleeding, or recurrent haemorrhage despite vasopressin, glypressin, or sclerotherapy
- To be inserted by experienced operators only
- Sedation, or an anaesthetic, to insert an endotracheal tube and secure the airway, may be necessary
- Insert a cooled, lubricated Sengstaken tube beyond 45 cm
- Inflate the gastric balloon with 250 ml tap water containing 10 ml of any intravenous X-ray contrast medium
- Traction with 0.5–1 kg over the head of the bed
- Aspirate gastric and oesophageal ports hourly, as well as connecting to a bag for continuous drainage
- Inflate the oesophageal balloon to 30 mmHg, measured by manometer, if oesophageal bleeding continues for 15 min after the gastric balloon has been inflated
- X-ray to check position
- Active bleeding is arrested in 90%. Continued bleeding usually means that the tube is misplaced or that there are gastric varices
- Deflate the oesophageal balloon after 6–24 h and the gastric balloon after 24 h, and leave the tube *in situ* for another 6 h in case of further bleeding
- Rebleeding after deflation occurs in 50% unless sclerotherapy is done, and may be due to varices in the gastric fundus
- Rebleeding is treated by reinflating the balloon, pending urgent sclerotherapy

1.4 Acute bleeding: upper gastrointestinal tract

• Complications include tracheal intubation, oesophageal rupture from inflating the gastric balloon in the oesophagus, mucosal necrosis from leaving the balloon inflated for too long, or obstruction of the airway by upwards displacement of the balloon

Definitive treatment of bleeding varices
• Injection sclerotherapy: at the time of bleeding, repeated at increasing intervals (days, then weeks), until all varices are obliterated
• Oesophageal transection with proximal gastric devascularization is indicated for persistent bleeding after three attempts at sclerotherapy, but revascularization may occur rapidly after surgery

Prophylaxis
• Sclerotherapy is not indicated unless varices have bled
• Varices recur after obliteration in 40%, usually within 1 year
• Propranolol 40 mg twice daily, or in a dose which reduces resting pulse rate by 25%, decreases the risk of bleeding by reducing portal pressure. It has little effect on mortality and is often poorly tolerated, but is worth trying in patients who bleed recurrently
• Surgical portal–systemic shunts may help in non-cirrhotic portal hypertension (p. 155)

Mallory–Weiss syndrome
A mucosal tear at the oesophagogastric junction, due to forceful vomiting, results in haematemesis. The features are:
• Initial vomitus does not contain blood
• Vomiting in young patients is often provoked by alcohol
• 90% settle with conservative treatment and H_2 receptor antagonists are unnecessary
• Surgery is rarely needed, unless severe bleeding continues

Acute gastric erosions and haemorrhagic gastritis
Erosions are diagnosed endoscopically, but may be obscured by oozing from haemorrhagic gastritis.

Causes
• NSAIDs
• Alcohol

1 Alimentary Emergencies

1.4 Acute bleeding: upper gastrointestinal tract

- Stress (trauma, major surgery, septicaemia, or patients in intensive care)

Specific treatment
- Ranitidine 50 mg intravenously in 20 ml over 2 min three times daily, probably prevents stress erosions and is indicated for initial treatment
- Omeprazole 40 mg/day intravenously is indicated for persistent bleeding
- Intravenous tranexamic acid 400 mg twice daily, or vasopressin 20 U/h, are indicated as well as omeprazole if bleeding continues in patients where the risks of total gastrectomy are exceptionally high (such as the elderly with cardiorespiratory disease)
- Medical treatment is effective in >95%
- Total gastrectomy is the last resort for continued bleeding after all medical treatment has been vigorously applied for 24–48 h, and should only be performed by an experienced surgeon

Gastric ulcer (Section 3.4, p. 85)
- Consider provoking causes (such as NSAIDs)
- Give ranitidine 300 mg/day for 12 weeks once bleeding has stopped. Misoprostol 200 µg three times daily may be appropriate for patients with NSAID-associated ulcers who cannot stop NSAIDs (p. 110)
- Arrange a repeat endoscopy after 12 weeks, to biopsy and take brushings for cytology from the ulcer site
- Billroth I gastrectomy is usually performed if surgery is needed for continued bleeding. Undersewing with a vagotomy and pyloroplasty is a simpler operation, but the ulcer cannot be examined histologically to exclude cancer. Wedge resection removes the ulcer, but long-term maintenance H_2 receptor antagonists are needed to prevent recurrent ulceration; it may be best for high-risk elderly patients, because it has the lowest morbidity

Duodenal ulcer (Section 3.8, p. 98)
- Give ranitidine 300 mg at night for 8 weeks
- Maintenance therapy (ranitidine 150 mg at night) is indicated for patients with concomitant diseases, or those at high risk of dying from the complications of recurrent ulceration (p. 103)

• NSAID-associated ulcers heal with H_2 receptor antagonists even if NSAIDs have to be continued (p. 110). There is no good evidence that misoprostol is effective for preventing NSAID-related duodenal ulcers
• Risk of repeat haemorrhage after one episode of bleeding is 20% over 5–10 years, but more likely if associated with NSAIDs

'No source of bleeding found'
Unfortunately this is quite common and can produce difficult management problems. Possible causes are:
• Lesion missed on endoscopy
• Mucosal lesion healed before patient endoscoped:
erosions
Mallory–Weiss tear
Dieulafoy lesion (bleeding vessel with no surrounding ulceration, usually on the lesser curve)
• Bleeding from third part of the duodenum, or beyond:
jejunum (ulcerative jejunitis)
Meckel's diverticulum
colon
• Other:
nose bleed
rare causes of bleeding (Table 1.1, p. 9)

Management
• Reassess the patient—no further action is necessary for lower-risk patients (p. 9)
• Repeat endoscopy in high-risk patients (p. 8)
• Investigate rare causes of bleeding (re-check coagulation, consider small bowel radiology, endoscopic retrograde cholangiopancreatography (ERCP), or ultimately laparotomy and peroperative endoscopy)
• Selective angiography during active bleeding (which must be at a rate of 1 unit/4 h) is indicated after two negative endoscopies, preferably in a specialist unit

Aorto-duodenal fistula
Consider this rare diagnosis in any patient with an aortic graft and gastrointestinal bleeding. Exsanguination at the first bleed is uncommon. Small 'herald' bleeds occur for up to 2 weeks. Aortography is usually unhelpful and careful endoscopy to the

fourth part of the duodenum, if possible, is the best investigation, but surgery should not be delayed if hypotension has occurred. Aggressive surgery is needed as soon as the diagnosis is made, preferably in a specialist unit.

1.5 Acute bleeding: lower gastrointestinal tract

Bleeding from the colon is recognized by the passage of fresh red, or reddish-brown altered blood, per rectum. It is usually readily differentiated from upper gastrointestinal bleeding, because it has neither the smell, nor the tarry-black appearance of melaena. Upper tract bleeding rapid enough to cause red rectal bleeding is very rare, and is invariably associated with haemodynamic disturbance.

Clinical approach
- Assess severity—as for upper tract bleeding
- Resuscitate
- First or recurrent episode?
- Establish the site of bleeding
- Specific treatment

Causes
See Table 1.2

Table 1.2 Causes of rectal bleeding

Common	Less common	Rare
Perianal conditions	Ischaemic colitis	Anorectal varices
haemorrhoids	Crohn's disease	Small intestinal
fissures, prolapse	Diverticular disease	diverticula
Colorectal polyps	Angiodysplasia	lymphoma
Colorectal carcinoma		Kaposi's sarcoma
Ulcerative colitis		

Investigations—first episode

Severe bleeding
- Full blood count, coagulation studies, crossmatch and check electrolytes
- Rigid sigmoidoscopy—blood is likely to prevent colonoscopy
- Gastroscopy—only to exclude brisk gastric or duodenal haemorrhage, although bright red rectal bleeding is not from the upper gastrointestinal tract
- Angiography—if bleeding continues in excess of 1 unit/4 h

1.5   Acute bleeding: lower gastrointestinal tract

Slight/moderate bleeding
- Blood tests as above
- Rigid sigmoidoscopy and proctoscopy
- Colonoscopy once the bleeding has stopped

Investigations—recurrent bleeding
When initial investigations prove negative consider:
- Repeat colonoscopy—angiodysplasia can be missed
- Small bowel enema—better than a follow-through for identifying mucosal lesions (p. 359)
- ^{99}Tc sulphur colloid red cell scan—during active bleeding
- ^{99}Tc pertechnate Meckel's scan—specificity is only 80%
- Angiography—during a subsequent episode of bleeding (1 unit/ 4 h). Colonoscopy by an experienced operator using an instrument with a wide suction channel may identify the site more successfully
- Self-induced rectal trauma is a rare cause of recurrent bleeding

Management
Severe bleeding stops spontaneously in 80% of cases after adequate blood replacement. Treatment of the cause (Table 1.2, p. 17) is then needed. In the remainder, bleeding is continuous or recurs, sometimes frequently over many months. Identifying the site of persistent or recurrent bleeding is one of the most difficult problems in acute gastroenterology. Once the site is identified, surgical resection is indicated. If the site cannot be found, treatment depends on the pattern of bleeding.

Continuous bleeding
Surgery is advisable if bleeding persists after replacement of 6 units of blood. The options are:
- Laparotomy with peroperative enteroscopy, using a fibreoptic endoscope. The physician is well advised to attend the laparotomy
- Segmental resection if the site can be identified
- 'Blind' right hemicolectomy if the site cannot be found and the patient is elderly, because in these patients the cause is often angiodysplasia in the proximal colon

Intermittent bleeding
- Referral to a specialist gastroenterology unit is advisable if the site of bleeding cannot be identified after three episodes of bleeding

1.6   Acute abdominal pain

Rectal bleeding in children
The differential diagnosis is:
- Intussusception—commonest at 6–12 months
- Foreign body
- Ulcerative colitis
- Juvenile polyps—usually in the descending colon
- Meckel's diverticulum
- Intestinal haemangiomas
- Child (sexual) abuse

1.6   Acute abdominal pain
Clinical diagnostic accuracy is about 50%. Consider the age and sex of the patient when making a diagnosis. Metabolic and extra-intestinal causes (Table 1.3) should be considered if the diagnosis is in doubt.

Table 1.3 Causes of acute abdominal pain

Common	Less common	Rare
Appendicitis	Ruptured aortic aneurysm	Necrosis
Biliary colic	Mesenteric infarction	hepatoma
Cholecystitis	Pyelonephritis	fibroid
Diverticulitis	Torsion	Splenic infarction
Intestinal obstruction	ovarian cyst	Pneumonia
Perforated viscus	testicle	Myocardial infarction
Pancreatitis	omentum	Diabetic ketoacidosis
Peritonitis	Rupture	Porphyria
Salpingitis	ovarian cyst	Addisonian crisis
Mesenteric adenitis	ectopic pregnancy	Lead poisoning
Peritonitis	Abscesses	Tabes dorsalis
'Non-specific'	Prolapsed disc	Inflammatory aneurysm
	Herpes zoster	
	Exacerbation of peptic ulcer	

Clinical approach
The type of pain, relieving factors and progress are so variable that they rarely discriminate between diseases causing acute pain (Tables 1.3 and 1.4).
   Discriminating questions are:
- Site
- Duration
- Severity

1.6 Acute abdominal pain

Table 1.4 Patterns of acute abdominal pain

	Appendicitis	Cholecystitis	Perforated viscus	Renal colic	Pancreatitis	Diverticulitis	Salpingitis	Intestinal obstruction
Site	C/RLQ	RUQ	UQs	R/L loin	UQs	LQs	LQs	Symm
Duration	12–48 h	Days	<12 h	<12 h	<48 h	Days	>24 h	<48 h
Severity	Moderate	Severe	Severe	Severe	Severe	Moderate	Moderate	Severe
Radiation	Nil	Shoulder, back	Nil	Groin	Nil	Nil	Groin, thigh	Nil
Aggravating factors	Movement cough	Inspiration	Movement cough	Nil	Movement	Movement cough	Nil	

C/RLQ: central or right lower quadrant; RUQ: right upper quadrant; UQs: upper quadrants; R/L: right or left; LQs: lower quadrants: Symm: symmetrical.

- Radiation
- Aggravating factors
Also ask about:
- Vomiting
- Time last ate or drank
- Bowel disturbance
- Urinary frequency
- Date of last menstrual period
- Previous abdominal surgery
Specifically examine for:
- Distension
- Visible peristalsis
- Rebound tenderness, guarding, or rigidity
- Pulsatile mass and peripheral pulses
- Hernial orifices and testicles
- Rectal tenderness or masses
- Bowel sounds
- Epigastric bruit (normally audible in about 10% of thin patients)

Investigations
Every patient with acute abdominal pain should have on admission:
- Full blood count—leucocytosis may be absent in the elderly
- Electrolytes
- Amylase—but many causes of slight elevation other than acute pancreatitis (p. 26)
- Group and save serum
- Blood cultures—if febrile
- ECG
- Urine examination—including pregnancy test if doubtful
- Erect chest X-ray—look for basal atelectasis and gas under diaphragms
- Supine abdominal X-ray—look for biliary and renal calculi, dilated bowel (>2.5 cm small intestine, >6.0 cm colon), air in the biliary tree (p. 358)

Management—general principles
- Analgesia—do not withhold opiates for severe pain 'pending a surgical opinion', if the diagnosis is clear
- Perforation, peritonitis, or obstruction need emergency surgery
- Observation overnight often clarifies a difficult diagnosis

1 Alimentary Emergencies

1.6 Acute abdominal pain

- 'Nil by mouth' until a decision about surgery has been made
- Specific management of common causes of abdominal pain are discussed below

Appendicitis
Section 7.4 (p. 235)

Biliary colic

Distinguishing features
- Recurrent right upper quadrant colic is a feature of chronic cholecystitis, but the pain may rarely be exclusively high epigastric in location. Biliary colic typically causes a few minutes' pain, with intervals of an hour, and subsides after several hours
- Fever, or pain lasting more than 12 h, are likely to be due to acute cholecystitis
- Murphy's sign (tenderness in the right upper quadrant on inspiration) is positive during pain
- Flatulence, distension, fat intolerance and nausea are frequent, but occur in other common conditions (such as non-ulcer dyspepsia)
- Daily pain is unlikely to be due to biliary colic, even if gall stones are present

Management
- Ultrasonography will detect gall stones although difficult in the obese and those with a fibrosed gall bladder. Repeat ultrasound after a fatty meal is a test of gall bladder function, and is abnormal (no contraction) in acute or chronic cholecystitis
- An isotope (HIDA) scan (p. 362), or an oral cholecystogram will identify a non-functioning gall bladder, which is likely to be due to chronic cholecystitis. Non-surgical options such as dissolution or lithotripsy are inappropriate in these circumstances
- Other laboratory investigations are usually unhelpful
- Cholecystectomy is appropriate if symptoms are typical. Non-surgical options are discussed on p. 191

Acute cholecystitis

Distinguishing features
- Fever and persistent pain distinguish acute from chronic cholecystitis

1.6   Acute abdominal pain

- Impaction of a gall stone in the cystic duct causes 96%
- Typical pain (Table 1.4, p. 20) occurs in <50%
- Pain may be provoked by a fatty meal and builds up to a peak over 60 min, unlike the short spasms of biliary colic
- Fever develops after 12 h due to bacterial invasion and pain then becomes continuous
- Murphy's sign is sensitive, but not specific
- Calcified calculi (15%) and very rarely gas within biliary tree due to *Clostridium welchii* infection may be visible on plain abdominal X-ray

Complications
- Recurrence (50%)
- Cholangitis due to associated common duct stones (10%)
- Mucocele, empyema or gangrene of the gall bladder (1%)
- Biliary peritonitis (0.5%, with a mortality of 50%)

Conservative management
- Confirm the diagnosis by ultrasound. Isotope (HIDA) scans are also accurate, but not universally available
- Analgesia—intramuscular pethidine 100 mg and hyoscine 20 mg, but not morphine, which can increase the pain
- Intravenous fluids
- Nasogastric suction may be helpful, to alleviate vomiting if present
- Antibiotics—intravenous amoxycillin 500 mg and gentamicin 80 mg, three times daily
- Cholecystectomy (see below)

Indications for surgery
- Optimum treatment during surgery in the same admission, on the next available list. The longer the interval between cholecystitis and surgery, the greater the risk of a recurrent attack; concern about an increased complication rate 7–14 days after an acute attack is probably unfounded
- Uncertainty about the diagnosis (when perforation or retrocaecal appendicitis cannot be excluded)
- Signs of peritonitis

Cholangitis
Section 6.4 (p. 199)

Diverticulitis
Section 9.4 (p. 302)

Perforated viscus
The commonest cause is a perforated duodenal ulcer, followed by sigmoid diverticula or carcinoma, Crohn's disease, and gastric ulcers.

Distinguishing features
• Sudden onset of severe, unremitting pain
• Temporary improvement 3–6 h later can trap the unwary
• Pain and peritonism may be absent in the elderly or those on steroids
• Abdomen fails to move with respiration
• Bowel sounds are usually absent
• Gas under the diaphragm on an erect chest X-ray is usual (70%), but not universal
• Lateral decubitus films for the very sick will also show free gas, but can be difficult to interpret
• Spontaneous sealing of the perforation occurs rarely

Surgical management
• Emergency surgery is almost invariably indicated
• Oversewing, omental patch and peritoneal lavage are customary for gastro-duodenal perforation
• Hemicolectomy is indicated for right-sided colonic perforation, but distal perforation is probably best managed by resection, colostomy and rectal closure (Hartmann's procedure)
• The late complication of subphrenic abscess is best detected by ultrasound, but an abscess may cause an immobile diaphragm which can be readily detected by X-ray screening

Conservative management
• Indicated for the few patients in whom the risks are too high, or who refuse surgery
• Intravenous fluids, antibiotics and nasogastric suction

___

• Some surgeons advocate starting intravenous fluids, antibiotics and suction for 4–6 h and operating on those who do not improve, since this may have a lower mortality than emergency surgery for all patients. Whilst pre-operative resuscitation is always advisable, this conservative surgical approach is not widespread

Peritonitis
Fever, guarding, rebound tenderness and rigidity may be minimal in patients on steroids and in the immunocompromised. Bowel sounds are absent.

Causes
• Perforated viscus
• Local:
  appendicitis
  cholecystitis
  diverticulitis
  pancreatitis
  salpingitis
• Primary infective peritonitis
• Tuberculous
• Rare:
  sclerosing peritonitis
  granulomatous peritonitis
  periodic (familial Mediterranean fever)

Treatment
• Intravenous resuscitation
• Intravenous antibiotics—cefuroxime 750 mg and metronidazole 500 mg three times daily, after blood cultures
• Laparotomy
• Primary infective peritonitis is usually due to *Escherichia coli* or *Str. pneumoniae* in cirrhotic patients with ascites. Ascitic fluid should be sent for immediate Gram stain (p. 150) and intravenous antibiotics (cefotaxime 1 g twice daily) started, pending the result of culture
• Tuberculous peritonitis is usually diagnosed at laparotomy, but can be suspected by a high ascitic adenosine deaminase level, although this is not widely available. Standard antituberculous chemotherapy for 9 months is advised (p. 334)

Acute pancreatitis
Initial symptoms are a poor indicator of prognosis. Complications
(p. 27) should be sought, because early recognition improves
prognosis and recovery is potentially complete.

Distinguishing features
• Abdominal pain with a serum amylase >4 times the upper limit
of normal is usually diagnostic, but late presentation (>12 h) of a
perforated duodenal ulcer, or ectopic pregnancy, may cause a
similar rise in amylase
• The severity, rather than the nature, of the symptoms (pain and
vomiting) characterizes pancreatitis
• Diabetic coma is occasionally caused by acute pancreatitis

Predisposing factors
• Small gall stones—40–50%, causing transient impaction at the
ampulla
• No predisposing cause is found in about 15%
• Alcohol—10–40%, more common in recurrent or chronic
pancreatitis
• Trauma—6%, postoperative, post-ERCP, or after blunt
trauma
• Other causes of acute pancreatitis are rare:
   drugs (steroids, azathioprine, sodium valproate, frusemide)
   viral (mumps, coxsackie B4)
   pancreatic, or ampullary carcinoma
   arteritis
   hypothermia
   hypercalcaemia
   hypertriglyceridaemia (>10 mmol/1)
Other abdominal causes of a moderately (<4-fold) raised serum
amylase are:
• Perforated peptic ulcer (see above)
• Ectopic pregnancy (amylase-secreting cells in the fallopian tube)
• Intestinal ischaemia, or infarction
• Aortic dissection
• Renal failure
• Consistent clinical features, a predisposing cause and an
associated abnormality (such as hypocalcaemia or hypoxia) help
discriminate acute pancreatitis from other causes of a moderately
raised serum amylase

Complications
* Local:
  pseudocyst (abdominal mass; persistently raised amylase, p. 113)
  abscess (swinging pyrexia 1 week after attack)
  jaundice (pancreatic oedema, or stones, can occlude the common
      bile duct)
* Paralytic ileus—exacerbates fluid and electrolyte imbalance
* Hypovolaemic shock—due to vomiting, hypoalbuminaemia,
ascites, or retroperitoneal haemorrhage (rare)
  Grey Turner's (flank) and Cullen's (periumbilical) signs of skin
      discolouration are caused by tracking of blood-stained fluid
* Hypoxia—(Pao_2 <8 kPa, or 60 mmHg) a prognostic factor and
clinically underdiagnosed
* Hypocalcaemia—(<2.0 mmol/1, corrected by adding 0.02
mmol/1 for every g/l of the serum albumin <40 g/l). Tetany is rare
* Acute renal failure—due to hypovolaemia, or disseminated
intravascular coagulation (rare)
* Effusions—ascitic and pleural exudates with a high amylase
* Death—6–28%, depending on severity
* Recurrent attacks occur in 30%, especially in alcoholics, or if
cholecystectomy for associated gall stones is delayed

Management
Establish the diagnosis:
* Serum amylase elevated >4-fold. Urinary amylase (spot sample)
remains elevated for longer than serum amylase, but is not widely
used
* Urgent ultrasound is often diagnostic and may reveal pancreatic
oedema and/or complications will also demonstrate gall stones if
present. A well-visualized, normal pancreas makes pancreatitis
most unlikely
* CT scan is indicated if the pancreas cannot be visualized by
ultrasound. Pancreatic underperfusion, visible on a contrast-
enhanced image, signifies a poor prognosis
  Assess the severity (Table 1.5, p. 28):
* Three or more factors present out of eight, indicates severe
disease (Glasgow Prognostic Score). Unfortunately none may be
abnormal in the early stages, but better predictive tests are being
developed
* C-reactive protein level >150 mg/l also discriminates between
mild and severe pancreatitis, and is easier to apply than a

27

Indications for surgery (p. 115)
• Treat predisposing causes
• Urgent ERCP and sphincterotomy if common bile duct stones are present
• Cholecystectomy if stones are identified in the gall bladder, immediately after recovery (p. 113)
• Abstinence from alcohol

Acute intestinal ischaemia
The superior mesenteric artery supplies the jejunum and intestine to mid-transverse colon (Fig. 9.4, p. 305). Acute intestinal ischaemia usually refers to mesenteric infarction and is uncommon. Colonic infarction can rarely be distinguished clinically from mesenteric infarction, but management is the same. The other three patterns of intestinal ischaemia (mesenteric angina, focal ischaemia and ischaemic colitis) are covered in Section 9.5 (p. 304). Causes of intestinal ischaemia are shown in Table 9.3 (p. 306)

Distinguishing features
• Severe abdominal pain in an elderly patient with arterial disease
• Atrial fibrillation, or vasculitis with abdominal pain
• Paucity of abdominal signs, compared with the severity of pain and general condition
• An epigastric bruit suggests the diagnosis if present, but is frequently absent
• Peritonism is a late sign, when the patient is usually beyond recovery
• Rectal bleeding or blood-stained mucus, after the onset of pain
• Marked leucocytosis ($20–30 \times 10^9$/l) is common, but not invariable
• Haematocrit >0.50 indicates dehydration

Management
Mesenteric infarction without resection is invariably fatal. Early liaison with an experienced surgeon is essential, because the situation is usually irretrievable by the time there is no clinical doubt about the diagnosis.
• Suspect the diagnosis in a sick, elderly patient with severe abdominal pain and few signs
• Plain abdominal X-ray—may be unremarkable or show decreased gas pattern, fluid levels, mucosal oedema (thickened small intestinal wall, or 'thumb printing' in the colon (Fig. 9.5, p. 308))

- Angiography does not help management of acute ischaemia, because non-obstructive infarction can occur and laparotomy is merely delayed
- Analgesia—intravenous morphine 10 mg, then 2.5 mg aliquots every 3–4 h to control pain
- Intravenous rehydration—monitor haematocrit, central venous pressure and urine output
- Check arterial gases—metabolic acidosis responds to rehydration
- Antibiotics—amoxycillin, gentamicin and metronidazole, after blood cultures, if hypotensive
- Laparotomy—for diagnosis and to remove infarcted gut. A 'second look' to remove further non-viable tissue after 24 h is often advisable
- Mortality is above 80% and morbidity after extensive resection is substantial (short bowel syndrome, p. 231)

Non-specific abdominal pain
No specific diagnosis is made in a third of patients with acute abdominal pain.

Distinguishing features
- Commoner in younger patients
- Type, site and relief of pain fail to fit a common pattern
- Vomiting occurs in 50%
- Constipation should not overlooked and can be diagnosed on plain abdominal X-ray
- Temperature, blood count, ESR and urine examination are normal

Management
- Observation with oral fluids and analgesics for 24 h will usually discriminate the non-specific from the pathological

Metabolic causes
Metabolic derangements can masquerade as acute abdominal emergencies.
- Diabetic ketoacidosis—severe pain occurs in 10%, but acute pancreatitis must be excluded
- Hypercalcaemia—constipation and vomiting can occur without acute pancreatitis (Ca >3.5 mmol/l)

1.6 Acute abdominal pain

• Acute adrenal insufficiency—with hyponatraemia, hyperkalaemia, elevated urea and hypotension
• Acute intermittent porphyria—neurological signs and abdominal pain, but no rash. Urine turns red on standing; porphobilinogen is detected by adding 2 ml Ehrlich's aldehyde to 2 ml urine. The pink colour is insoluble in chloroform
• Lead poisoning—ask about constipation, water supply and look at the gums for a fine blue line. Basophilic stippling and red cell lead are diagnostic
• Tabetic crisis—'lightning' pain; look for Argyll–Robertson pupils and at posterior column function. It is extremely rare

Extra-intestinal causes
Referred pain is more common in children and young adults.
• Lobar pneumonia—especially basal
• Testicular torsion—do not forget to look, especially in teenagers
• Inferior myocardial infarction
• Herpes zoster—before the rash appears
• Spinal arthritis
• Root compression—classically with a thoracic meningioma; pain radiates from back to front

Munchausen's syndrome
Psychiatrically disturbed patients who manipulate recurrent admission to hospital by simulating an acute medical condition, often describe acute abdominal pain in a convincing manner. Features that should raise suspicion are:
• 'Textbook' story of an acute abdominal condition (renal colic, peptic ulcer, biliary colic), with normal investigations
• History of surgery, or admission to hospitals in other parts of the country. Recent admissions are frequently concealed (look for signs of venesection)
• Psychiatric history, or inappropriate affect
• Neuropsychiatric disorders and acute abdominal pain can occur in acute porphyria, lead poisoning, or syphilis (see above)

Previous hospital admissions should be pursued. The patient is often well known to hospitals in one area. Once the diagnosis is documented, a description should be circulated to local hospitals, but self-discharge is usual before a photograph can be taken.

1.7 Intestinal obstruction

Mechanical intestinal obstruction or failure of peristalsis (ileus) is life threatening.

Clinical features

The cardinal features are:

- Pain
- Distension
- Vomiting
- Constipation

The pain is colicky, but once strangulation occurs the pain becomes continuous and rebound tenderness is present. Vomiting can be the only feature of high jejunal obstruction. Subacute obstruction means incomplete occlusion of the lumen and diarrhoea occasionally occurs.

Visible peristalsis may be seen. Hernial orifices must be examined carefully and previous abdominal surgery noted. Bowel sounds are increased in mechanical obstruction, but decreased in ileus.

Causes

Mechanical

- External herniae
- Adhesions
- Malignant colonic strictures

The above three causes account for 75% of intestinal obstructions.

Less common mechanical causes

- Luminal:
  ingested foreign bodies
  fibrous food bolus
  gall-stone ileus
  intussusception
- Mural:
  sigmoid diverticular disease
  Crohn's disease
  NSAID-induced small intestinal strictures
  ileocaecal tuberculosis

- Extrinsic:
  volvulus (sigmoid, caecal, gastric)
  internal herniation (through mesenteric foramina)

Ileus
- Following laparotomy
- Retroperitoneal lesions:
  pancreatitis
  haemorrhage
  ureteric obstruction
- Drugs:
  anticholinergics and opiates, among others
- Metabolic:
  diabetic ketoacidosis
  acute renal failure
  hypokalaemia
- Intestinal infarction
- Pseudo-obstruction

Investigations
- Plain abdominal X-ray—the upper limit of normal diameter of the small intestine is 2.5 cm and of the colon is 6.0 cm. An occasional fluid level is normal. Look for air under the diaphragms, in the bowel wall and in the biliary tree
- Blood tests—look for hypokalaemia and a high urea. Leucocytosis suggests strangulation. Crossmatch 2 units prior to surgery
- Arterial gases—metabolic alkalosis occurs with severe vomiting

Management
- Nasogastric suction
- Replace fluid and electrolytes—5 l 0.9% saline and 200 mmol KCl are commonly needed in the first 24 h. Sequestered fluid in obstructed bowel is not measured, so adjust the infusion rate according to the urine output
- Assess concomitant medical problems—drugs may not have been absorbed
- Relieve the obstruction—the site governs the type of operation. Suspicion of strangulation demands urgent surgery. Non-operative manoeuvres are initially indicated for ileus, pseudo-obstruction, volvulus, or intussusception

- Monitor:
urine output
nasogastric aspirate
central venous pressure in the shocked or elderly
daily electrolytes

Ileus
- Nasogastric suction, maintaining serum potassium at 4.0–4.5 mmol/l, intravenous fluids and patience are usually sufficient
- Check that anticholinergic drugs are not prescribed and decrease opiate analgesia to a minimum
- Try metoclopramide 10 mg intravenously three times daily, or cisapride 30 mg per rectum three times daily if ineffective, as prokinetic agents
- Confirm by contrast radiology that mechanical obstruction is not present, if obstruction persists after a few days

Volvulus
- Sigmoid volvulus—common in elderly males, the mentally handicapped and patients in developing countries. Plain X-ray shows massive sigmoid distension. Sigmoidoscopy and a deflating rectal tube should be attempted before surgery
- Caecal volvulus—obstruction is often incomplete initially but recurs without surgery, so laparotomy is advisable
- Gastric volvulus—associated with diaphragmatic eventration, visible on plain chest and abdominal X-rays. Distinguish from 'acute gastric dilatation' which is a misnomer for gastric ileus, caused by poor attention to nasogastric suction and electrolyte balance. Surgery is needed for gastric volvulus, with repair of the diaphragm

Intussusception
- Usually idiopathic in infants, due to a Meckel's diverticulum in adolescence, and a polyp or carcinoma in adults
- Intermittent pain, followed by rectal bleeding, with small intestinal fluid levels and an absent caecal gas shadow on X-ray, suggest the diagnosis. Facial pallor during pain occurs in infants
- Barium enema is diagnostic and may be therapeutic in the early stages

---

Pseudo-obstruction
• Clinical features of intestinal obstruction without a mechanical cause. The motility disorder commonly affects the whole gastrointestinal tract, although it is colonic distension that is often most prominent
• Consider the diagnosis in the elderly and mentally handicapped, or when obstruction is associated with other disorders (myocardial infarction, pneumonia, Parkinson's disease)
• An urgent barium enema is often necessary to distinguish pseudo- from mechanical obstruction, and may have a therapeutic effect
• Stop causative drugs (phenothiazines, tricyclic antidepressants) and treat associated disease. Rectal cisapride 30 mg three times daily may be helpful
• 90% resolve spontaneously, but colonoscopic decompression is warranted if pain is severe, or the caecum >10 cm. Surgery should be avoided if at all possible

1.8 Toxic dilatation of the colon
Dilatation of the colon with signs of systemic upset ('toxic') is becoming less common as acute attacks of ulcerative colitis are recognized and appropriately treated (p. 270). The danger if surgery is inappropriately delayed is colonic perforation, which still carries a very high mortality.

Clinical features
• Colitis—usually caused by severe ulcerative colitis, but can occur in Crohn's colitis, and rarely in ischaemic or infective colitis (*Yersinia enterocolitica, Campylobacter* sp., *Cl. difficile*)
• Fever >38.5°C
• Neutrophils $>10 \times 10^9/l$
• Tachycardia >90 bpm
• Radiological colonic dilatation (widest diameter >6.0 cm, Fig. 1.3)
• Clinical appearance can be deceptive due to steroids

Management
The diagnosis must be recognized and the response to medical treatment carefully assessed after 24 h. A decision to continue for a

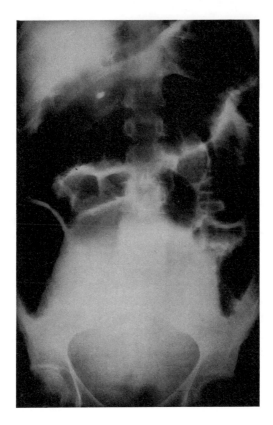

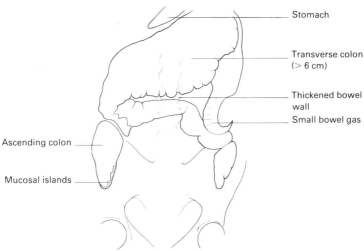

Stomach

Transverse colon
(> 6 cm)

Thickened bowel
wall

Small bowel gas

Ascending colon

Mucosal islands

Fig. 1.3 Toxic dilatation of the colon in ulcerative colitis. Plain abdominal X-ray in toxic megacolon showing a grossly dilated transverse colon with mucosal islands in the ascending colon. Concomitant gas in the small bowel is associated with the need for colectomy.

further 24 h or proceed to emergency colectomy must then be made by a senior physician in consultation with the surgeons.

Diagnosis
• Always take a daily plain abdominal X-ray in patients with severe colitis (p. 268). Mucosal islands (polypoid mucosal swellings projecting into the colonic lumen, Fig. 1.3), in addition to dilatation indicate very severe ulceration and predict the need for colectomy
• Stool culture and faecal *Cl. difficile* toxin assay
• Blood cultures
• Colonoscopy and barium enema (but not rigid sigmoidoscopy) are dangerous

Supportive
• Involve the surgeons as soon as the diagnosis is made
• Nil by mouth
• Intravenous fluids and electrolyte supplementation (serum K 4.0–4.5 mmol/l)
• 2-hourly observation of pulse and temperature, 4-hourly blood pressure, as well as fluid balance and stool charts
• Examine the patient at least twice daily (check pulse, blood pressure, abdominal girth and tenderness)
• Monitor daily full blood count, ESR, electrolytes and maximum colonic diameter on plain abdominal X-ray

Specific
• Stop antidiarrhoeal agents
• Intravenous hydrocortisone 100 mg four times daily, for ulcerative colitis or Crohn's disease
• Rectal hydrocortisone 100 mg in 100 ml twice daily (p. 271)
• There is no evidence that antibiotics alter the outcome

Indications for emergency colectomy
The decision can be difficult, but delayed surgical intervention increases mortality, even in young patients. If the situation is stable after 24 h, a further 24-h trial of medical treatment may be justified. This decision should be taken by a senior physician, jointly with the surgeons. Indications for colectomy are:
• Increasing tachycardia, fever
• Failure to improve clinically (no change in stool frequency, tachycardia, or abdominal pain) or radiologically within 24 h

- Signs of perforation (may be minimal, due to steroids)
- Mucosal islands as well as dilatation (because such severe ulceration and oedema are very unlikely to respond to steroids)

1.9   Acute hepatic failure

Acute hepatic failure occurs in a previously normal liver and is either fulminant or late-onset (subacute). The time of onset and mortality distinguish the two types, although other features and management are the same.

The main differential diagnosis is between acute and acute-on-chronic liver failure (Table 1.7, p. 40). The potential for complete recovery distinguishes acute failure, although it has a worse prognosis.

Clinical features

Fulminant hepatic failure
- Encephalopathy 0–8 weeks after symptoms of the initial illness
- Encephalopathy includes all stages from personality change to coma
- The grade may change rapidly (Table 1.6)

Table 1.6 Grade of hepatic encephalopathy

Grade	Features
1	Altered mood or behaviour
2	Drowsy
3	Stupor
4	Coma
5	Coma with no response to painful stimuli

Late onset
- Encephalopathy after an interval of 9–26 weeks

Associated features
- Fetor—the smell of pear drops
- Jaundice—may be minimal in the early stages
- Liver size—usually small, due to hepatic necrosis. If enlarged, acute-on-chronic liver failure (Table 1.7, p. 40) is more likely
- Spleen—usually impalpable
- No single feature entirely discriminates between acute and acute-

1.9   Acute hepatic failure

Table 1.7 Acute versus acute-on-chronic hepatic failure

	Acute	Acute-on-chronic
History	Short	Long
Nutrition	Good	Poor
Liver	Small	Usually enlarged
Spleen	Impalpable	Enlarged
Spider naevi	Absent	Many
Encephalopathy	Early	Late
Jaundice	Late	Early
Ascites	Late	Early

on-chronic hepatic failure, although the history is the best guide

Causes

Viral hepatitis and paracetamol overdose are the commonest causes in Britain. Presentation a few days after apparent recovery from paracetamol poisoning is typical.
• Viral—hepatitis B, C (non-A, non-B) or D (delta agent). Rare after hepatitis A or E (community-acquired non-A, non-B), yellow fever, or leptospirosis
• Drugs—paracetamol (especially associated with alcohol), halothane, isoniazid
• Alcohol—occasionally without underlying liver disease, but usually acute-on-chronic
• Wilson's disease
• Budd–Chiari syndrome—ascites is often prominent
• Fatty liver of pregnancy—third trimester

Investigations

Blood tests

• Coagulation studies, glucose and potassium immediately and creatinine as soon as possible
• Full blood count, group and save, bilirubin, albumin, aspartate aminotransferase, amylase
• Hepatitis serology, paracetamol levels, serum copper and caeruloplasmin, and 24-h urinary copper where appropriate

---

Radiology
* Chest X-ray
* Ultrasound of liver and pancreas. Hepatic vein Doppler studies if Budd–Chiari syndrome is suspected

Other
* Blood cultures—even if afebrile
* Electroencephalogram—may be diagnostic when there is doubt and may be prognostic, but seldom necessary

Management

General
* Intensive care nursing
* Monitor urine output, blood glucose and vital signs, every hour
* Check serum potassium twice daily, full blood count, creatinine, albumin and coagulation daily
* Do not give intravenous saline

Encephalopathy
* Limit oral protein
* Lactulose, starting at 90 ml/day and increasing until mild diarrhoea develops (neomycin is of little additional benefit)
* No sedation if possible

Hypoglycaemia and hypokalaemia
* 10% dextrose 100 ml/h with KCl 40 mmol/l, but 20–50% dextrose may be needed if hypoglycaemia is severe

Bleeding
* Avoid arterial punctures
* Fresh frozen plasma if bleeding occurs, but coagulation studies seldom fully correct. Vitamin K will not work
* Ranitidine 50 mg, in 20 ml intravenously over 2 min, three times daily (to reduce stress-induced erosions)
* Disseminated intravascular coagulation can cause bleeding as well as clotting factor deficiency due to liver failure

Renal failure
- 55% develop renal impairment. Serum urea is falsely low in severe liver disease, so creatinine should be measured
- Haemofiltration or dialysis is indicated if serum potassium >6.0 mmol/l, HCO_3 <15 mmol/l or creatinine >400 μmol/l

Infection
- Meticulous care of intravenous and urinary catheters
- Blood, urine and catheter cultures are essential and must be performed before starting antibiotics
- Antibiotics are recommended, because patients are critically ill and common signs of sepsis are often absent. Intravenous cefotaxime 1 g twice daily is an appropriate broad-spectrum antibiotic, until culture results are available

Artificial hepatic support
- No controlled trials have shown a reduction in mortality

Indications for transplant
Deciding when the chance of spontaneous recovery is less than the risks of a liver transplant is difficult. Discuss the situation with the nearest transplant centre at an early stage (Appendix 1). Table 1.8 shows the criteria used for transplantation in fulminant hepatic failure at King's College Hospital, but it is too late to transfer a patient at this stage. Hepatitis B or alcohol are not absolute contraindications.

Table 1.8 Criteria for liver transplant in fulminant failure

Paracetamol cases	Non-paracetamol cases
Arterial pH <7.30	Prothrombin time >100 sec
or all of the following:	*or 3/5 of the following:*
Prothrombin time >100 sec	Aetiology non-A, non-B or drug reaction
Creatinine >300 μmol/l	Age <11 or >40 years
Grade 3 encephalopathy	>7 days between onset of jaundice and encephalopathy
	Prothrombin time >50 sec
	Bilirubin >300 μmol/l

Take into account:
- Age (<60 years)
- Previous liver function (should have been normal)
- Ability to cope with post-transplant regimen

During transfer:
- Give 20% glucose 100 ml/h with 40 mmol/l KC1 to prevent hypoglycaemia or hypokalaemia
- 20% mannitol 20 ml/h if grade 2 encephalopathy or worse, because cerebral oedema is exacerbated by movement

See Appendix 1 for addresses and telephone numbers.

Prognosis

Factors
- Grade of encephalopathy—15% survival without transplant when grade 3–4
- Age:
  >40 years 15% survival
  <30 years 40% survival
- Albumin:
  >35 g/l 80% survival
  <30 g/l 20% survival
- Cause—drug reactions and non-A, non-B (hepatitis C) induced failure have a worse prognosis than other causes
- Onset—late-onset has a worse prognosis than fulminant failure

Transplant in acute liver failure
- 65% survive, but this is improving
- Auxiliary liver transplantation is under trial

2 Oesophagus

2 Oesophagus

2.1 Dysphagia

2.1 Dysphagia

Acute or progressive dysphagia demands urgent investigation. Oral, pharyngeal and oesophageal causes are recognized (Table 2.1). Bolus obstruction is covered in Section 1.2, p. 4.

Table 2.1 Causes of dysphagia

	Oral	Pharyngeal	Oesophageal
Common	Aphthous ulcers Candidiasis	Stroke	Oesophagitis Peptic stricture Carcinoma oesophagus cardia
Unusual	Xerostomia Parkinson's disease	Globus hystericus Pseudobulbar palsy Motor neurone disease Pharyngeal pouch	Muscular achalasia diffuse spasm systemic sclerosis External pressure bronchial carcinoma mediastinal nodes aortic aneurysm Post-cricoid web Schatzki ring Radiation stricture
Rare	Oral tumours	Syringobulbia Bulbar poliomyelitis Muscular dystrophy	Cricopharyngeal bar Aberrant vessels Left atrial enlargement Retrosternal goitre Chagas' disease

Clinical features

• Ask whether dysphagia is for liquids (usually pharyngeal), or solids (oesophageal cause more likely)
• The interval between swallowing and food sticking distinguishes upper from lower obstruction. Where the patient points to is no help
• Short (<3 months), progressive history indicates malignancy
• Weight loss confirms that an organic cause is probable, but lack of weight loss is of no diagnostic value
• Associated reflux suggests a peptic stricture

- Cough indicates spillover into the bronchial tree, or, very rarely, an oesophagobronchial fistula
- Odynophagia (pain during swallowing) often accompanies dysphagia in achalasia, diffuse oesophageal spasm, or oesophagitis
- A 'lump in the throat' as the only symptom is unlikely to have a mechanical cause
- Examine the mouth and teeth or dentures, and feel for supraclavicular nodes (from carcinoma of the cardia)
- Look for signs of systemic disease (anaemia, systemic sclerosis or neurological disorders)

Urgent investigations
A telephone call to the radiologist or gastroenterologist is appropriate, to arrange urgent investigation of any patient with dysphagia. Confirmation by request form or letter can follow.
- Chest X-ray—look for a hilar tumour, mediastinal fluid level, absent gastric bubble, or right lower lobe consolidation (aspiration)
- Barium swallow—within 48 h. A smooth, tapering stricture is often benign. Irregularity or asymmetry suggests malignancy (see Fig. 2.3, p. 57)
- Endoscopy—usually after a barium swallow, although can be the initial investigation by experienced endoscopists. Allow 12 h for barium to clear; it can block the endoscope
- Blood tests—anaemia may be due to malignancy, poor nutrition, bleeding, or Brown Kelly–Paterson syndrome (p. 63). A high urea usually reflects dehydration

Later investigations
- Cine or bread barium swallow, or oesophageal manometry may be appropriate if the barium swallow is normal (p. 66 and 67)
- Lung function tests (spirometry and transfer factor) establish a baseline in patients with systemic sclerosis
- ENT assessment is indicated for most pharyngeal causes of dysphagia

2.2 Oesophagitis and hiatus hernia
Gastro-oesophageal reflux does not always cause symptoms. Abnormal reflux results in prolonged exposure of the oesophageal mucosa to refluxate and causes oesophagitis. Abnormal reflux is caused by dysfunction of the lower oesophageal sphincter. Severe

reflux is usually, but not necessarily, associated with a hiatus hernia. It is associated with obesity and, to a lesser extent, smoking. Posture (lying down) provokes reflux, which is why there is an association with nocturnal asthma. Peptic stricture of the oesophagus is an unusual complication, in view of the high prevalence of oesophageal reflux.

Clinical features
• Heartburn—retrosternal pain related to meals, lying down, stooping, straining and occasionally to exercise
• Water brash—regurgitation of acid or bile. Patients often have difficulty in describing the taste as bitter or sour
• Excess salivation during pain
• Relief by antacids
• Pain during swallowing (odynophagia) is unusual unless there is severe oesophagitis or a stricture (when dysphagia is also present)
• Chest pain, related to posture or exercise (both of which increase intra-abdominal pressure), can be difficult to distinguish from angina (p. 66)
• Nocturnal asthma (cough, or wheeze) may be the only symptom, and can be relieved by treatment of reflux
• Oesophagitis is sometimes asymptomatic

Hiatus hernia
Hiatus hernia is compatible with normal lower oesophageal sphincter function and is not necessarily pathological. Reflux may be encouraged when the gastro-oesophageal junction is in the thorax, owing to the lower intrathoracic pressure, and symptoms occur due to oesophagitis.

Features
• About 30% of patients over 50 years have a hiatus hernia
• Commoner in obese women
• 50% of these have symptomatic gastro-oesophageal reflux
• Endoscopy detects fewer hiatal herniae than barium X-rays, but is better at detecting oesophagitis if it is present

Types of hiatus hernia (Fig. 2.1)
All types may be complicated by oesophagitis or a peptic stricture.
• Sliding—the commonest type

2 Oesophagus

2.2 Oesophagitis and hiatus hernia

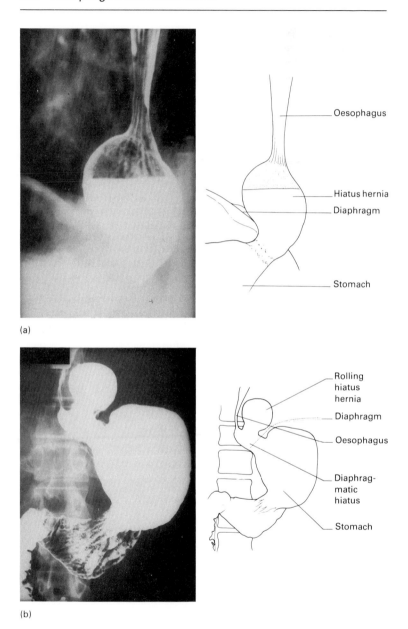

(a)

(b)

Fig. 2.1 Different types of hiatus hernia. (a) Barium meal showing a sliding hiatus hernia. (b) Barium meal showing a rolling hiatus hernia.

2.2   Oesophagitis and hiatus hernia

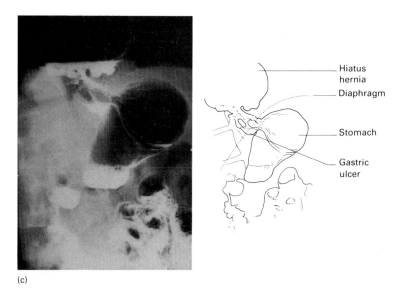

(c)

Fig. 2.1 (*continued*) Different types of hiatus hernia. (c) Barium meal showing an incarcerated hiatus hernia with a gastric ulcer above the diaphragmatic hiatus.

- Rolling (para-oesophageal):
  —dysphagia relieved by a change in posture is classic
  —strangulation of the herniated fundus is rare
- Incarcerated:
  —chest X-ray shows an air fluid level behind the heart
  —management is no different from other types

Investigations
- Isolated symptoms of gastro-oesophageal reflux do not require investigation
- Endoscopy is indicated if symptoms are not relieved by general measures (below), in preference to a barium meal, because oesophagitis is more reliably detected
- Macroscopic oesophagitis (erythema, erosions, linear and then confluent or circumferential ulcers) indicates reflux, but the severity does not always correlate with symptoms
- Microscopic oesophagitis within 5 cm of the gastro-oesophageal junction occurs in some normal subjects. More proximal changes occur in symptomatic reflux, even when the mucosa looks normal
- Iron deficiency anaemia should not be attributed to oesophagitis

• 24-h oesophageal pH monitoring is indicated when it is difficult to distinguish symptomatic reflux from other causes of chest pain (p. 66), but is not part of routine management

General measures
General measures to reduce reflux are more important than drugs in most patients.
• Weight reduction (height/weight charts: Appendix 3; weight-reducing diet: p. 383)
• Stop smoking
• Raise head of bed by about 10 cm, using blocks or bricks
• Small, regular meals
• Allow 3 h between last meal and retiring at night
• Avoid hot drinks or alcohol before bed
• Avoid drugs that adversely affect oesophageal motility (nitrates, anticholinergic agents, antidepressants, theophylline compounds), or that damage the oesophageal mucosa (NSAIDs, slow-release potassium)

Management
There is no evidence that one antacid is better than another for relief of symptoms. Neither antacids nor alginates (Gaviscon, Gastrocote) will heal oesophagitis, but may reduce reflux and associated symptoms. The plan outlined in Fig. 2.2 is suggested.

Difficult cases
Oesophagitis often relapses after stopping drug treatment. Overweight, smoking drinkers characteristically continue to have symptoms. If symptoms persist despite dieting, stopping smoking, or whilst still on drug treatment *and* the diagnosis has been confirmed by a repeat endoscopy and biopsy, then:
• Prescribe omeprazole 20–40 mg at night. >90% effective and concerns about long-term sequelae appear unfounded
• Prokinetic drugs (such as cisapride 10 mg or metoclopramide 10 mg three times daily) with H_2-receptor antagonists are better than either alone, but are more expensive and less effective than omeprazole
• Relapse after complete healing remains common when treatment is stopped. Intermittent treatment of recurrent symptoms is necessary

2 Oesophagus

2.2 Oesophagitis and hiatus hernia

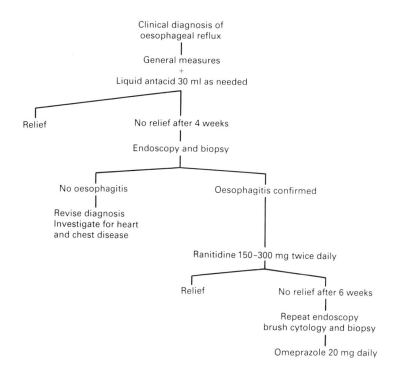

Fig. 2.2 Management plan for symptomatic gastro-oesophageal reflux.

- Maintenance treatment may be necessary in patients with severe, recurrent symptoms.
- Surgery is rarely indicated. Persistent, severe symptoms despite all medical treatments vigorously applied *and* objective evidence of gross reflux (radiological, or pH monitoring) are required before surgery can be considered, in patients <60 years.

Alkaline reflux
Bile, pancreatic enzymes and bicarbonate due to duodenogastric reflux, as well as acid and pepsin, can cause oesophagitis. Biliary reflux at endoscopy is normal if the patient is retching.
Oesophagitis with a pH >4 at all times during ambulatory monitoring is necessary for diagnosis. Gastric surgery predisposes to bile and bicarbonate reflux.

General measures and antacids should be tried. Dilute hydrochloric acid BP (0.1 ml in 10 ml water) would be logical and is said to be better than placebo for heartburn in pregnancy, but is not in general use. Surgical (Roux-en-Y) revision is reserved for severe, intolerable symptoms.

Barrett's oesophagus

Features
• Endoscopic biopsy evidence of gastric columnar epithelium >2.5 cm proximal to the gastro-oesophageal junction
• Oesophageal adenocarcinoma develops in 2–5% and dysplasia in 10% over 5 years

Management
• Standard anti-reflux therapy is indicated
• Annual surveillance endoscopy to detect dysplasia has not yet been shown to reduce mortality, but repeat endoscopy after 3–6 months is indicated if early dysplasia is detected

Oesophageal ulcers

Features
• Associated with severe oesophagitis and Barrett's oesophagus
• Endoscopy, biopsy and brush cytology are needed to exclude malignancy

Management
• Check that biopsies and brushings for cytology have been taken at endoscopy
• Prescribe omeprazole 20 mg at night for 6 weeks
• Repeat the endoscopy, biopsy and brushings at 6-week intervals until healing occurs
• Refer for surgery if high-grade dysplasia is detected in ulcers that persist or recur despite treatment

Infections
Oesophageal infections occur in the debilitated and immunocompromised (Section 11.4, p. 343). Underlying disease should be sought and treated.

2 Oesophagus

Candidiasis
- Painful dysphagia (odynophagia) with oral candidiasis is typical
- Barium swallow, or endoscopy with biopsy, is diagnostic
- Nystatin suspension 2 ml four times daily for 10 days is as effective and has fewer side effects than amphotericin (200 mg lozenges four times daily for 10 days)
- Oral fluconazole 50 mg daily or ketoconazole 200 mg daily for 14 days are better for patients with AIDS. Maintenance therapy may be needed

Cytomegalovirus
- Oesophageal biopsy is diagnostic
- Ganciclovir 5 mg/kg intravenously over 1 h, twice daily for 14—21 days is only appropriate for severe infection

Herpes simplex virus
- Vesicles are rarely seen endoscopically
- Electron microscopy of brushings transported in 4% glutaraldehyde is diagnostic
- Intravenous acyclovir 5 mg/kg three times daily, until tablets (200 mg 5 times daily for 5 days) can be swallowed

2.3 Benign strictures

Causes
- Peptic—95%
- Anastomotic—following a surgical procedure
- Radiotherapy—for carcinoma of the breast or bronchus. Stenosis after radiotherapy for oesophageal carcinoma is almost always malignant
- Corrosives—bleach and drugs (such as slow-release potassium tablets). Patients taking NSAIDS have a higher incidence of strictures
- Mucocutaneous disorders—Behçet's disease, epidermolysis bullosa

Clinical features
Dysphagia is the main symptom and reflux is usually present. The main differential diagnosis is carcinoma. Dysphagia for <3 months or rapid weight loss favour carcinoma.

Investigations and management

Initial investigations
• As for dysphagia (p. 48 and Fig. 2.3)
• Check the results of biopsies and brushings

Dilatation
• Endoscopic dilatation as an outpatient procedure is safe in experienced hands. The technique is beyond the scope of this book (Appendix 2)
• A subsequent chest X-ray is not necessary unless pain occurs or perforation is suspected
• Repeat dilatations (two or three) are often needed
• Encourage the patient to make appointments direct with the Endoscopy Unit if dysphagia recurs, to save time
• Recurrent symptoms <4 weeks after dilatation suggest a carcinoma

Other advice
• Omeprazole 20 mg at night for 4 weeks for recurrent strictures.
• Prevention of oesophageal obstruction (p. 5)

2.4 Oesophageal carcinoma
Oesophageal carcinoma accounts for 2% of all cancers. Whilst only 30% are resectable and 5-year survival is 10%, palliation is vital because inability to swallow saliva after oesophageal obstruction is a miserable way to die. Carcinoma of the cardia may mimic carcinoma of the lower third oesophagus, or achalasia (p. 61).

Causes
The cause is usually unknown. The importance of different factors varies in different parts of the world. Associations are:
• Alcohol
• Tobacco
• Barrett's oesophagus (p. 54)—the degree of risk is debated

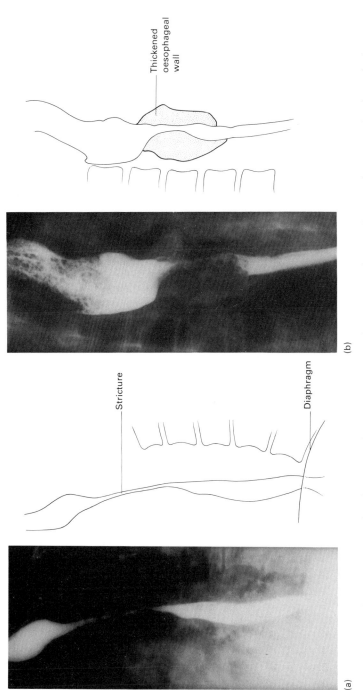

Fig. 2.3 Radiological appearances of benign and malignant oesophageal strictures. (a) Barium swallow showing a smooth stricture in the mid-oesophagus. Negative biopsies and cytology from the stricture confirmed its benign nature. (b) Barium swallow showing irregular stricturing in the lower oesophagus due to a carcinoma. The oesophageal wall is thickened by the tumour.

57

- Achalasia (p. 60)—the risk (<1%) is less than previously considered
- Iron deficiency anaemia and post-cricoid web, with high oesophageal carcinoma (Brown Kelly–Paterson syndrome)—10 times commoner in women, often aged 40–50 years
- Geographical:
  Caspian littoral (Iran)—commonest malignancy
  northern China—20 times more common than in Britain
  Transkei (South Africa)
  molybdenum deficiency, aflatoxin contamination of cereals and
      nitrosamines are postulated reasons for this variation
- Familial tylosis (palmar hyperkeratosis) is exceedingly rare

Clinical features
Progressive dysphagia and weight loss are typical, but pain and hoarseness of the voice may occur due to local spread. Patients are usually aged 60–80 years. Rapidly recurrent dysphagia after dilatation should be considered malignant until proven otherwise.

Pathology
- 90% are squamous
- Dysplasia may precede carcinoma
- Adenocarcinoma is due to spread from the gastric fundus, or malignant change in Barrett's oesophagus. It is becoming more common

Spread
- Local invasion is the rule
- Oesophago-bronchial fistula, recurrent laryngeal nerve palsy and atrial fibrillation may occur
- Death usually precedes distant metastases

Investigations

Diagnostic
- Barium swallow (Fig. 2.3, p. 57)
- Endoscopy, biopsy *and* brushings (98% detection rate), for a tissue diagnosis

2   Oesophagus

2.4   Oesophageal carcinoma

Look for complications
- Chest X-ray—mediastinal lymphadenopathy, evidence of aspiration
- ECG—atrial fibrillation

Surgical assessment
- Thoraco-abdominal CT scan
- Take into account age, cardiorespiratory disease and nutrition
- Lung function tests (including arterial gases), to estimate respiratory reserve
- Oesophageal endosonography is useful for assessing local invasion, but not generally available

Management
The objectives of treatment are to relieve dysphagia, prolong survival and to cure a minority. There is no single ideal treatment; the site and stage of the carcinoma and the general health of the patient determine the approach. Operability is the first decision.

Surgery
- Indicated for fit patients under 70 years without evidence of local invasion, when satisfactory resection can be achieved. This is less than a third of patients with oesophageal cancer
- Staging CT scan, preoperative nutritional supplementation and physiotherapy are important
- Subtotal oesophagectomy and formation of a gastric tube is usually appropriate, requiring separate thoracic and abdominal incisions
- Operative mortality is 10%

Palliation
- For most (70%) patients
- Surgical palliation is effective in experienced hands
- Endoscopic dilatation may be sufficient and should be tried initially for unresectable tumours, but can be complicated by oesophageal perforation
- Obstructing tumours can be relieved endoscopically by alcohol injection into the tumour through a sclerotherapy needle. This is cheap, safe and effective, but repeat treatments are often necessary. Laser photocoagulation is also effective, but not widely available

• Intubation—with a Celestin or Atkinson tube—is indicated for middle or lower third tumours when dilatation becomes unacceptable. Perforation, tube migration, blockage and persistent discomfort from proximal tubes are disadvantages
• Palliative radiotherapy is ineffective for long tumours or adeno-carcinomas and inappropriate for advanced disease. It can be used as an adjunct to endoscopic palliation, but the benefit is uncertain
• Radical radiotherapy is indicated for post-cricoid, upper third and short tumours. It is commonly converted into 'palliative' therapy because of side effects. Radiotherapy alone relieves dysphagia in <50%

Terminal care (p. 132)
Treatment should be carefully considered after assessing the patient, seeing the family and discussing with senior colleagues. Hydration, but not alimentation or antibiotics, is usually appropriate. Good mouth care, pharyngeal suction and liaison with the nursing staff are vital. Aspiration pneumonia is the usual cause of death.

Prognosis
• Mean survival is 10 months after diagnosis
• 5-year survival (apparent cure) is 11% after surgery

2.5   Achalasia
Achalasia is a motility disorder characterized by increased lower oesophageal sphincter pressure (>40 mmHg) and failure of relaxation during swallowing. Peristalsis in the body of the oesophagus is absent. It is due to degeneration of the myenteric plexus of unknown cause. Carcinoma of the cardia must be excluded.

Clinical features
• Occurs at any age
• Dysphagia—all patients; slowly progressive and often associated with a trick movement of the head, or Valsalva manoeuvre to help swallowing
• Weight loss—quite common
• Regurgitation—30%; undigested food, with aspiration
• Pain—substernal cramps may be severe and precede dysphagia
• Symptoms for <1 year and age >50 years, with weight loss, suggest carcinoma

2.5 Achalasia

• Megaoesophagus is a late manifestation of achalasia and there is an increased risk of oesophageal carcinoma in these patients
• Carcinoma of the cardia, gastric lymphoma, diffuse spasm, systemic sclerosis, Chagas' disease (South American trypanosomiasis) and amyloidosis can simulate achalasia

Investigations
• Chest X-ray—an oesophageal fluid level at the aortic knuckle and right lower lobe consolidation, or fibrosis may be present. The gastric air bubble is characteristically absent
• Barium swallow—food debris in the oesophagus with a smooth, tapered distal narrowing and aperistaltic contractions when recumbent, are characteristic (Fig. 2.4). Oesophageal dilatation

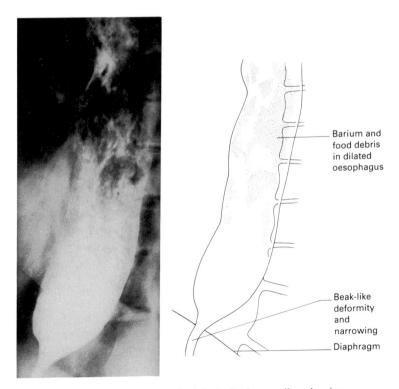

Barium and food debris in dilated oesophagus

Beak-like deformity and narrowing

Diaphragm

Fig. 2.4 Radiological appearance of achalasia. Barium swallow showing achalasia with dilatation of the oesophagus. Barium is mixing with food residue in the oesophagus. The oesophagus narrows to a typical beak-like deformity at the level of the cardia.

develops later. A cine- or bread barium swallow may elucidate difficult cases
- Endoscopy must always be performed to exclude a stricture and to examine the fundus for carcinoma. Once food debris is negotiated the endoscope easily passes the lower oesophageal sphincter
- Manometry may be the only way to distinguish oesophageal spasm from achalasia and should be performed if dysphagia persists despite a normal barium swallow (p. 66)

Management
The choice is between endoscopic dilatation and surgery (Heller's cardiomyotomy). Dilatation is often preferred by the patient, with surgery reserved for recurrent symptoms.

Dilatation
- Balloon dilatation with X-ray screening is effective in 70%, but repeat dilatations are often required
- Dilatation should only be performed by experienced endoscopists and the patient should be admitted overnight
- A chest X-ray in expiration is necessary 1 h after dilatation, before the patient eats, to look for mediastinal gas or pneumothorax. Perforation occurs in 2%

Surgery
- Indicated when symptoms recur after three attempts at dilatation, or if the patient prefers a definitive procedure at the outset
- Cardiomyotomy is effective in 90% and gives long-term relief

Complications
- Megaoesophagus is now rare
- Aspiration pneumonia can be chronic, or the presenting feature
- Carcinoma may occur in untreated achalasia, but probably not after treatment. It is less common (<1%) than previously thought
- Treatment (dilatation or surgical) may lead to:
    reflux
    stricture
    failure to relieve symptoms
    persistent pain, even after apparent relief of obstruction

---

2.6   Other conditions (Fig. 2.5)

Diffuse oesophageal spasm

Symptoms are caused by high-amplitude, aperistaltic oesophageal contractions without a demonstrable organic lesion.

Symptoms
• Dysphagia—intermittent but associated with pain
• Chest pain—may mimic cardiac pain and be provoked by stress

Investigations
• Barium swallow—a corkscrew appearance is classic but unusual. Aperistaltic 'tertiary' contractions are common when recumbent, but stasis does not occur, unlike achalasia (Fig. 2.5). Similar asymptomatic changes can occur in the elderly
• Manometry—is diagnostic if positive. Repetitive contractions, high-amplitude waves and periods of normal peristalsis are typical. Negative results do not exclude the diagnosis

Treatment
Symptoms are difficult to relieve totally. Reassurance that the pain is not cardiac is essential, also explaining that the drugs prescribed are often used for angina.
• Nifedipine 10 mg three times daily should be tried first, with isosorbide dinitrate 10 mg four times daily as an alternative, but side effects are common. Prokinetic agents may make symptoms worse
• Pneumatic dilatation should be reserved for the most severe cases, because the outcome is unpredictable

Oesophageal webs

Features
• Not circumferential, unlike rings (Fig. 2.5)
• Demonstrated radiologically, but difficult to see at endoscopy
• Check for iron deficiency anaemia, associated with a post-cricoid web and high oesophageal carcinoma (Brown Kelly–Paterson syndrome)
• Exclude carcinoma of the upper third of the oesophagus by careful radiology and endoscopy. ENT advice may be necessary

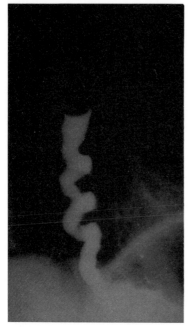

(a)

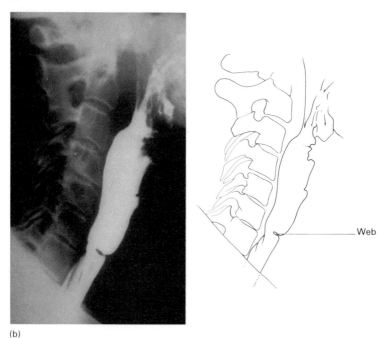

Web

(b)

Fig. 2.5 Radiological appearances of unusual causes of dysphagia. (a) Barium swallow showing diffuse oesophageal spasm with a typical 'corkscrew' deformity. (b) Barium swallow showing a clearly defined web arising from the anterior wall of the oesophagus and partly encircling it. A jet of barium is passing through the narrowed lumen at the level of the web.

2.6   Other conditions

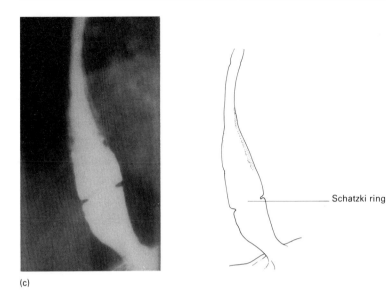

(c)

Fig. 2.5 (*continued*) Radiological appearances of unusual causes of dysphagia. (c) Barium swallow showing a narrow ring in the lower oesophagus. This is typical of the appearance of a Schatzki ring. The ring is often visible only when the oesophagus is fully distended by barium.

Schatzki ring
• Circumferential contraction in the middle or lower third, usually diagnosed radiologically rather than by endoscopy (Fig. 2.5)
• Often asymptomatic and of no significance
• If dysphagia is present, dilatation is justified after biopsy

Diverticula
• Pharyngeal pouches (Zenker's diverticulum) present with intermittent dysphagia and regurgitation in the elderly
• An ENT opinion is advisable after diagnosis by barium swallow (taking care to show the upper oesophagus)
• Endoscopy is not indicated and may be dangerous
• Surgical excision with or without cricopharyngeal myotomy is the treatment of choice for symptoms
• Mid-oesophageal diverticula are an endoscopic hazard, but of no other consequence

---

Systemic sclerosis
- Dysphagia with Raynaud's phenomenon is characteristic
- Recurrent strictures caused by reflux and stasis are the principal problem
- CREST syndrome (digital calcinosis, Raynaud's phenomenon, dysphagia, sclerodactyly and telangiectasia) should be distinguished clinically from systemic sclerosis, because it has a better prognosis
- Omeprazole 20–40 mg/day is the best treatment, because standard anti reflux treatment is ineffective. Cisapride 5–10 mg three times daily may help oesophageal emptying
- Endoscopic dilatation is necessary for strictures
- Other gastrointestinal complications (constipation, bacterial overgrowth) should be treated as well

2.7   Clinical dilemmas
General advice for diagnostic dilemmas is given in Appendix 5.

Chest pain ?cause
40% of patients with chest pain and a normal exercise ECG have an oesophageal disorder
- Confirm the history—especially the duration and type of pain, precipitating and relieving factors
- Oesophageal reflux and diffuse oesophageal spasm most commonly mimic angina
- Endoscopy is indicated to exclude oesophagitis
- Oesophageal manometry and 24-h pH monitoring with symptom recording should be performed after referral to a specialist centre. Provocation tests (edrophonium for spasm and acid perfusion (Bernstein test) for reflux) occasionally help (p. 366)
- A cine barium swallow in the recumbent position or a barium swallow with bread (since spasm sometimes only occurs with food) are alternative investigations
- Coronary angiography is indicated if no oesophageal lesion can be demonstrated and symptoms are disabling

Dysphagia with a 'normal' barium swallow
Globus hystericus is not the only cause. Diffuse spasm, achalasia and strictures may be overlooked.
- Confirm the history—especially whether dysphagia is for solids or liquids and the duration of symptoms

- Document the present weight and any loss
- Check the films:
  is it the correct patient?
  do they show *all* the oesophagus?
- Arrange a bread barium swallow recorded on video, after discussion with the radiologist
- Referral for manometry (p. 366) is indicated for persistent symptoms. Obscure cases of diffuse spasm or achalasia may be detected

3 Stomach and Duodenum

3.1 Dyspepsia

Dyspepsia (indigestion) is a non-specific group of symptoms related to the upper gastrointestinal tract. Organic disease must be detected and distinguished from 'non-ulcer dyspepsia', so that specific treatment can be given. Table 3.1 shows the differential diagnosis of post-prandial epigastric pain.

Causes
See Table 3.1

Table 3.1 Differential diagnosis of post-prandial epigastric pain

Common	Uncommon*	Rare
Non-ulcer dyspepsia	Biliary colic	Chronic pancreatitis
Duodenal ulcer	Gastro-oesophageal	Small intestinal stricture
Gastric ulcer	reflux	Mesenteric ischaemia
Gastritis	Oesophagitis	Myocardial ischaemia
Duodenitis		

* Although these conditions are common, they do not usually present with epigastric pain after meals.

Clinical features

Common symptoms
• Epigastric, upper abdominal, or retrosternal discomfort related to eating, specific foods, hunger or time of day
• Heaviness, unease, bloating or fullness are common descriptive terms, often associated with heartburn, flatulence, or borborygmi

Pointers to organic disease
• Age >40 years (but duodenal ulcers are most common at age 20–40 years)
• Symptoms for >8 weeks
• Weight loss
• Symptoms in smokers
• Symptoms at night

Examination
• Epigastric tenderness is non-specific
• Palpate carefully for an upper abdominal mass

• Feel for supraclavicular nodes and hepatomegaly

Investigations
Not all patients need investigation. A therapeutic trial of antacids is indicated if the patient is aged <40 years and symptoms are of short duration. Magnesium trisilicate mixture 20 ml as needed is cheap and as good as any (p. 76)

Indications for investigation
• Age >40 years
• Symptoms for longer than 8 weeks
• Relapsing symptoms
• Persistent symptoms despite antacids
• Weight loss

Specific investigations
• Blood tests—anaemia, a high platelet count or ESR and abnormal liver function tests point to an organic cause
• Barium meal or endoscopy (below)
• Ultrasound of the gall bladder and pancreas, if the endoscopy is normal

Barium meal or endoscopy?
Endoscopy is usually preferable for the initial investigation of dyspepsia because:
• Mucosal lesions (oesophagitis, gastritis, erosions, duodenitis and superficial ulceration) can be seen
• Biopsies can be taken to exclude malignancy and for identification of *Helicobacter pylori*
• It is generally well tolerated, especially by the elderly, with light sedation
    A barium meal is indicated if:
• Endoscopy is difficult or impossible—young drinkers tolerate the procedure poorly
• Oesophagogastric anatomy needs elucidating—cup and spill deformity or anastomoses can confuse endoscopists (Fig. 3.1). It is often easier to evaluate pyloric stenosis, or tumour infiltrating the stomach wall, by barium meal
• The choice may be determined by local availability

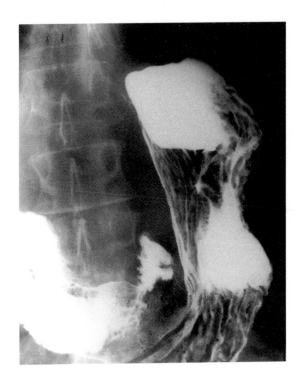

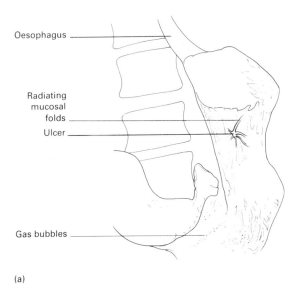

Oesophagus

Radiating
mucosal
folds

Ulcer

Gas bubbles

(a)

Fig. 3.1 Radiological appearances of peptic ulceration. (a) Barium meal showing a benign gastric ulcer in the body of the stomach, with gastric folds radiating from the edge of the ulcer crater.

73

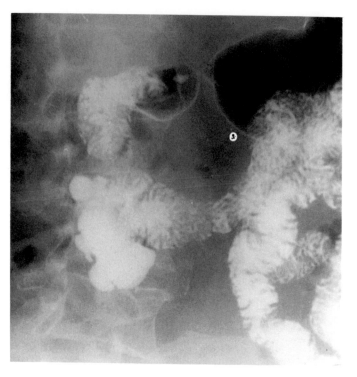

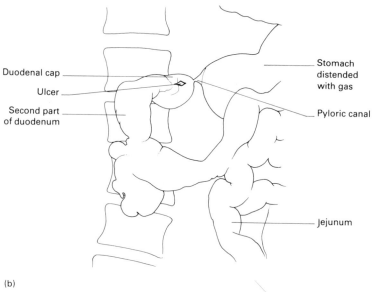

Duodenal cap	Stomach distended with gas
Ulcer	
Second part of duodenum	Pyloric canal
	Jejunum

(b)

Fig. 3.1 (*continued*) Radiological appearances of peptic ulceration. (b) Barium meal showing an ulcer in the first part of the duodenum.

3 Stomach and Duodenum

3.1 Dyspepsia

Organic dyspepsia
Dyspepsia due to lesions readily identified on routine investigation:
• Peptic ulcer
• Gastric cancer
• Reflux oesophagitis
• Gastritis
• Duodenitis
• Cholelithiasis
Management of organic disease is discussed in the appropriate sections.

Non-ulcer dyspepsia
Defined as upper abdominal or retrosternal discomfort related to meals, lasting for more than 4 weeks and for which no cause can be found after investigation. Rational investigation and management is helped by identifing one of three symptom patterns.

Dysmotility
• Upper abdominal pain:
  poorly localized
  may be several types
  not at night
  continuous, not periodic
• Abdominal distension
• Premature satiety
• Nausea—but vomiting is unusual
• Food intolerance:
  variable
  multiple

Reflux-type
• Retrosternal discomfort:
  on stooping
  after large meals
  on lying flat
  temporary relief from antacids
• Recent weight gain
• Cyclical severity
• No endoscopic or microscopic evidence of oesophagitis

3.1   Dyspepsia

Ulcer-type
- Epigastric pain:
  occasionally at night
  relieved by antacids or food
  episodic
- No ulcer, past or present
There remain some patients who have upper abdominal pain after meals that does not follow one of these patterns. Features common to all patients with non-ulcer dyspepsia are:
- The patient remains well
- Weight is steady, or fluctuating
- Normal investigations

Treatment of non-ulcer dyspepsia
- Explanation and reassurance are essential
- Lifestyle changes (regular meals, weight loss, stopping smoking) often help
- Drugs should only be used when symptoms are intolerable. Antacids should always be tried first. The following recommendations are made, but controlled trials have not shown clear benefits from drug treatments, or have not been performed with some agents
- Dysmotility type—antispasmodic or prokinetic agent (mebeverine 135 mg or cisapride 5–10 mg three times daily, for example)
- Reflux-type—H_2 receptor antagonist or prokinetic agent (cimetidine 400 mg twice daily, cisapride 5–10 mg three times daily, for example)
- Ulcer-type—H_2 receptor antagonist. Eradication of *H. pylori* (p. 83) is not indicated unless chronic gastritis has been histologically proven and symptoms are not relieved by other treatment
- Other patients often respond poorly to treatment. An exclusion diet (p. 390) may help

Which antacid?
There are 70 antacid preparations in the British National Formulary (BNF), not all of which are prescribable on the NHS. Efficacy, peripheral effects and cost need to be considered.

Efficacy
- *In vitro* neutralizing capacity is greatest with magnesium hydroxide/aluminium hydroxide mixtures (Maalox, Mucaine)
- Alginates (Gastrocote, Gaviscon) have low neutralizing capacity

but may be better for symptoms of gastro-oesophageal reflux
• Liquids act more quickly than tablets, but the latter are more convenient

Peripheral effects
• Sodium content is important in patients with cardiovascular, renal, or hepatic disease. Magnesium trisilicate mixture ('Mist. mag. trisil.') has 6.3 mmol/10 ml whereas Maalox has 0.1 mmol/10 ml. Gastrocote has half the sodium content of Gaviscon
• Aluminium compounds bind bile salts and may be more effective in biliary reflux. They also cause constipation and can be absorbed, which contributes to osteodystrophy and encephalopathy in chronic renal failure
• Magnesium compounds cause diarrhoea
• Absorption of other drugs (iron, antibiotics, phenothiazines) may be impaired by antacids
• Rebound hyperacidity can occur after regular antacid treatment has been stopped. This may contribute to stress ulcers

Cost
• Magnesium trisilicate, Maalox and aluminium hydroxide tablets are the cheapest (20–30p for 20 tablets)
• Gaviscon or Gastrocote tablets cost about 75p for 20 tablets and Gaviscon mixture costs 5 times as much as magnesium trisilicate mixture.

Recommendations
• Magnesium trisilicate tablets or mixture for routine use
• Maalox if a low-sodium antacid is required
• Aluminium hydroxide mixture for biliary reflux

3.2 Nausea and vomiting
The timing, amount and content of the vomitus are important. Associated symptoms often indicate the cause, since isolated nausea or vomiting is rarely organic.

Causes
• Abdominal:
gastroenteritis
gastric or duodenal ulcer
pyloric stenosis

3.2   Nausea and vomiting

---

ileus
intestinal obstruction
cholecystitis
pancreatitis
• Metabolic:
diabetic ketoacidosis
hypercalcaemia
hyponatraemia
uraemia
• Drugs:
opiates, chemotherapy, sulphasalazine, digoxin and many others
alcohol
• Cerebral:
migraine
raised intracranial pressure
brain stem lesions
• Vestibular:
Menière's disease
motion sickness
viral (rarely bacterial) labyrinthitis
• Endocrine:
pregnancy
Addison's disease
• Other organic:
myocardial infarction
autonomic neuropathy
• Non-organic:
non-ulcer dyspepsia
bulimia, anorexia nervosa
self-induced
psychogenic
motion sickness

Investigations and management

Assessment
• Look for signs of dehydration
• Listen for a gastric splash and feel for a mass
• Examine the vomitus for volume, blood, bile (indicates patent pylorus)
• Check the urine—osmolality, sugar and a pregnancy test

3.2 Nausea and vomiting

- Request serum electrolytes, urea, random sugar and calcium
- Metabolic alkalosis (pH >7.44, Pa_{CO_2} >45 mmHg or 6.0 kPa) only occurs in severe vomiting
- Arrange an endoscopy if vomiting is persistent

Drugs
- Metoclopramide 10 mg three times daily (parenterally) for gastrointestinal causes other than intestinal obstruction
- Prochlorperazine 25 mg suppository or 12.5 mg intramuscular, but not intravenous, for metabolic or drug-induced vomiting. A digoxin level within the therapeutic range may still cause vomiting
- Cinnarizine 15 mg or promethazine 25 mg orally for vestibular disorders
- Domperidone 20 mg oral or 60 mg suppository has fewer extrapyramidal side effects than metoclopramide and is preferable in the elderly. Cisapride 30 mg suppository three times daily is an alternative

Pregnancy
- Avoid drugs if at all possible
- Promethazine 25 mg oral/injection may be given, even in the first trimester if really necessary

Chemotherapy
- Intravenous dexamethasone 8 mg with lorazepam 2 mg before chemotherapy
- Domperidone 60 mg suppositories four times daily help persistent nausea
- 5-HT$_3$ antagonists (such as ondansetron 8 mg three times daily, oral or parenteral, for a few days) may also be helpful

Persistent vomiting
- Review the diagnosis, especially considering cerebral, brain stem (fourth ventricle), metabolic and mechanical causes
- Arrange an endoscopy if not already performed
- Gastric emptying studies (p. 363) occasionally identify gastroparesis due to autonomic neuropathy
- Combination therapy occasionally helps when single drugs fail
- Methotrimeprazine 100 mg by continous subcutaneous infusion daily is useful in terminal care

3.3 Gastritis

Inflammation of the gastric mucosa (gastritis) represents the stomach's response to injury. Whether gastritis is transient or related to peptic ulcer or gastric cancer depends on the site, type and cause of inflammation.

Classification

Many classifications have been proposed, but the Sydney (1990) system is the most acceptable, because it combines topographical and morphological details (Table 3.2).

Three types of gastritis are now recognized—acute, chronic and special forms. These are then qualified by site, morphology and associated aetiology, if known.

Table 3.2 Summary of the Sydney classification of gastritis

Type	Site	Morphology	Aetiology
Acute	Antrum	Inflammation	Microbial (*H. pylori**)
Chronic	Body	Activity	Non-microbial
Special forms	Pangastritis	Atrophy	autoimmune
granulomatous		Metaplasia	alcohol
eosinophilic		*H. pylori* numbers	post-gastrectomy
lymphocytic			NSAID
hypertrophic			chemical
reactive			Unknown

* Other microbial causes are very rare

Site

• The stomach is divided into two topographical areas—antrum and body. Gastritis in both sites is termed pangastritis

Morphology

The five principal features (inflammation, activity, atrophy, intestinal metaplasia and numbers of *H. pylori*) are graded none, mild, moderate, or severe.

• Inflammation means the number of chronic inflammatory cells in the lamina propria

• Activity means the presence of neutrophil polymorphs, which characterize acute gastritis

---

• Atrophy evaluates the depth of gastric glands, which is positively related to cancer and negatively associated with ulcers
• Intestinal metaplasia is fairly common in chronic gastritis and in association with gastric ulcers or cancer. It may precede early gastric cancer, but is not necessarily premalignant
• Numbers of *H. pylori*, detected by Giemsa or Gram stain (culture and urease techniques only indicate presence or absence of the organism), indicate the density of infection
• Other morphological features of gastritis are the presence of erosions (common in acute gastritis), or diagnostic features of special forms (granulomas, eosinophils, cytomegalovirus) which are not graded

Aetiology
• Microbial—*H. pylori* (Fig. 3.2, p. 84) causes almost all antral chronic gastritis (>95%). *Gastrospirillum hominis*, another spiral bacterium, cytomegalovirus, or herpes virus are very rare causes
• Non-microbial causes are mentioned in Table 3.2. Autoimmune-associated chronic gastritis is largely confined to the body of the stomach, where it causes atrophy, anacidity, vitamin B_{12} deficiency and predisposes to cancer
• Unknown factors cause up to 50% of gastritis in the body of the stomach

Previous terms for gastritis
Previous descriptive terms include Types A (autoimmune, in the gastric body, associated with atrophy), B (bacterial, in the antrum), AB (pangastritis), or C (chemical, drug-induced).

Chronic superficial gastritis (acute-on-chronic gastritis), chronic atrophic gastritis (distinct from gastric atrophy due to autoimmune causes) are other terms that have been used, but lack specificity.

Clinical features and investigations
Gastritis can only be reliably diagnosed by histology and can only be adequately classified when biopsies have been taken from both the body and antrum of the stomach. Histological gastritis, however, does not always correlate with either endoscopic appearances or symptoms, and consequently does not always need treatment.

3.3 Gastritis

Acute gastritis
- Caused by drugs (salicylates), alcohol, or as a response to trauma (stress erosions). *H. pylori*-associated acute gastritis is rarely seen, although it is a common cause of acute-on-chronic gastritis
- Often asymptomatic, but dyspepsia, retching or haematemesis may occur
- Endoscopic appearances range from erythema to erosions which may be obscured by haemorrhagic oozing (haemorrhagic gastritis, p. 14)

Chronic gastritis
- Common worldwide, especially in developing countries, or in patients of low socio-economic status. Prevalence increases with age (about 50% have some chronic gastritis when aged >60 years)
- Usually caused by *H. pylori*, but occasionally autoimmune
- Frequently antral, asymptomatic and remains stable for many years
- Chronic gastritis sometimes heals spontaneously, but it is associated with peptic ulcers. A small proportion (about 3% at each stage) develop intestinal metaplasia, progress to atrophy, and then to cancer
- Parietal cell antibodies occur in 10% with chronic gastritis. Pernicious anaemia (in about 10% with antibodies, but up to 80% when titre >1:40) is associated with autoimmune thyroiditis, adrenal disorders, vitiligo and insulin-dependent diabetes mellitus

Special forms
- Granulomatous gastritis is a rare feature of sarcoidosis or Crohn's disease
- Eosinophilic gastritis is extremely rare and may indicate vasculitis
- Hypertrophic gastritis (Ménétrier's disease) may cause weight loss due to a protein-losing enteropathy. Hypertrophic mucosal folds on a barium meal must be distinguished from lymphoma
- Lymphocytic gastritis causes a varioliform pattern in the fundus
- Reactive gastritis refers to reflux (post-gastrectomy) or drugs

Management
Asymptomatic gastritis, whether endoscopic or histological, does not need treatment. General measures such as avoiding provoking

factors (alcohol, NSAIDs and smoking, although the latter is not proven) are appropriate for all symptomatic patients. Symptomatic treatment with antacids or drugs for non-ulcer dyspepsia (p. 76) are suitable when a specific cause cannot be identified, or for mild symptoms from *H. pylori*-associated gastritis.

Helicobacter pylori (Fig. 3.2)
• Indiscriminate use of antibiotics to treat *H. pylori* should be avoided, because resistance to metronidazole is already developing, especially in women in emergent countries
• The aim of treatment must be eradication of *H. pylori* rather than suppression or clearance, if the natural history of chronic gastritis (and ulcers) is to be altered
• Treatment is indicated when chronic gastritis is associated with recurrent duodenal ulcers, or when severe symptoms are unrelieved by symptomatic treatment and *H. pylori* is identifiable. Eradication may also be attempted when more than one cause of ulceration is present
• Treatment is not indicated for mild symptoms from chronic gastritis, non-ulcer dyspepsia, gastric ulcers (whether or not the organism is present), or when *H. pylori* cannot be identified
• Treatment means triple therapy (bismuth compound and two antibiotics), to minimize resistance. Bismuth subcitrate (De-Nol) 1 tablet and tetracycline 500 mg four times daily with metronidazole 400 mg three times daily for 2 weeks are appropriate. Ampicillin may be substituted for tetracycline
• This eradicates infection in >90%, but side effects (nausea, abdominal discomfort) are common, and may result in poor compliance. Bismuth subcitrate 2 tablets twice daily with metronidazole 400 mg three times daily for 4 weeks, causes fewer side effects, but may not be as effective

Specific treatment for other types of gastritis
• Acute gastritis, with bleeding from erosions, is treated with H_2 receptor antagonists or omeprazole (p. 15)
• Autoimmune-associated—serum vitamin B_{12} should be measured and if <150 ng/l, intramuscular hydroxycobalamin 1000 μg is needed every 3 months for life

3.3 Gastritis

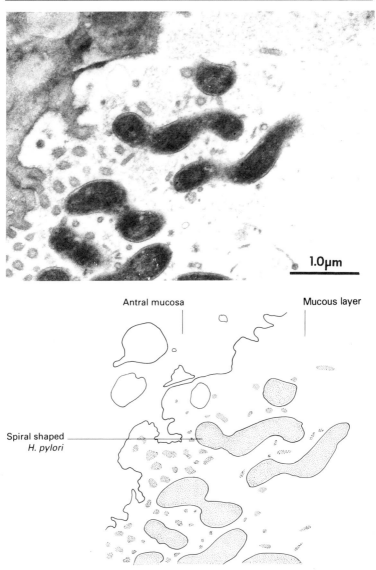

Fig. 3.2 Transmission electron micrograph of antral mucosa in a human patient, illustrating the spiral shape of *Helicobacter pylori*.

• Hypertrophic gastritis (Ménétrier's disease)—oral probanthine 15 mg four times daily until symptoms resolve
• Intestinal metaplasia alone is not an indication for treatment, or repeat endoscopy, unless associated with a gastric ulcer

3.4 Gastric ulcer

Benign gastric ulcers occur predominantly in the elderly, on the lesser curve (Fig. 3.1 p. 74). Ulcers on the greater curve, fundus and in the antrum are more commonly malignant. Gastric ulcers are less common than duodenal ulcers before age 40 years, but become more common in the elderly. Features and treatment for gastric and duodenal ulcers are compared in Section 3.8 (p. 101).

Causes

The cause is usually multifactorial and there is often no obvious provoking factor.

• Chronic, benign ulceration is more strongly associated with smoking than alcohol. Environmental stress may be weakly associated. Chronic antral gastritis is also associated

• Drug-related (NSAID) ulcers may be a separate entity, often causing few symptoms before a complication occurs. The risk of ulceration in patients on steroids has probably been exaggerated

• Acute ulcers or erosions are related to stress (Cushing's or Curling's ulcers, after neurosurgery or burns, respectively)

• Proposed mechanisms include impairment of the mucus–bicarbonate barrier, deficient gastric mucosal blood flow (possibly related to prostaglandin E_2 (PGE_2)) and acid–pepsin damage. Duodenogastric reflux of bile may also damage the mucosa. Although the dictum 'no acid, no ulcer' is valid, acid secretion in patients with chronic gastric ulcers is frequently in the low–normal range.

Clinical features

Ulcers cannot be diagnosed by history or physical examination, nor can gastric or duodenal ulcers be differentiated on clinical grounds. 'Typical' ulcer pain (epigastric, related to meals and relieved by antacids) is non-specific (Table 3.1, p. 71).

• Vomiting, weight loss, or unremitting pain sometimes predominate in elderly patients with a gastric ulcer, but malignancy *must* be excluded by biopsy and brush cytology. Some may be asymptomatic, especially drug-induced ulcers. If a gastric ulcer is found during investigation of asymptomatic iron deficiency anaemia, it is usually the cause

• Complications (haematemesis or perforation, p. 88) may be the presenting feature in a third of patients

3.4 Gastric ulcer

Investigations

Blood tests
• Serum iron and total iron-binding capacity should be measured if the patient is anaemic. A microcytic anaemia can also be caused by thalassaemia-trait, chronic disease, or sideroblastic anaemia, as well as iron deficiency. Serum ferritin is the best marker of iron stores, if there is doubt

Endoscopy
• Multiple rim and crater biopsies as well as brush cytology are mandatory, except for gastric ulcers that have recently bled
• When gastric ulcers are diagnosed at emergency endoscopy for bleeding, a further endoscopy should be arranged after the bleeding has stopped, to allow biopsies and brushings to be taken
• Repeat endoscopy after 8–12 weeks' treatment should be booked at the time of diagnosis to confirm healing. The ulcer site must be biopsied, even if the ulcer has healed. Further endoscopies, with more brushings and biopsies, are necessary for persistent ulcers until complete healing has occurred
• Symptomatic relapse after a gastric ulcer has been diagnosed is an indication for repeat endoscopy

Barium meal
• When a gastric ulcer is shown on a barium meal (Fig. 3.1, p. 74), endoscopy should be arranged for biopsies and brushings

Management

General
• Stop smoking—this increases the healing rate and decreases relapse rates
• Alcohol intake—should be curtailed if excessive (this means >14 units/week for women, >21 units/week for men), but abstinence is unnecessary
• Diet—does not affect healing, but common sense advice to ensure adequate nutrition and to avoid foods that exacerbate symptoms is appropriate
• Lifestyle—regular meals can assist symptom control

3.4   Gastric ulcer

• Drugs—stop NSAIDs, aspirin, or steroids (gradually) if possible, but healing is still likely if it is necessary to continue treatment. Small doses of aspirin (75–150 mg/day) are unimportant

Which H_2 receptor antagonist?
• All H_2 receptor antagonists heal 75–90% benign gastric ulcers in 6–8 weeks
• Cimetidine is preferable to ranitidine in young patients, because it is as effective but cheaper
• Ranitidine is preferable to cimetidine in those with liver disease or those taking anticonvulsants or anticoagulants, since it does not interfere with hepatic metabolism. It may cause less confusion in the elderly and heal more ulcers, but the advantage over cimetidine is not very great
• Famotidine and nizatidine are very similar to ranitidine

Dose, frequency and duration
• Cimetidine 800 mg/day, or ranitidine 300 mg/day are recommended
• A single dose at 6 p.m. is as effective in healing ulcers as divided doses
• 8 weeks' initial treatment for gastric ulcers is advisable, although treatment may need to be continued for 12–16 weeks if the ulcer has not healed at the repeat endoscopy
• NSAID-associated gastric ulcers are healed by H_2 receptor antagonists, even if NSAIDs have to be continued, but maintenance treatment is needed

Maintenance treatment
• Indicated for patients with cardiorespiratory disease, or any disorder that would affect survival in the event of developing complications of a recurrent ulcer
• Indicated for patients on NSAIDs with a past (or current) history of ulceration. Misoprostol 200 μg three times daily may prevent gastric ulcers in patients on NSAIDs, but there are no indications for prescribing this drug routinely. Misoprostol is believed to be cytoprotective, but may cause diarrhoea
• Ranitidine 150 mg at night is recommended, since most patients are elderly. H_2 receptor antagonists can be continued indefinitely in elderly patients on NSAIDs, or those with medical complications

---

Alternatives to H₂ receptor antagonists
- The side effects of carbenoxolone, pirenzepine, or high-dose antacids usually limit treatment, although all have been shown to be as effective as cimetidine
- Sucralfate 1 g four times daily or 2 g twice daily works best in an acid medium, so antacids should be avoided
- Omeprazole 20 mg at night is little better than H₂ receptor antagonists after 6–8 weeks' treatment, although it heals gastric (and duodenal) ulcers more rapidly. It does not alter the relapse rate and is not recommended for first-line or long-term treatment. It has a place in treating resistant ulcers (see below)
- Bismuth compounds have no place in the current treatment of gastric (as opposed to duodenal) ulcers, even though many gastric ulcers are associated with *H. pylori*

Resistant ulcers
- Ulcers that have not healed after 8 weeks' treatment must be rebiopsied and brushed for cytology
- In unhealed ulcers, double the dose of H₂ receptor antagonists for a further 8 weeks (cimetidine 800 mg twice daily, or ranitidine 300 mg twice daily) and arrange a repeat endoscopy
- Poor compliance is probably the commonest cause of failure to heal
- Failure of a gastric ulcer to heal after 12–16 weeks' treatment may be due to malignancy (which can be missed, even with biopsies and brushings), and is often an indication for surgery
- Early relapse after apparent healing suggests malignancy and should be fully investigated
- Omeprazole 20 mg at night can be tried in those unfit for surgery

Indications for surgery
- Complications:
  bleeding (p. 15)
  perforation (p. 24)
- Failure to heal after 12–16 weeks' treatment, unless the risks of operation are very high
- Relapse on maintenance therapy

A Billroth I partial gastrectomy is the standard operation, carrying a <2% operative mortality and 10–30% incidence of long-term sequelae (p. 104)

Special categories

Giant ulcers
• >2.5 cm diameter carry no special risk of malignancy

Antral ulcers
• 20% are malignant

Prepyloric ulcers
• Behave like duodenal ulcers

Pyloric channel ulcers
• Vomiting and weight loss are common
• If ulceration extends through to the duodenum, consider lymphoma

Combined gastric and duodenal ulcers
• Bleeding and obstruction are said to be more common

Complications
Complications of gastric ulcers may occur without any preceding symptoms, especially in those taking NSAIDs or steroids.
• 50% recur
• 25% bleed (p. 15)
• 10% perforate (p. 24)
• Fibrosis causing deformity ('hour-glass', or 'tea-pot' stomach) is rare. Pyloric stenosis may complicate pre-pyloric ulceration
• Carcinoma at the site of a 'benign' ulcer is the result of an initial misdiagnosis, rather than a complication, even if the ulcer has responded to conventional treatment

3.5   Gastric carcinoma
Gastric cancer is the fourth most common cause of cancer deaths. There is widespread geographical variation in incidence and prognosis, but the incidence in the West is falling. It is twice as common in men as in women.

Causes
No single factor can be implicated. Gastritis and *H. pylori* commonly coexist with cancer, but the risk is debated. Chronic

benign gastric ulcers do not predispose to cancer.

Well-differentiated early gastric cancer may develop at sites of intestinal metaplasia, but metaplasia is not definitely premalignant, nor is it an indication for repeat endoscopy and biopsy unless an ulcer is present. Gastric adenomatous polyps are unusual, but have the same malignant potential as in the colon (p. 290).

• Diet—may explain the high incidence in Japan, China and Central America, since the incidence declines in migrant populations. *N*-nitrosamines have been implicated. The prevalence of *H. pylori* is also high in these populations

• Genetic—blood group A is associated with a 20% increase in risk patients with familial adenomatous polyposis (p. 292) have an increased risk of upper gastrointestinal malignancy

• Low socio-economic class—the incidence is 5 times higher in labourers than professionals. There is also a high prevalence of *H. pylori* infection, acquired at a young age, in this group

• Gastric surgery—the increased incidence 15 years after partial gastrectomy is small, but probably real

• Pernicious anaemia—the risk (about 1%) is increased

Clinical features

General

• Dyspepsia is usual, but is non-specific, poorly related to meals and relief by simple antacids is common

• Anorexia and weight loss often indicate incurable disease

• Haematemesis is an unusual presentation

• Signs are absent until incurable disease exists

• Metastases to the lungs (lymphangitis carcinomatosa), bone or brain may be the presenting feature. A supraclavicular (Troissier's) node, or migratory phlebothrombosis (Trousseau's sign) are uncommon

• Dermatomyositis and acanthosis nigricans are most frequently associated with gastric carcinoma

• H_2 receptor antagonists or omeprazole can temporarily relieve symptoms and heal malignant ulcers

---

Pathology
No classification is satisfactory, but there is a spectrum from polypoid lesions, through ulcers, to diffuse infiltrating cancer (linitis plastica). All types are adenocarcinomas. The degree of differentiation, local and remote spread affect the prognosis, but not histological type (mucinous, signet ring). Tumours are multiple in 10%.

Early gastric cancer
Early gastric cancer is distinguished by an excellent prognosis (90% 5-year survival) after resection. It means a gastric cancer that is recognized endoscopically at a curable stage when it is intramucosal, and is probably a distinct entity rather than an early stage of the more common variety. Early gastric cancer is often asymptomatic unless it ulcerates, when dyspepsia occurs. Endoscopy shows a superficial excavated or slightly protuberant lesion which may look insignificant. Biopsy of any gastric lesion is therefore essential if early gastric cancer is to be diagnosed. Local venous or lymphatic metastases are sometimes present.

Investigations
Dyspepsia lasting more than 8 weeks after the age of 40 years demands investigation (p. 71). Once the diagnosis has been made, a search for clinically silent metastases is indicated, before a decision about treatment strategy is made.

Diagnosis
• Endoscopy—antral ulcers, or rolled and irregular edges of an ulcer crater favour malignancy, but multiple biopsies and brushings must be taken from all gastric ulcers
• Barium meal—blunting, fusion, and tapering of mucosal folds radiating from the ulcer favour malignancy (Fig. 3.3). Endoscopy, biopsy and brush cytology are *always* indicated after radiological diagnosis of a gastric ulcer

Looking for metastases
• Chest X-ray—look for a pleural effusion, solitary metastasis, or reticular shadowing from lymphangitis

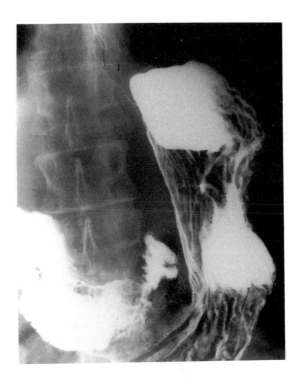

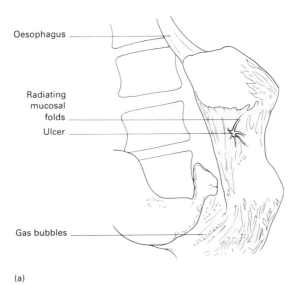

(a)

Fig. 3.3 Radiological appearances of benign and malignant gastric ulcers.
(a) Barium meal showing a benign gastric ulcer with gastric folds radiating from the edge of the ulcer crater.

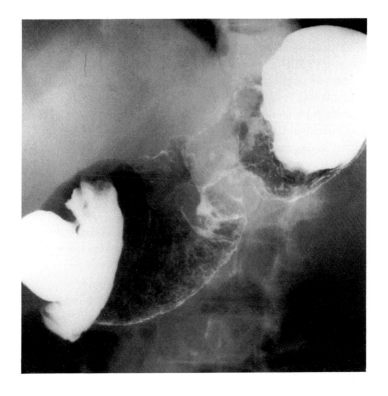

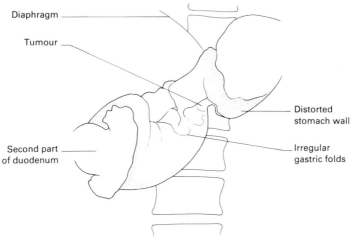

Diaphragm

Tumour

Second part
of duodenum

Distorted
stomach wall

Irregular
gastric folds

(b)

Fig. 3.3 (*continued*) Radiological appearances of benign and malignant gastric
ulcers. (b) Barium meal showing a large cancer arising from the greater curve
and distorting the stomach wall. The abnormal, irregular folds often do not
reach the edge of the cancer.

- Blood tests—leucoerythroblastic anaemia or abnormal liver function tests (LFTs) suggest incurable disease. Elevated alkaline phosphatase may be due to bony metastases if the γ-glutamyl transferase (γGT) is normal
- Ultrasound scan of the liver
- An abdominal CT scan is not routine, but may be useful in assessing local or hepatic metastases if the ultrasound is normal but spread is still suspected (abnormal LFTs, for instance)
- Laparotomy may still be needed to assess resectability

Early diagnosis

An early diagnosis programme is part of the reason for the better outcome in Japan where incidence is high and intramucosal lesions are common (25% overall 5-year survival). Public awareness and early investigation of dyspeptic symptoms in patients aged >40 years are essential to early diagnosis. Screening asymptomatic individuals (even those with pernicious anaemia or previous gastric surgery) is not justifiable in the United Kingdom.

Management

Curative surgery
- Indicated for patients aged <75 years with no signs of metastases and otherwise in good health—about a third of all patients
- Radical surgery has a mortality of 10%, but post-gastrectomy sequelae are more common (p. 104)
- The operation rate, curative resection rate and survival are appreciably higher in Japan than the UK, probably as a result of population screening and more aggressive surgery

Palliative surgery
- Indicated for obstruction, pain, or bleeding

Adjuvant therapy
- Neither radiotherapy nor chemotherapy affects survival and they do little for the quality of life

Supportive therapy
- Pain can be relieved by cimetidine 800 mg or omeprazole 20 mg daily, unless it is due to infiltration, when opiates are usually

necessary. It is debatable whether cimetidine improves survival
• Explanation to the family, home support and liaison with the general practitioner are vital aspects of terminal care (p. 132)

Prognosis
Local recurrence is the main cause of failure. The prognosis will only be improved by earlier detection followed by effective surgery.
• The 5-year survival for all patients is 9%
• Following curative surgery the 5-year survival in the United Kingdom is 23%
• Median survival for inoperable disease is 4 months

3.6   Other gastric tumours

Lymphoma
The stomach is the most common extranodal site for lymphoma, but it remains rare. Prognosis is much better than for gastric cancer.

Clinical features
Gastric lymphoma cannot be distinguished clinically from a benign ulcer or gastric cancer. Weight loss, nausea and vomiting are said to occur earlier than in gastric cancer and haematemesis may be more common. An epigastric mass is palpable in about 30%, but splenomegaly and peripheral lymphadenopathy are unusual. Patients are aged 50–70 years.

Diagnostic investigations
• Blood tests—a microcytic anaemia and raised ESR are common
• Endoscopy—appearances may be similar to a carcinoma. Multiple ulcerated nodules, transpyloric infiltration and giant rugae favour lymphoma. Deep, multiple biopsies (best performed by snaring a mucosal fold, with diathermy for haemostasis) are necessary, but still may not be positive. Diagnostic laparotomy and frozen section biopsies may then be needed
• Barium meal—polypoid ulcerated lesions on the greater curve and extension into the duodenum favour lymphoma, but none are specific

Further investigations
- Bone marrow—infiltration indicates stage IV disease
- Abdominal CT scan—for staging (Table 3.3)
- Histological type—the distinction between 'high grade' and 'low grade' is more helpful than the type of malignant cell when planning treatment
- Frozen sections (as well as formalin-fixed biopsies) are often necessary, and need to be planned with the pathologist before surgery

Table 3.3 Staging of intestinal lymphoma

Stage*	Interpretation
I	Disease in a single extralymphatic organ
II	Localized involvement of an extralymphatic organ as well as lymph nodes on the same side of the diaphragm
III	Localized involvement of an extralymphatic organ and lymph nodes on both sides of the diaphragm
IV	Diffuse or disseminated involvement of more than one extralymphatic organ, with or without lymph node involvement

* The suffix 'E' may be used to denote extralymphatic lymphoma

Treatment
Regimens are complex and evolving. Specialist oncological advice is recommended. General guidelines are as follows:
- Surgery for:
  stage I disease
  complications (haemorrhage or obstruction)
- Radiotherapy for:
  stage II disease, often with chemotherapy
- Chemotherapy for:
  stage III or stage IV disease

Polyps
Hyperplastic polyps are regenerative and the commonest epithelial lesions (70%). They are of no significance. It is good endoscopic practice, however, to biopsy all mucosal lesions, because early gastric cancer may look insignificant (p. 91).
    True adenomatous polyps are unusual but have the same

malignant potential as colonic adenomatous polyps. Endoscopic removal or resection is indicated. They may be associated with colonic polyps, so check for large bowel symptoms or blood loss.

Leiomyoma
Account for 50% of benign gastric tumours. Haemorrhage due to ulceration at the apex is the main clinical problem. Because they arise from the muscle of the gastric wall they cannot be removed endoscopically, so surgery (wedge resection) is indicated. Leiomyosarcomas probably arise *de novo* rather than from an existing leiomyoma.

Other tumours
Submucosal lipomas may reach a large size and bleed. Gastric carcinoid tumours may be more common in patients with pernicious anaemia. Secondary deposits and heterotopic pancreas are extremely rare.

3.7 Duodenitis
Duodenitis is an endoscopic diagnosis and it is often difficult to determine whether it is causing the patient's symptoms. It can represent the healing phase of duodenal ulceration.

Causes
• Almost always caused by *H. pylori*
• Very occasionally caused by Crohn's disease, cytomegalovirus, ectopic pancreatic tissue, nematodes, or sarcoidosis

Clinical features
Duodenitis causes very variable symptoms which may be provoked by alcohol or drugs. Ulcer-type pain, dysmotility symptoms (p. 75) or no symptoms may be present. Duodenitis never causes anaemia, but is sometimes the only abnormality found at endoscopy for haematemesis.

Duodenal inflammation is recognized endoscopically as patchy erythema or superficial erosions (salt-and-pepper or 'salami' duodenitis) in the first part of the duodenum. The mucosa can be nodular, but the second part of the duodenum is usually normal.

Histology does not always correlate with the endoscopic appearance, but biopsies almost always show *H. pylori*.

Management

Asymptomatic patients
• Duodenitis can be ignored

Symptomatic patients
• Antacids are often disappointing, but should be tried before H_2 receptor antagonists
• Dysmotility symptoms (bloating, fullness, poorly localized pain) may be treated with metoclopramide 10 mg, cisapride 5–10 mg, or mebeverine 135 mg three times daily
• Eradication of *H. pylori* (p. 83) is not indicated unless duodenitis is associated with recurrent duodenal ulcers or severe symptoms unrelieved by other treatment

3.8 Duodenal ulcer
Duodenal ulcers are 4 times more common than gastric ulcers below the age of 40 years and are more common in men. Although the overall incidence is falling, the incidence in women is increasing. The natural history of ulcers is a relapsing one; 80% relapse within 1 year of healing. Symptoms are said to remit after 10 years, but little is known about the long-term pattern of duodenal ulceration.

Causes
Interactions between acid, pepsin, *H. pylori*, genetic and environmental factors cause duodenal ulcers. Localization of ulcers to the first part of the duodenum reflects acid exposure, or colonization of gastric metaplastic islands by *H. pylori*, but does not mean that acid initiates mucosal damage.

Acid and pepsin
• Basal, peak and nocturnal acid secretion are increased in many, but not all, patients
• Pepsinogen (precursor of pepsin) secretion is increased in 60%
• The number and sensitivity of parietal cells influence the tendency to hypersecretion of acid
• Faster gastric emptying in duodenal ulcer patients may decrease duodenal pH

3.8   Duodenal ulcer

Helicobacter pylori
- 96% of patients have associated antral *H. pylori* (compared to 15% of young asymptomatic controls, but increasing with age)
- Eradication of *H. pylori* decreases the relapse rate

Genetic
- Blood group O (relative risk 1.25)
- Non-secretors of blood group substances
- First-degree relatives are affected in about 20%, compared to a 10% prevalence of duodenal ulcers in the UK, but this may be due to environmental influences

Environmental
- Smoking retards healing and increases the likelihood of relapse
- Drugs (NSAIDs, aspirin and possibly steroids) are associated with bleeding and perforation, but not necessarily with uncomplicated ulcers. The elderly are more at risk and may be asymptomatic before presenting with a complication
- Stress is often said to be related to duodenal ulceration, but this cannot be quantified. It may contribute to the non-specific association with chronic renal failure, lung disease and cirrhosis

Clinical features
- Young men are most often affected. Incidence increases in post-menopausal women
- Epigastric pain classically occurs before meals (hunger pain), wakes the patient at night and recurs several times a year for a few weeks. It may radiate to the back
- Vomiting and weight loss are unusual without pyloric stenosis
- Examination, apart from epigastric tenderness, is unremarkable in the absence of complications
- Symptoms frequently fail to fit this pattern and all conditions that may cause dyspepsia (Table 3.1, p. 71) are included in the differential diagnosis

Investigations

Initial presentation
- Endoscopy is the most appropriate method of diagnosis (p. 72) because it can be difficult on a barium meal to distinguish active from past ulceration causing distortion of the duodenal cap

---

• Biopsies are unnecessary unless unusual causes are suspected (Crohn's disease, lymphoma, ectopic pancreatic tissue)
• Routine determination of *H. pylori* status is not necessary
• Blood tests to detect anaemia or hepatic dysfunction should be performed. An elevated ESR does not occur in uncomplicated ulceration and raises the possibility of Crohn's or other disease elsewhere

Subsequent presentations
• The first recurrence of the same symptoms, in a patient who has had an endoscopically diagnosed duodenal ulcer in the previous 2 years, can be treated without further investigation
• Further recurrence or persistent pain are indications for repeat endoscopy and biopsies to exclude unusual causes
• Gastrin concentrations should be measured (p. 368) if ulcers are postbulbar (p. 103), recurrent, resistant to treatment (p. 101), or recur after surgery

Management

General
• The guidelines for gastric ulcers (stopping smoking, reducing alcohol intake, regular meals, p. 86) apply equally to duodenal ulcers. A summary of the differences between gastric and duodenal ulcers is shown in Table 3.4 (p. 101)
• Repeat endoscopy to confirm healing is not needed, unless symptoms persist at the end of treatment (resistant ulcers, p. 101)

Healing treatment
• H_2 receptor antagonists are the best treatment at present (p. 87)
• Cimetidine 800 mg or ranitidine 300 mg at night are safe and effective; about 90% of ulcers are healed after 6 weeks' treatment
• *H. pylori* eradication should not be attempted unless duodenal ulcers are recurrent and not readily managed by H_2 receptor antagonists. If eradication is indicated, triple therapy using bismuth and two antibiotics is recommended (p. 83), because the risk of resistance is decreased. The optimal combination and duration of treatment has not yet been determined, but bismuth subcitrate 1 tablet with tetracycline or ampicillin 500 mg four times daily and metronidazole 400 mg three times daily for 2 weeks is highly

3.8 Duodenal ulcer

Table 3.4 Practical differences between duodenal and gastric ulcers

	Duodenal	Gastric
Clinical*		
age	Young	Elderly
gender	Male	Either
pain	Nocturnal or before meals	Soon after eating
vomiting	Unusual	Common
appetite	Normal, increased or afraid to eat	Anorexia
weight	Stable	Loss
Endoscopy	Only for diagnosis	Repeat required after 8 weeks and until healing confirmed
Biopsies	None	Multiple biopsies and brushings
Treatment	Ranitidine 300 mg nocte or cimetidine 800 mg nocte	Ranitidine 300 mg nocte or cimetidine 800 mg nocte
Duration	6 weeks	8–12 weeks
Relapse	No endoscopy if <2 years Triple therapy for *H. pylori* (p. 83)	Repeat endoscopy always needed Surgery
Maintenance	Frequent relapses, elderly, NSAIDs Cardiorespiratory disease	Patients on NSAIDs, unacceptable operative risk

* None of the differences are diagnostic without endoscopy.

effective, although side effects are common. Bismuth subcitrate (De-Nol) 2 tablets twice daily and metronidazole 400 mg three times daily for 4 weeks causes fewer side effects, but may be less effective
• Omeprazole 20 mg/day works faster than ranitidine, but results after 6–8 weeks' treatment are similar. Faster healing can also be achieved with high-dose ranitidine (300 mg twice daily), but is of doubtful clinical benefit. Omeprazole is indicated for ulcers that are difficult to heal

Resistant ulcers
• Patients with persistent symptoms after 6 weeks' treatment should be reviewed. Drug compliance, smoking habits or alternative causes of dyspepsia (Table 3.1, p. 71) should be considered

---

• Repeat endoscopy is necessary to diagnose a resistant ulcer, but a further 4 weeks' treatment with high-dose H_2 receptor antagonists (such as ranitidine 300 mg twice daily) is reasonable before further endoscopy
• Biopsies must be taken from the ulcer at the repeat endoscopy and fasting gastrin concentrations checked
• Omeprazole 20–40 mg/day will heal most ulcers that are resistant to H_2 receptor antagonists. Failure to heal on omeprazole suggests poor compliance, or an unusual cause (such as Crohn's disease or lymphoma)

Relapse
• Eradication of *H. pylori* (p. 83) may decrease the relapse rate to about 20% at 1 year, but is only necessary if relapses occur more than once a year
• Infrequent relapses (less than once a year) can be treated with intermittent courses of H_2 receptor antagonists
• Frequent relapses (more than 1 every 6 months) are an indication for maintenance therapy with H_2 receptor antagonists, if eradication of *H. pylori* is ineffective. Tests to confirm eradication of *H. pylori* (urea breath test, or antral biopsies for histology, culture and urease test) are advisable 1 month after treatment

Maintenance therapy
• Indicated for elderly patients, frequent relapses, those with cardiorespiratory disease and those needing NSAIDs after diagnosis of a duodenal ulcer
• Half the treatment dose (ranitidine 150 mg or cimetidine 400 mg) given at night, reduces the relapse rate from 80% to 30% at 1 year
• Patients with severe symptoms and recurrent ulceration sometimes request surgery, but the chance of post-operative sequelae (p. 104), including recurrent ulceration, must be considered

Indications for surgery

Complications
• Continuing, recurrent or major haemorrhage (p. 12)
• Perforation (p. 24)

- Pyloric stenosis
- Relapse after recovery from a complication

Resistant ulcers
- Ulcers causing severe symptoms that persist despite aggressive medical treatment (including omeprazole)
- Frequent relapse, or relapse during maintenance treatment, if the patient prefers surgery to vigorous medical treatment (p. 101)

Type of operation
- Vagotomy and pyloroplasty are safer than partial gastrectomy, but the recurrence rate is higher (p. 105). Highly selective vagotomy is an alternative, but results depend on the experience of the surgeon
- Risks of recurrent ulceration (1–10%), unwanted sequelae (10–15%, p. 105) and mortality (1%) should be discussed with the patient

Postbulbar ulcers
Ulcers more than 3 cm beyond the pylorus are atypical (<2%) and require a search for underlying disease. Crohn's disease, Zollinger–Ellison syndrome, carcinoma, ectopic pancreatic tissue, lymphoma and tuberculosis are differentiated by biopsies and measurement of fasting plasma gastrin concentration.

Complications

Relapse
- 80% after 1 year, 90% after 2 years
- Asymptomatic relapse occurs in 25%, but does not require treatment unless the patient is taking NSAIDs or is due for major surgery

Haemorrhage
- 20% over 5–10 years

Perforation
- 10% over 5–10 years
- Pancreatitis or aorto-duodenal fistula (p. 16) are very rare sequelae

Pyloric stenosis
• Profuse post-prandial vomiting is characteristic, with an audible succussion splash, but is rare in the United Kingdom (1% over 5–10 years)
• Metabolic alkalosis and uraemia are less common than hypokalaemia
• Antral malignancy must be excluded by endoscopic biopsies
• Intravenous fluids and nasogastric suction before surgery is the standard approach
• Endoscopic balloon dilatation is under evaluation

Gastrinoma (Zollinger–Ellison syndrome)
Gastrin-secreting neuroendocrine tumours present with recurrent duodenal ulceration and diarrhoea, due to excess acid and inactivation of pancreatic lipase; 25% have other endocrine tumours (p. 131)

Gastrin concentrations (p. 368) are elevated. H_2 receptor antagonists, omeprazole and hypochlorhydria may also cause hypergastrinaemia. The secretin test (>100% rise in gastrin with a gastrinoma) is not always reliable and gastric acid studies (increased basal and peak acid output) can also give false positive results. Localization is difficult because multiple tumours and metastases are common. Referral to a specialist centre is strongly advised, where treatment with omeprazole 40 mg/day, sometimes without resection of the tumour, is the usual practice. Streptozotocin is reserved for advanced malignancy.

Outpatients should have their blood pressure, calcium, electrolytes and liver function checked regularly to detect associated endocrinopathies. Gastrin levels are uninterpretable in those on maintenance omeprazole or H_2 receptor antagonists. Gastrinomas grow very slowly and prolonged survival is possible even after hepatic metastases have occurred.

3.9   Sequelae of gastric surgery
The incidence of gastric surgery was declining before the introduction of H_2 receptor antagonists, but has declined greatly since. Indications for gastric surgery are given in the appropriate sections (pp. 12, 88, 94, 102)

Derangement of gastric function causes symptoms in nearly all patients after surgery, but adaptation occurs within weeks. After

3.9   Sequelae of gastric surgery

6 months only 10–15% have persistent symptoms (Table 3.5.). A combination of problems is common in those affected and few are specific to the type of surgery.

Vagotomy and antrectomy have the lowest risk of recurrent ulcers, but other complications are commoner after drainage, or resection and total vagotomy. Highly selective vagotomy has the lowest rate of complications but a higher incidence of recurrent ulceration (Fig. 3.4).

Table 3.5 Unwanted sequelae of gastric surgery

Common	Less common
Diarrhoea	Late dumping
Gastric stasis	Malabsorption
Early dumping	Reflux oesophagitis
Recurrent dyspepsia	Afferent loop syndrome*
Bilious vomiting	Small reservoir*
Weight loss	Retained antrum*
	Carcinoma*
	Dysphagia (transient)†

* Specifically after partial gastrectomy
† Specifically after vagotomy

Diarrhoea
• More common after truncal vagotomy than after gastric resection
• Rapid gastric emptying and fast intestinal transit are the usual mechanisms, but coeliac disease, immunoglobulin deficiency and bacterial overgrowth should also be considered
• Treatment with smaller, more frequent meals, codeine phosphate up to 120 mg/day or loperamide up to 16 mg/day in divided doses, is indicated

Gastric stasis
• Persistent postoperative nasogastric drainage, or later post-prandial vomiting, may be due to mechanical obstruction or disordered motility
• A barium meal will confirm stasis and may give more information than endoscopy, but both investigations are often needed to demonstrate patency of the anastomosis and to exclude a stomal ulcer

3.9   Sequelae of gastric surgery

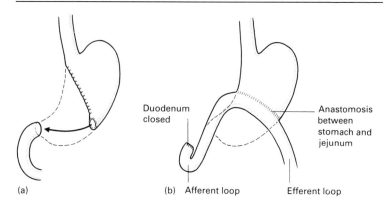

Duodenum closed

Anastomosis between stomach and jejunum

(a)

(b)   Afferent loop   Efferent loop

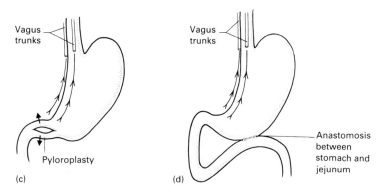

Vagus trunks

Pyloroplasty

(c)

Vagus trunks

Anastomosis between stomach and jejunum

(d)

Fig. 3.4 Anatomy of gastric operations. (a) Billroth I partial gastrectomy. (b) Polya (Billroth II) gastrectomy. (c) Vagotomy and pyloroplasty. (d) Vagotomy and gastroenterostomy.

• A prokinetic agent (such as cisapride 10 mg orally or 30 mg rectally three times daily) is worth trying for gastric stasis without mechanical obstruction
• Surgical revision is necessary for outlet obstruction

Dumping

Early dumping
• Rapid gastric evacuation results in a hypertonic load to the small intestine, triggering autonomic reflexes and release of vasoactive peptides
• Characteristic symptoms are epigastric fullness, sweating,

faintness and palpitations 30 min after eating, and avoided by fasting
• Helpful advice includes eating smaller meals that are low in sugar and high in fibre, to decrease the osmotic load and slow gastric emptying. Drinking before or after, rather than during, meals may help
• Surgical revision is a last resort

Late dumping
• Rebound hypoglycaemia 2–3 h after eating is the cause, because rapid carbohydrate absorption stimulates excessive or asynchronous insulin secretion
• Relief by eating and the timing of symptoms, are the main differences between late and early dumping; symptoms can be similar

Recurrent dyspepsia
Endoscopy is the first investigation, to determine if the dyspepsia is associated with recurrence of the ulcer.

Recurrent ulcer present
• Recurrent ulcers are not always near the stoma
• All ulcers should be biopsied
• Gastrin concentrations need checking, but very few recurrent ulcers are due to the Zollinger–Ellison syndrome (p. 104)
• High-dose H_2 receptor antagonists followed by maintenance treatment are generally appropriate. Smoking and NSAIDs should be avoided
• Omeprazole 20 mg daily usually heals ulcers that are resistant to H_2 receptor antagonists, but ulceration may be due to the effect of bile or pancreatic enzymes rather than acid damage
• Surgical revision should not be attempted until fasting gastrin concentrations have been measured. Unfortunately vagotomy, H_2 receptor antagonists and omeprazole all cause hypergastrinaemia and results must be discussed with the laboratory. The completeness of vagotomy should be checked by cephalic-stimulated acid secretion studies (p. 363), but this may also be difficult to interpret due to alkaline reflux

No recurrent ulcer
• Exclude cholelithiasis (ultrasound) and consider early dumping or bilious vomiting as a cause of pain

• Treat for non-ulcer dyspepsia (p. 76) if no cause is found

Bilious vomiting
• Free biliary reflux into the stomach is usually asymptomatic
• Burning discomfort with morning bile-stained vomiting can be treated with a prokinetic agent (such as metoclopramide or cisapride 10 mg three times daily), cholestyramine 4–12 g/day, or aluminium-containing antacids (aluminium hydroxide mixture, 10–20 ml as needed)
• Severe bilious vomiting may be an indication for surgical revision

Miscellaneous problems

Anaemia
• Inadequate dietary intake or bleeding recurrent ulcer are the most common causes of iron deficiency. Malabsorption of iron should only be diagnosed after other (colonic) causes have been excluded by barium enema or colonoscopy, especially in those aged >50 years
• Vitamin B_{12} deficiency after partial gastrectomy (usually presenting as macrocytosis) is due to bacterial overgrowth, ileal malabsorption, or autoimmune gastritis, since sufficient parietal cells usually remain to produce intrinsic factor
• Osteomalacia due to mild steatorrhoea and calcium chelation is very rare. Steatorrhoea is probably due to rapid transit in the upper gut and poor mixing of food with pancreatic enzymes

Afferent loop syndrome
• Rapid emptying of a kinked afferent loop after a meal causes sudden vomiting. Treatment is surgical, after radiological demonstration
• Bacterial overgrowth in the loop after a Polya gastrectomy is rare. Metronidazole 400 mg three times daily is indicated for 1 week, but repeated courses of antibiotics or surgical revision to decrease stasis are often needed

Cancer
• The incidence of gastric cancer 15–25 years after resection (but not vagotomy) is increased about 4-fold

---

• Prospective endoscopic surveillance is not indicated, but post-operative dyspepsia needs investigating

Retained antrum
• A very rare cause of recurrent ulceration and hypergastrinaemia, which has to be distinguished from the Zollinger–Ellison syndrome

Post-vagotomy dysphagia
• Dysphagia is transient (lasting a few days or weeks) and due to trauma and oedema rather than denervation. No special treatment is needed

3.10 Clinical dilemmas

Persistent dyspepsia despite treatment
Persistent dyspepsia after an identifiable cause has been treated is usually due to a concomitant motility disorder (non-ulcer dyspepsia). A definitive diagnosis of non-ulcer dyspepsia and explanation assists management. Treatment (p. 76) aims to provide symptomatic relief.

First steps
• Careful history and re-examination
• Repeat endoscopy to confirm healing of the original lesion

Subsequent investigations
• If the endoscopy, full blood count, ESR and liver function tests are normal, further investigations are not indicated in most patients
• Abdominal ultrasound to exclude gall stones and pancreatic lesions, or a small bowel enema to exclude Crohn's disease, are necessary in a minority
• Outpatient review after 3 months is often better than further invasive investigations if the pain persists without other signs
• Oesophageal pH monitoring, or mesenteric angiography (if there is post-prandial pain and weight loss), occasionally allow a diagnosis of reflux or mesenteric ischaemia (very rare) to be made in difficult cases

3.10 Clinical dilemmas

Dyspepsia and NSAIDs

NSAIDs should be taken with milk or meals. Dyspepsia is a common side effect, but is a poor guide to the presence or absence of an ulcer, especially in elderly patients taking NSAIDs. Identification of high-risk groups is difficult. Furthermore, ulcers may bleed or perforate without causing preceding symptoms and elderly women taking NSAIDs seem particularly vulnerable. The following approach is suggested.

Initially
• Critically assess the need for NSAIDs. Stop the drug and substitute paracetamol if possible, or try decreasing the dose of NSAIDs and avoid long-acting preparations
• Reassess the symptoms after 2 weeks (a pain and stiffness chart, scored out of ten each morning, may help)

Continued requirement for NSAIDs
• Arrange an endoscopy if dyspepsia has not resolved on stopping the NSAID, or if dyspepsia persists and NSAIDs cannot be stopped
• Restart the NSAID with H_2 receptor antagonists twice daily during NSAID treatment (p. 87). Misoprostol 200 μg three times daily can be tried if a 6-week course of H_2 receptor antagonists has failed to achieve healing of either gastric or duodenal ulcers. Misoprostol may cause diarrhoea, although this often settles, and is not very effective at relieving pain. It is more effective at preventing NSAID-associated gastric ulcers than duodenal ulcers. Omeprazole 20 mg/day is useful if H_2 receptor antagonists or misoprostol are ineffective
• Use the smallest effective does of NSAID and avoid sustained-release formulations
• There is no convincing evidence that different NSAIDs, pro-drugs (such as nabumetone), slow-release formulations (such as diclofenac), or rectal administration reduce the incidence of peptic ulcer complications
• Routine prescription of prostaglandin analogues (such as misoprostol) with NSAIDs is not advisable, even in the elderly

4 Pancreas

4.1 Acute pancreatitis

The distinguishing features of acute pancreatitis, predisposing factors, other causes of a raised serum amylase, complications and management are covered in Section 1.6 (p. 26).

Subsequent investigations
- All patients should have an ultrasound scan within 24 h of the diagnosis, to look for gall stones and to assess pancreatic size, although the pancreas may initially be obscured by bowel gas
- Repeat ultrasound should be performed if the first scan did not visualize the biliary tree clearly, and to exclude a pseudocyst if there is persistent pain or pyrexia, or if the amylase has not returned to normal after 5 days
- An ERCP is indicated urgently by an experienced endoscopist if common bile duct stones are detected, or if jaundice or cholangitis occur, so that sphincterotomy can be performed. A dilated common duct can be caused by pancreatic oedema, as well as by obstructing stones
- ERCP is also appropriate if acute pancreatitis recurs without a provoking factor, but is contraindicated in the presence of a pseudocyst. It appears to be safe to obtain a pancreatogram in acute pancreatitis

Pseudocysts
Pseudocysts are not related to the severity of the attack. Pain that persists or a serum amylase that remains elevated suggests the diagnosis, but an abdominal mass is palpable in only 50%. Ultrasound is the simplest method of diagnosis, but a CT scan (Fig 4.1) may be needed if the pancreas cannot be clearly seen due to overlying bowel gas.

Management
- Pain control and nutritional support are initially indicated
- Enteral nutrition (p. 376) should replace parenteral feeding, which is usually needed during a severe attack of acute pancreatitis (pp. 26–30), once ileus resolves
- Cysts <6 cm diameter measured by ultrasound usually resolve spontaneously, but larger cysts may need surgery, or aspiration. Size should be monitored by ultrasound scans every few days during the early stages

4.1 Acute pancreatitis

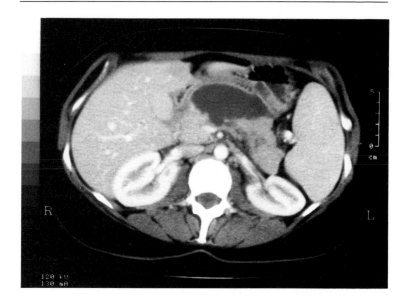

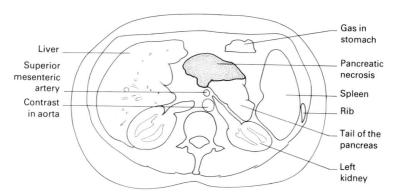

Fig. 4.1 Contrast enhanced CT scan in a 35-year-old woman showing pancreatic necrosis shortly after developing pancreatitis.

• Indications for surgery (usually an internal drainage procedure) are persistent pain after 6 weeks, or the development of complications
• Percutaneous aspiration under ultrasound control is an alternative method of treatment and pain control, but recurrence is common

4   Pancreas

4.1   Acute pancreatitis

Complications
- Jaundice—due to compression of the bile duct
- Infection—abscess may develop spontaneously, or follow ERCP or aspiration
- Haemorrhage into the cyst—causes collapse with an acute abdomen, but may present with haematemesis if the cyst erodes into the stomach, or if blood enters the duodenum through the ampulla
- Painless ascites—high amylase and protein content, exacerbated by hypoalbuminaemia. Leakage of cystic fluid is occasionally chronic
- Rupture—rare but catastrophic

Recurrence
The first attack of acute pancreatitis is usually the most severe, but 30% of all patients have a recurrent episode. Recurrence is common in alcoholics, or if gall stones have not been treated, but uncommon in idiopathic acute pancreatitis.

Management
- Gall stones should have been removed at cholecystectomy, immediately after recovery from the first attack
- An ERCP is indicated to exclude or remove retained stones, pancreatic or ampullary tumours
- Consider hypercalcaemia, hypertriglyceridaemia and drug-induced causes of acute pancreatitis (p. 26)
- Counsel absolute abstinence from alcohol, whatever the cause
- Frequent recurrence is almost invariably due to alcohol abuse and progresses to chronic pancreatitis. Recurrent pancreatitis due to very small gall stones very rarely progresses to chronic pancreatitis

Indications for surgery
Early surgery does not increase survival and should be avoided if possible during the acute phase, but surgery is indicated for gall stones, or local complications that fail to resolve.

Gall stones
- Cholecystectomy is indicated immediately after recovery from the acute attack, preferably on the same admission

• Exploration of the common bile duct is not necessary if an ERCP and sphincterotomy have recently been performed. Whilst retained stones are the most common cause of recurrent pancreatitis after cholecystectomy, these can usually be removed at ERCP
• Cholecystectomy should be performed if pancreatitis is diagnosed during emergency laparotomy for an acute abdomen in the elderly. Peripancreatic drains should be inserted for peritoneal lavage and the abdomen closed

Local complications
• Collections of fluid (pseudocyst), pus (abscess), or necrotic tissue can be visualized by ultrasound or CT scan (Fig. 4.1, p. 114) and cause persistent pain, elevated amylase, leucocytosis, or fever
• Delayed surgical drainage of a collection (6 weeks) is recommended in the absence of fever or jaundice, because 40% resolve and surgery is easier in collections that persist
• Abscesses need earlier operation if antibiotics (intravenous cefuroxime 750 mg and metronidazole 500 mg three times daily) are to be effective
• Cystogastrotomy is most likely to prevent reaccumulation of fluid

4.2 Chronic pancreatitis
Irreversible glandular destruction may follow episodes of acute pancreatitis, or occur without an identifiable attack. The prevalence is increasing in Europe, where it is more common in men and due to alcohol. Acini are replaced by fibrous tissue causing ductular distortion and later atrophy of the islets with subsequent calcification.

Causes
• Alcohol—commonest factor (80%)
• Gall stones—very uncommonly cause chronic pancreatitis
• Cystic fibrosis (p. 123)
• α_1-antitrypsin deficiency
• Congenital—pancreas divisum or annular pancreas possibly predisposes to chronic disease. A hereditary form has been described
• Malnutrition is no longer thought to be a cause, but the high prevalence among young adults in Southern India remains unexplained

4 Pancreas

4.2 Chronic pancreatitis

Clinical features

Early disease is asymptomatic, but pain, exocrine and endocrine insufficiency supervene in many patients. 90% loss of exocrine function is necessary before steatorrhoea develops. Acute attacks, with attendant complications, may still occur in chronic disease.

Pain

- Frequent abdominal pain, which may be anterior and radiate into the back, or primarily posterior, is characteristic and may be the only feature
- Food or alcohol may exacerbate the pain
- Painful attacks resolve as inflammation is replaced by fibrosis, but this takes many years. The pain sometimes becomes continuous, when it should be distinguished from pancreatic cancer in which symptoms and weight loss are more rapidly progressive
- Painless chronic pancreatitis occurs in a few patients, who present with exocrine insufficiency

Weight loss

- Malabsorption and small meals, because of associated pain, lead to malnutrition

Exocrine insufficiency

- Steatorrhoea (pale, bulky, offensive stools with visible fat globules after flushing) is often massive, but may be minimal if patients unconsciously reduce fat intake
- Defective secretion of lipase and bicarbonate cause fat malabsorption, but malabsorption of fat soluble vitamins rarely results in clinical osteomalacia, bleeding tendency, or other signs of deficiency (p. 373)
- Hypocalcaemia is common, because unabsorbed fat chelates calcium
- Weight loss is exacerbated by protein catabolism, because deficient pancreatic proteases (trypsin) cause protein malabsorption
- Serum vitamin B_{12} concentrations are often low because proteases are required to release R-proteins which bind to vitamin B_{12} before absorption. Pancreatic enzyme supplements are effective and vitamin B_{12} replacement is unnecessary

---

Endocrine insufficiency
- Impaired glucose tolerance and, eventually, frank diabetes occur in 30%
- Insulin requirements are often low due to the lack of glucagon

Miscellaneous
- Jaundice may be caused by distortion of the common bile duct or associated cirrhosis, but pancreatic carcinoma is a more common cause
- Portal hypertension due to splenic or portal vein thrombosis is rare, but needs to be distinguished from associated alcoholic cirrhosis (about 10% of patients with chronic pancreatitis), because surgical decompression occasionally helps
- The risk of cancer is probably not increased, but can be difficult to distinguish from chronic pancreatitis in the early stages. Rapidly progressive symptoms and weight loss are likely to be due to cancer
- Haemorrhage from associated varices, ulcers or periductular vessels is rare
- Pancreatic duct strictures cause stasis and pancreatic calculi. These can cause recurrent acute pancreatitis which is difficult to treat. Endoscopic balloon dilatation of strictures and lithotripsy of calculi are potential alternatives to surgery. Referral to a specialist centre is advisable

Investigations

Diagnostic
- Plain abdominal X-ray—30% have pancreatic calcification in the later stages
- Ultrasound—better than a CT scan for detecting tumours, cysts and assessing duct diameter, especially in thin patients
- ERCP—the 'gold standard', revealing duct distortion and side branch dilatation (Fig. 4.2). 'Minimal change pancreatitis' is an indication for repeat ERCP after an interval of 6 months if symptoms persist, or to perform pancreatic function tests (p. 121)

Blood tests
- Serum amylase may be elevated in acute-on-chronic episodes of pain, but is often normal in between
- Albumin and clotting studies may be abnormal, due to associated cirrhosis or malabsorption. Low calcium or serum vitamin B_{12}

4.2   Chronic pancreatitis

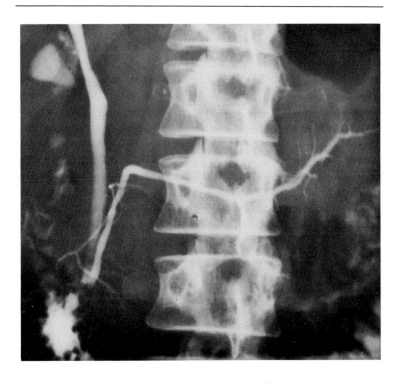

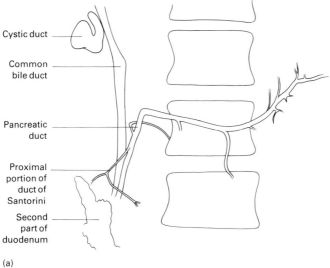

Cystic duct

Common
bile duct

Pancreatic
duct

Proximal
portion of
duct of
Santorini

Second
part of
duodenum

(a)

Fig. 4.2 ERCP in chronic pancreatitis. (a) Normal ERCP showing the pancreatic duct, duct of Santorini and the common bile duct entering at the papilla.

4.2 Chronic pancreatitis

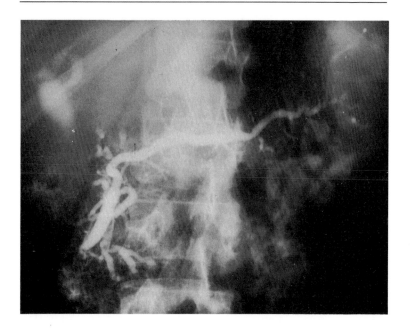

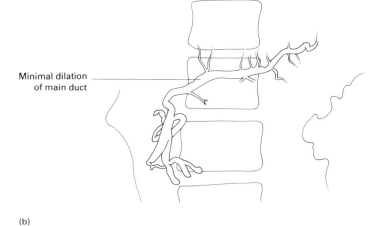

Minimal dilation
of main duct

(b)

Fig. 4.2 (*continued*) ERCP in chronic pancreatitis. (b) ERCP showing moderate chronic pancreatitis (major irregularity of all side branches and minor irregularity of main duct).

suggest malabsorption. Elevated alkaline phosphatase reflects biliary obstruction (if the γ-glutamyl transferase is elevated) or, rarely, osteomalacia
• 2-h post-prandial blood glucose >8 mmol/l indicates impaired glucose tolerance and >11 mmol/l diagnoses diabetes

Functional assessment
• Assessment of pancreatic exocrine function is not routinely performed, especially when clinical malabsorption is present because management is rarely altered
• Function tests are indicated to help interpret minimal changes on ERCP and to assist diagnosis when ERCP is not readily available
• Fat globules in stools indicate malabsorption, but their absence is unhelpful. Few laboratories quantify faecal fats (normal <5 g/day), because they do not distinguish pancreatic from intestinal causes
• Direct tests (Lundh test meal with duodenal intubation) are more accurate, but less convenient than indirect tests (fluorescein dilaurate or btPABA) which lack specificity (p. 364)

Pain control
• Pancreatic enzyme supplements and avoiding alcohol help alleviate pain
• Dihydrocodeine 60 mg four times daily is sometimes sufficient
• Opiates (pethidine) are often required during severe pain, but dependence is common, possibly because of a susceptible personality in those who also abuse alcohol
• Repeat ultrasound and ERCP are indicated for persistent pain, because duct strictures or calculi may be the cause
• Coeliac plexus block provides temporary relief, sometimes for months. Early hypotension and later impotence or total visceral anaesthesia are potential complications. Recurrent blocks are often necessary, but relief can sometimes be permanent. Coeliac plexus excision by surgery can be valuable in patients who need recurrent anaesthetic blocks
• The assistance of a psychologist to teach coping strategies for pain is helpful for patients with unrealistic expectations
• Referral to a pain clinic helps both patients and physicians
• Surgery is indicated for localized chronic pancreatitis or pancreatic calculi causing severe intractable pain, but should only be performed by an experienced pancreatic surgeon. Total

pancreatectomy for diffuse chronic pancreatitis has an unacceptable morbidity and a substantial number still have persistent pain

Exocrine insufficiency
• A low-fat diet (30–40 g/day, p. 388) is helpful, even with pancreatic supplements. A dietitian's advice is necessary
• Pancreatic enzyme supplements, taken during meals, are a convenient way of replacing deficient enzymes. No one type (Creon, Nutrizym, Pancrease, Pancrex) is of proven superiority to another and anything from 5–50 capsules/day may be needed. Enzyme preparations are unpalatable when sprinkled on food
• Creon is convenient, because H_2 receptor antagonists are not needed unless steatorrhoea persists despite a low-fat diet. Other preparations usually need H_2 receptor antagonists to prevent acid hydrolysis of the enzymes in the stomach
• Persistent steatorrhoea may be due to:
poor dietary compliance
insufficient enzyme supplements
taking the capsules at the wrong time (before or after, rather than during, meals)
misdiagnosis (consider Crohn's disease, coeliac disease and thyrotoxicosis)
• Medium-chain triglyceride supplements (Trisorbon) are not very palatable but may help to improve fat absorption if a low-fat diet, enzyme supplements and H_2 receptor antagonists fail to control steatorrhoea

Endocrine insufficiency
• Oral hypoglycaemics are usually ineffective
• Insulin requirements are usually modest, but control is often difficult. 'Brittle' (labile) diabetes needs careful monitoring of blood sugars and close liaison between patient and diabetic team

Indications for surgery
The decision balancing the quality of life with persistent pain against the complications of surgery is always difficult. Surgery is more likely to be successful when ERCP demonstrates localized chronic pancreatitis or focal lesions (such as strictures or calculi), and is rarely indicated when there is diffuse disease. Postoperative steatorrhoea and diabetes that is difficult to control are common,

depending on the amount of pancreas resected. An experienced pancreatic surgeon is essential. A joint decision by the physician, surgeon and patient is indicated for:
• Intractable pain
• Pancreatic cysts or pseudocyst
• Recurrent gastrointestinal bleeding

Prognosis
80% with alcoholic chronic pancreatitis survive 10 years if drinking stops, but this falls to less than half if drinking continues.

Death occurs from the complications of acute-on-chronic attacks, the cardiovascular complications of diabetes, associated cirrhosis, drug dependence, or suicide.

4.3 Cystic fibrosis
Cystic fibrosis (CF) is the commonest autosomal recessive inherited disorder in Caucasians (1:2000 births) and is due to defective regulation of chloride transport. The gene and its product (CF transmembrane regulator) were identified in 1989. Children with CF invariably have bronchiectasis and pancreatic insufficiency, but adults may rarely present with exocrine pancreatic malfunction.

Clinical features (Table 4.1)
Respiratory and pancreatic complications are the most important.
• Abdominal pain in adolescents with CF may be due to acute or

Table 4.1 Clinical features of cystic fibrosis

Infants	Children	Young adults
Meconium ileus	Bronchiectasis	Bronchiectasis
Rectal prolapse	Cor pulmonale	Chronic pancreatitis
Respiratory infections	Pancreatitis	Cholelithiasis
Failure to thrive	acute	Biliary strictures
Steatorrhoea	chronic	Aspermia
Malnutrition	Diabetes	Intestinal obstruction
	Biliary cirrhosis	Duodenal ulcer
	Portal hypertension	
	Hypersplenism	
	Gall stones	
	Heat exhaustion	

chronic pancreatitis, intussusception, faecal impaction ('meconium ileus equivalent'), gall stones, or duodenal ulceration
• Sufficient pancreatic exocrine function for normal digestion is present in <10% of adolescents
• Pancreatic exocrine insufficiency causes steatorrhoea, hyperphagia, deficiency of fat-soluble vitamins (A, D, E, K) in children. Malnutrition is less common in adolescents, but steatorrhoea persists
• Impaired glucose tolerance is common (50%), but rarely causes ketoacidosis
• Hepatic disease due to inspissated secretions blocking bile ductules causes pericholangitis, periportal fibrosis or cirrhosis in 5%

Management (for adults)

Diagnosis
• A sweat sodium >60 mmol/l after pilocarpine iontophoresis is diagnostic in children, but unreliable after adolescence
• There is no reliable test after adolescence, so the diagnosis is usually clinical. DNA analysis is restricted to prenatal diagnosis at present, but is likely to become more widely available

Pancreatic malfunction
• Low-fat diet (palatability must be maintained, p. 388)
• Pancreatic enzyme supplements (p. 122) during meals
• Fat-soluble vitamin supplements are rarely needed if steatorrhoea is controlled
• Nutritional supplements (enteral feeds, medium-chain triglycerides) are prescribable items, but 'ACBS' (Advisory Committee on Borderline Substances) should be written on NHS prescriptions (see BNF)

Intestinal obstruction
• Gastrografin enema is diagnostic and may be therapeutic for intussusception. Surgery should only be performed in a specialist unit because of respiratory complications
• Acetylcysteine 200 mg three times daily after recovery stimulates secretions and prevents recurrent pain due to faecal impaction. NHS prescriptions should be endorsed 'S3B' (or 'S2B' in Scotland, see BNF)

Other aspects
- Joint management with a respiratory physician is essential
- Genetic counselling for parents and young adults is necessary

Prognosis
- CF used to be a purely paediatric disease, but 80% now live to be older than 20 years, although all have respiratory complications and 90% have pancreatic exocrine insufficiency
- Adults who present with chronic pancreatitis probably have a similar prognosis to chronic pancreatitis from other causes

4.4 Pancreatic cancer
The incidence of pancreatic adenocarcinoma is increasing in Europe and does not appear to be due to better diagnosis. Men are more commonly affected than women. Only 1% survive for longer than 5 years. Pancreatic cancer should be distinguished from ampullary carcinoma, which has a much better prognosis (40% 5-year survival).

Causes
The cause is unknown. The following are considered to be risk factors:
- Smoking—occurs at a younger age in smokers
- Alcohol—any association is weak, and chronic pancreatitis not related to alcohol does not increase the risk of pancreatic cancer
- Diabetes—may double the risk

Clinical features
Tumour site determines the presentation. Cancers of the body or tail cause pain, anorexia and weight loss, and have usually disseminated before diagnosis; jaundice occurs earlier when the tumour is in the head of the pancreas. Multifocal tumours are common.

Symptoms
- Mean age 66 years
- Epigastric pain is the presenting feature in 75%. It typically radiates to the back, but may be intermittent, provoked by food and relieved by posture
- Painless obstructive jaundice is the other common presentation

- Non-specific features, including anorexia, weight loss, depression or lassitude, occur in most patients by the time of diagnosis
- Diabetic patients may present with ketoacidosis
- Recurrent attacks of acute pancreatitis occasionally herald cancer, due to intermittent duct obstruction
- Delayed diagnosis is common because early symptoms are non-specific and weight loss may not have occurred. Chronic pancreatitis is the main differential diagnosis, but rapid progression of symptoms or weight loss indicate carcinoma

Paraneoplastic features
- Rare
- Tender, subcutaneous nodules (like erythema nodosum) and polyarthritis are due to metastatic fat necrosis. Recurrent venous thrombosis (thrombophlebitis migrans), abacterial endocarditis, hypercalcaemia and Cushing's syndrome are other features
- Local spread to the peritoneum causes ascites. Obstruction of the splenic or renal vein can cause portal hypertension, or nephrotic syndrome

Physical signs
- Usually indicate an unresectable tumour
- The exception is isolated jaundice, which may be due to an ampullary carcinoma (p. 128). Courvoisier's 'law' states that jaundice in the presence of a palpable gall bladder is unlikely to be due to stones
- Exceptions to Courvoisier's law are impacted stones in both the cystic and common bile ducts, or a stone in Hartman's pouch causing oedema of the bile duct (Mirizzi's syndrome)
- Hepatomegaly, splenomegaly, ascites, supraclavicular nodes, or an abdominal mass are present in 40% at diagnosis

Investigations
The suggested sequence of investigations is shown in Fig. 4.3.
- Percutaneous needle cytology (obtained by an automatic sampling instrument) can be difficult to interpret. Laparotomy and biopsy may still be required in younger patients to differentiate chronic pancreatitis from cancer, with the option of palliative or radical surgery at the time.

4   Pancreas

4.4   Pancreatic cancer

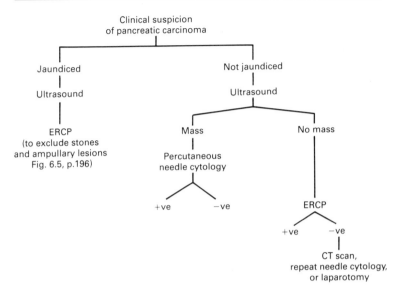

Fig. 4.3 Investigation of suspected pancreatic cancer.

• CT scan is only necessary when ultrasound is impracticable (pancreas obscured by bowel gas) or when ERCP fails to provide a definitive diagnosis

Management
Although a cure is impossible in most patients, it is important not to take a despairing approach. There is much that can be offered by expert palliation. The small proportion (<10%) who might benefit from radical surgery should be identified first.

Radical surgery
Pancreatoduodenectomy (Whipple's procedure) should only be considered by experienced pancreatic surgeons if:
• Patient is fit
• Tumour <3 cm
• No metastases detected
Operative mortality is <5% in expert hands, but much higher amongst occasional operators. Morbidity after pancreatectomy is substantial.

Palliation of jaundice

- Endoscopic (ERCP) stent insertion by an experienced endoscopist is preferable in the elderly, because the morbidity is lower and hospital stay substantially shorter than after surgery
- A combined percutaneous radiological and endoscopic approach in difficult cases gives a success rate of up to 90%
- Percutaneous drainage alone is unsatisfactory, because the displacement and infection rates are too high
- Recurrent jaundice after stenting is usually due to obstruction by biliary sludge rather than tumour. The stent should be replaced endoscopically as necessary
- Surgery is indicated if there is evidence of duodenal obstruction or ERCP is unsuccessful. Choledochoduodenostomy and gastroenterostomy are appropriate

Palliation of pain

- Pain can be effectively relieved. It is important to tell this to the patient and family, and to ensure that it is achieved
- Opiate analgesics—start with morphine sulphate (MST Continus) 20 mg twice daily—cannot be introduced too early once the diagnosis is made. The dose is increased by the patient until symptoms are controlled (p. 132)
- Coeliac plexus infiltration with alcohol at the time of palliative surgery should be considered. Percutaneous coeliac plexus block is more difficult and often needs to be repeated after 2 months
- Radiotherapy can relieve intractable pain
- NSAIDs, benzodiazepines and patient-controlled infusions of opiates also have a place (p. 132)

Ampullary tumours

Any maligant lesion that appears at endoscopy to arise from the ampulla of Vater is called an ampullary tumour, but such tumours are rare. They behave very differently from cancer in the rest of the pancreas because they present earlier, but they have no unique histological features.

- 10 times less common than pancreatic cancer
- 90% present with painless obstructive jaundice
- 80% are resectable by local excision
- 5-year survival after local excision is 40%, with an operative

mortality of 7%. Proximal pancreatectomy has a similar mortality
and probably further improves survival

Prognosis
- Mean survival after diagnosis is <6 months
- Overall 5-year survival is 0.5–1%
- 5-year survival after pancreatoduodenectomy is 4–15%

4.5 Neuroendocrine tumours

Functioning neuroendocrine tumours produce clinically interesting
syndromes but are extremely rare. The incidence of all tumours is
about 1 per million population. All patients should be referred to a
specialist centre for treatment, but outpatient follow-up may be
arranged locally. For this reason, management details concentrate
on procedure at routine review, rather than definitive treatment.
Evidence of recurrent disease is an indication for re-referral.

Carcinoid

45% of carcinoid tumours arise in the appendix, 30% in the small
intestine and 20% in the rectum. Clinically silent tumours are often
diagnosed incidentally at appendicectomy. Intussusception may
occur with ileal tumours. Metastases must occur before the
carcinoid syndrome develops, in 2%. 5-hydroxytryptamine (5-HT,
or serotonin) accounts for only some of the effects; kinins,
prostaglandins and other vasoactive substances may also be
secreted.

Carcinoid syndrome
- Flushing and cyanosis, often provoked by anxiety or alcohol
- Tears, excess nasal secretion
- Diarrhoea, may be episodic
- Hepatomegaly
- Skin sclerosis over the shins
- Cardiac involvement, fibrosis, tricuspid or pulmonary
incompetence

Diagnosis and treatment
- The association of diarrhoea with hepatomegaly and flushing
should suggest carcinoid syndrome
- 24-h urinary 5-hydroxyindoleacetic acid (5-HIAA) excretion

>0.3 mmol/24 h. Borderline tests should be repeated after excluding foods rich in 5-HT (walnuts, bananas, avocados)
• Chest X-ray, liver ultrasound, small bowel radiology and echocardiography are necessary to establish the extent of disease
• Surgical resection of the primary tumour is curative if the tumour <2 cm and has not metastasized. Resection will also decrease systemic effects in metastatic disease. Serotonin antagonists (methysergide, cyproheptadine) have largely been replaced by octreotide (a synthetic analogue of somatostatin). Octreotide, starting at 50 μg subcutaneously twice daily, should be started only by a specialist, but is usually effective

Outpatient checks
• Ask about flushing and diarrhoea
• Palpate for hepatomegaly and record the blood pressure
• Look for an elevated jugular venous pressure
• Measure 24-h urinary 5-HIAA annually to monitor progress in patients who have had the carcinoid syndrome, but not in other patients unless symptoms develop

Insulinoma

Syndrome
• Spontaneous hypoglycaemia
• Provoked by fasting or exercise and relieved by eating
• Neuroglycopenia may present with confusion, focal neurological deficit, or psychiatric abnormalities

Diagnosis and treatment
• 72-h fast under observation in hospital. Blood is taken for glucose, insulin and C-peptide concentrations when symptoms develop. Intravenous glucose must be readily available
• Normal C-peptide concentrations (from the laboratory) exclude exogenous insulin administration, but not sulphonylurea ingestion, which are the main differential diagnoses
• Treatment is surgical because metastases are rare (5%), but localization needs expert imaging

Outpatient checks
• Ask about recurrence of presenting symptoms

• Examine visual fields and check calcium levels annually to detect multiple endocrine adenomatosis (MEA type I; pancreatic endocrine tumour, pituitary tumour and hyperparathyroidism)
• Plasma insulin and C-peptide levels do not need checking unless symptoms recur

Glucagonoma

Syndrome
• Necrotizing migratory erythema (superficial bullous eruption that moves from one area to another)
• Mild diabetes (insulin secretion compensates for excess glucagon)
• Wasting

Diagnosis and treatment
• Elevated plasma glucagon levels are diagnostic
• Initial treatment is surgical if the tumour is localized. Octreotide improves the rash and streptozotocin may be of benefit in metastatic disease

Outpatient checks
• Ask about polyuria, diarrhoea and fatigue
• Examine the skin, check visual fields, serum calcium and glucose (in case of recurrence, or MEA type I)

VIPoma (Werner–Morrison syndrome)

Syndrome
• Watery diarrhoea (profuse, but may be intermittent)
• Hypokalaemia (<3.0 mmol/l)
• Metabolic acidosis (50% also have gastric anacidity)

Diagnosis and treatment
• Elevated plasma vasoactive intestinal polypeptide (VIP) concentrations may come from a tumour in the pancreas, or rarely from a retroperitoneal neuroma
• Treatment is surgical if localized, but octreotide relieves diarrhoea should the tumour be unresectable

---

Outpatient checks
- Ask about diarrhoea and fatigue
- Measure serum potassium and VIP levels at annual visits

4.6 Terminal care
Terminal care is an important part of management in patients dying from any disease, but especially in pancreatic cancer when the prognosis is so poor. The essential features are symptom control, communication and supportive care.

Symptom control

Pain
- Best relieved by morphine sulphate (MST) Continus. Start at 20 mg twice daily (20 mg daily is equivalent to 8 aspirin/day) and increase by 20 mg/day until symptoms are controlled. The correct dose is that which controls symptoms
- Breakthrough pain between doses can sometimes be treated by increasing the frequency of doses (three or four times a day) rather than the total amount
- Patient-controlled continuous subcutaneous infusions of morphine are useful when pain cannot be effectively controlled by other means
- Benzodiazepines (diazepam 2 mg three times daily) or chlorpromazine (25 mg three times daily) have a synergistic effect with MST Continus for very anxious patients, but excessive sedation must be avoided. Anxiety usually has a cause and is aggravated by ignorance or fear
- Bone pain due to metastases often responds to indomethacin 25 mg three times daily, or slow-release diclofenac 100 mg once daily, with or without MST Continus. Radiotherapy is also effective
- Local pain (arm, leg, chest, abdomen) from metastases may be amenable to anaesthetic nerve blocks, which may need to be repeated
- When oral therapy is no longer possible, subcutaneous morphine by infusion pump (dose/h = oral dose/24) is best combined with methotrimeprazine 100 mg/24 h as an anti-emetic. Intramuscular morphine is never justified. Morphine and NSAIDs are available as suppositories

___

Vomiting
• Consider hypercalcaemia, intestinal obstruction, cerebral metastases and, most important, drug-induced causes
• Standard drugs (p. 79) can be tried. Dexamethasone 2 mg three times daily is frequently helpful
• Methotrimeprazine 100–200 mg/24 h subcutaneous infusion can stop vomiting caused by intestinal obstruction

Irritability
• Consider pain, constipation, or urinary retention when consciousness is impaired

Secretions
• Atropine 0.6 mg by intravenous or intramuscular injection (max. 2.4 mg/day) will dry noisy pharyngeal and bronchial secretions

Communication

With the patient
• Discussion of the diagnosis should wait until it has been definitely established and a plan of action made
• Not all patients wish to know that they have 'cancer', but the diagnosis should be explained if a direct question is asked
• All patients should be given the opportunity to ask questions, told that symptoms can be treated even if a cure is not possible, and given a contact telephone number (GP, medical secretary) if there are problems

With the family
• May precede or influence discussion with the patient, but it is always useful to talk to both patient and family together. This avoids future confusion about what has been said to individuals and helps cut down communication barriers within the family
• Explain what support is available in the later stages and whom to call

With the general practitioner
• Telephone prior to discharging the patient from hospital
• Say what the patient/family have been told
• Explain what supportive arrangements have been made

• Offer immediate access to hospital if symptoms become intolerable

Supportive care

Home
• Liaise with family, general practitioner, district nurse, MacMillan (terminal care) nurses, hospital support team, home help, or meals on wheels, as appropriate (Appendix 1)

Hospice
• The general practitioner and the patient should agree before a hospice is contacted
• Early referral is advisable. It is poor practice to transfer a patient a few days before death, because the hospice team have no time to apply their skills, or to gain the necessary rapport

5 Liver

5.1 Jaundice

Jaundice is clinically detectable when the serum bilirubin is >50 μmol/l. Classification into three predominant types (pre-hepatic, hepatic and extra-hepatic) is convenient, but there is considerable overlap in the clinical and biochemical features. A basic knowledge of bilirubin metabolism is necessary to understand the investigation of jaundice (Fig. 5.1).

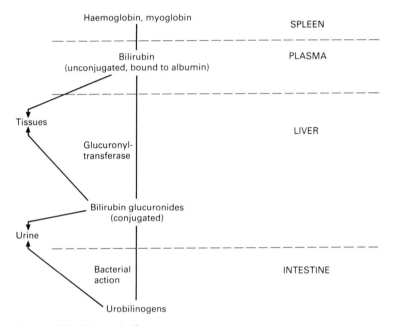

Fig. 5.1 Bilirubin metabolism.

Causes (Table 5.1)

• The predominant type of bilirubin must occasionally be identified before a diagnosis is made. A mixed pattern of conjugated and unconjugated bilirubin is usually present, unless there is an enzyme deficiency or transport defect
• Predominant unconjugated hyperbilirubinaemia occurs in:
  haemolysis
  Gilbert's syndrome
  Crigler–Najjar syndrome (children)
  'physiological' (neonatal)
  dyserythropoiesis (such as megaloblastic anaemia) or resorption

of a large post-traumatic haematoma may cause an elevated bilirubin, but not clinically detectable jaundice
- Predominant conjugated hyperbilirubinaemia occurs in: cholestasis (intra- or extrahepatic, see Tables 6.3 and 6.4, p. 193) Dubin–Johnson syndrome (without cholestasis)

Table 5.1 Causes of jaundice—main types

	Pre-hepatic	Hepatic	Extra-hepatic
Common	Neonatal	Viral hepatitis Cirrhosis Alcoholic hepatitis Hepatic metastases Primary biliary cirrhosis	Common duct stones Pancreatic cancer
Uncommon	Haemolysis Gilbert's syndrome	Drug-induced Leptospirosis Liver abscess	Cholangiocarcinoma Sclerosing cholangitis Benign stricture Pancreatitis
Rare	Crigler–Najjar syndrome	Budd–Chiari syndrome Cardiac failure Pregnancy Benign recurrent Post-cardiac surgery Wilson's disease Hodgkin's disease Dubin–Johnson syndrome	Chronic pancreatitis Portal lymphadenopathy Biliary atresia Choledochal cyst

Clinical features
A systematic clinical approach is important.

History
- Occupation (alcohol-related, animal contact, industrial exposure)
- Travel abroad, past or recent (hepatitis-endemic areas, malaria)
- Contact with jaundiced patients
- Injections, especially abroad (drug abuse, transfusions of blood or plasma factors, tattoos)
- Drugs (prescribed, over-the-counter or 'alternative' medicines such as herbal teas)
- Sexual relations
- Shellfish consumption (hepatitis A)

5 Liver

5.1 Jaundice

- Associated symptoms (the time sequence of symptoms is often helpful in distinguishing hepatitis from extrahepatic causes):
  anorexia, nausea, distaste for cigarettes (hepatitis)
  right upper quadrant abdominal pain (gall stones)
  weight loss (malignancy)
  dark urine, pale stools, pruritus (cholestasis)
  pyrexia, rigors (cholangitis, abscess)

Examination

Good light is essential to detect early jaundice. Icterus is first detectable in the sclerae when the eyes are downturned (although usually preceded by a change in colour of the urine) but may be visible in the hard palate, especially in patients with discoloured sclerae (elderly, black patients).
- The depth of jaundice is not a reliable indicator of the cause
- Look for signs suggesting acute or chronic liver disease (Table 5.2), or cholestasis (see Table 6.5, p. 193)
Other signs to be noted:
- Age (young adults may have Epstein–Barr virus (EBV) hepatitis)
- Portal–systemic encephalopathy (personality change, confusion)
- Fetor (sweet, sickly smell in hepatic failure)
- Asterixis (flapping tremor of outstretched hands, with fingers splayed)
- Dilated periumbilical veins are very rare. They either:
  flow radiating away from umbilicus (portal hypertension, 'caput medusae'), or
  flow towards the head only (inferior vena cava obstruction)

Table 5.2 Physical signs in hepatic jaundice

Acute*	Chronic*	Either
Well-nourished	Leuconychia	Palmar erythema
Tender hepatomegaly	Loss of muscle bulk	Bruising
	Telangiectases	Splenomegaly
	(spider naevi)	Small or large liver
	Splenomegaly	Facial telangiectases
	Ascites	
	Peripheral oedema	
	Loss of axillary/pubic hair	
	Testicular atrophy	
	Dupuytren's contracture	

* No clinical sign is invariably associated with either acute or chronic liver disease

5   Liver

5.1   Jaundice

• An arterial bruit over the liver is rare (hepatoma or acute alcoholic hepatitis)
• Rectal examination for stool colour (pale in cholestatic jaundice)

Investigations—all patients

Blood tests
• Typical values that help distinguish different types of jaundice are given in Table 5.3

Table 5.3 Blood tests in jaundice

Test	Normal	Pre-hepatic	Hepatic	Extra-hepatic
Bilirubin (μmol/1)	3–17	50–150	50–250	100–500
AST (IU)	<35	<35	300–3000	35–400
ALP (IU)	<250	<250	<250–700	>500
γGT (IU)	15–40	15–40	15–200	80–600
Albumin (g/1)	40–50	40–50	20–50	30–50
Hb (g/dl)	12–16	<10	12–16	10–16
Reticulocytes (%)	<1	10–30	<1	<1
INR	1.0–1.2	1.0–1.2	1.0–3 +	1.0–3.0*
Prothrombin time (sec)	13–15	13–15	15–45	15–45*

* Falls in response to parenteral vitamin K 10 mg

• Liver enzymes, aspartate transaminase (AST, previously SGOT) and alkaline phosphatase (ALP) are markers of liver dysfunction rather than 'liver function tests'. Alanine transaminase (ALT, previously SGPT) is more specific than AST, but is not as commonly measured by automated assays
• γ-glutamyl transferase (GGT) is elevated when a high ALP is of hepatic, rather than bony, origin. It is an unreliable test for alcohol abuse and a raised mean corpuscular volume (MCV) is more suggestive. Any change in GGT does, however, reflect alcohol consumption
• Serum albumin and coagulation—prothrombin time, international normalized ratio (INR)—are better markers of liver function, but serum albumin may also be altered by redistribution of body fluids

Urine
• Urine testing is less commonly performed now that biochemical tests are readily available, but should not be overlooked

5 Liver

5.1 Jaundice

- Bilirubin (tested with Ictotest tablets) is absent in pre-hepatic causes (the urine is clear, not orange, 'acholuric jaundice')
- Urobilinogen (Dipstix testing) is absent in complete cholestasis

Other tests

- Ultrasound—to look for bile duct dilatation or hepatic metastases. Also helpful to assess hepatic size, splenomegaly, the pancreas, portal blood flow, or lymphadenopathy and ascites. It is not a reliable method for detecting cirrhosis, but much depends on the skill of the operator
- Chest X-ray—look for bronchial carcinoma or metastases

Subsequent investigations

Further investigations depend on the type of jaundice, determined from the results of blood tests and ultrasound. Investigation of extrahepatic and cholestatic jaundice is summarized in Fig. 6.4 (p. 194)

Pre-hepatic jaundice:
- Serum haptoglobin (decreased in haemolysis)
- Direct antihuman globulin (Coomb's) test
- Discuss with haematologists (bone marrow, or Ham's test to exclude paroxysmal nocturnal haemoglobinuria)

Hepatic jaundice:
- Viral titres (HBsAg, anti-HAV IgM; also Table 5.9, p. 156)
- Monospot (Paul–Bunnell, for infectious mononucleosis)
- Anti-smooth muscle, antinuclear and antimitochondrial antibodies, if viral titres are negative, to look for evidence of chronic active hepatitis or primary biliary cirrhosis
- Liver biopsy if diagnosis remains uncertain, chronic disease is suspected, or hepatic enzymes remain abnormal 6 months after acute viral hepatitis. Biopsies should be stained for iron and copper
- Serum iron, iron binding capacity and ferritin (haemochromatosis), serum copper, caeruloplasmin and 24-h urinary copper (Wilson's disease), if viral titres and autoantibodies are negative

Drug-induced liver damage

The list of drugs causing jaundice is long, but drug-induced jaundice is not common. Drug-induced liver damage usually

presents as asymptomatic elevation in liver enzymes (p. 180).
Hepatotoxic effects are divided into those that occur in most
patients given a sufficiently high dose of the drug (dose-related),
and idiosyncratic (dose-independent) reactions.

The diagnosis is suspected from a history of liver dysfunction or
jaundice within 3 months of starting any new drug. Peripheral
eosinophilia is uncommon, although eosinophils in a liver biopsy
raise the possibility of drug-induced damage.

Dose-related hepatotoxicity
- Paracetamol (>10 g/24 h, but less in alcoholics)
- Tetracycline (>4 g/24 h)
- Anabolic steroids (should only be used by specialists)
- Halothane-induced liver damage is partly related to dose; it
should be avoided for anaesthetics less than 6 weeks apart.
- Methotrexate causes dose-dependent cirrhosis but not jaundice
until the terminal stages; liver biopsy is necessary after a total dose
of 2 g. Alcohol potentiates the hepatotoxic effect

Dose-independent hepatotoxicity (Table 5.4)
- For a complete list of causes, refer to other textbooks (Appendix 2)

Table 5.4 Dose-independent hepatotoxicity

Liver lesion	Common culprits
Hepatitis	Isoniazid Sodium valproate Rifampicin
Cholestasis	Chlorpromazine Prochlorperazine Fusidic acid Glibenclamide
Chronic active hepatitis	Methyldopa
Alcoholic hepatitis-like	Verapamil
Granulomas	Hydralazine Allopurinol Phenylbutazone

Management
- Minor elevations in AST (up to 3-fold) after starting potentially hepatotoxic drugs (especially isoniazid, rifampicin) are not an indication for stopping the drug, since improvement usually occurs
- Stop all possible drugs if enzymes deteriorate or jaundice occurs
- Exclude other causes of jaundice and liver dysfunction (Table 5.1, p. 138)
- Severe, fulminant hepatitis is managed as for other causes (p. 39)
- Monitor liver enzymes until they return to normal—usually over several weeks. Most hepatotoxic effects resolve completely after the drug is withdrawn, unless liver dysfunction is unrecognized for several months (methotrexate, methyldopa)
- Liver biopsy is not necessary if the drug is well known to cause liver dysfunction, unless liver enzymes have not returned to normal after 8 weeks. Liver biopsy is essential if the history is uncertain

Prescribing in liver disease
- Most drugs are safe to prescribe in stable liver disease
- Dose should be decreased by 25–50% of the normal starting dose in patients with hypoalbuminaemia, disordered coagulation, or recent encephalopathy
- High-risk drugs are:
  sedatives (including chlormethiazole and benzodiazepines)
  opiates (decreased first-pass metabolism enhances the effect)
  diuretics (overdiuresis can provoke encephalopathy)
  drugs known to cause dose-related or dose-independent hepatotoxicity (the threshold for hepatotoxicity is decreased)

Postoperative jaundice
Possible causes are:
- Drugs—scrutinize each prescription. Prochlorperazine is often implicated
- Anaesthetic—repeated exposure to halothane within 4–6 weeks. Enflurane is preferable for repeated anaesthetics
- Septicaemia—cholestatic pattern
- Pancreatitis—pancreatic oedema can obstruct the common bile duct

5 Liver

5.1 Jaundice

- Latent liver disease—perioperative hypotension may provoke decompensation of cirrhosis
- Hepatitis:

  transfusion-acquired HCV (non-A, non-B), or HBV (1–6 months after operation)

  operation during the incubation period of hepatitis (shorter interval)
- Post-cardiac surgery—benign and rare
- Resorption of a large haematoma (p. 137)—jaundice only occurs if there is an associated metabolic disorder, such as Gilbert's syndrome
- Surgical mishap:

  common bile duct stones overlooked

  oedema, or (later) stricture of the common duct

  inadvertent ligation of common duct

Investigations
- Blood cultures—low-grade sepsis may not cause a fever
- Serology—hepatitis B, C and A, as well as antimitochondrial antibodies, or liver–kidney–microsomal antibodies if halothane hepatitis is suspected
- Measure unconjugated bilirubin—>75% suggests haemolysis, or resorption of a large haematoma
- Ultrasound—looking for dilated bile ducts and at the pancreas. CT scan is better for detecting common bile duct stones, but if the common bile duct is dilated, ERCP is indicated whether a stone is visible or not
- Contact blood transfusion laboratory to trace donors if hepatitis is diagnosed; sexual partners should be traced and offered hepatitis B vaccination if appropriate (p. 161)

Jaundice with normal liver enzymes
Bilirubin may be disproportionately elevated compared to the AST or ALP when there is very severe liver disease (acute hepatitis or end-stage cirrhosis), because there are few hepatocytes to produce the enzymes. In these cases the albumin is low and coagulation disordered.

Isolated hyperbilirubinaemia is uncommon. Consider:
- Haemolysis—blood film, reticulocyte count, haptoglobins
- Gilbert's syndrome—unconjugated bilirubin
- Dubin–Johnson or Rotor syndromes—conjugated bilirubin

***

Gilbert's syndrome
- Slight elevation of unconjugated bilirubin is quite common (up to 5% of the population)
- Liver enzymes are otherwise normal
- Bilirubin increases on fasting (rarely necessary to establish)
- Jaundice is rare, except in concomitant illness with anorexia
- No treatment other than reassurance is necessary

Crigler–Najjar syndrome (glucuronyl transferase deficiency) very rarely affects adults, although some with the milder (type II) form survive from childhood.

Dubin–Johnson and Rotor syndromes are very rare causes of isolated conjugated hyperbilirubinaemia that can present with jaundice in adults.

Very occasionally other causes of diffuse hyperpigmentation (carotenaemia, melanosis) may be confused with jaundice, but these do not cause scleral discolouration and the bilirubin is normal.

5.2   Hepatic decompensation
Hepatic decompensation is often reversible in chronic liver disease, except in chronic cholestasis when it marks the terminal phase. An acute exacerbation of chronic hepatic failure is far more common than acute (fulminant) liver failure (p. 39).

Causes
Every patient who presents with decompensation of chronic liver disease should be investigated for a provoking factor:
- Intestinal bleeding:
  from varices, ulcer or erosions
- Infection:
  urinary tract, chest
  spontaneous bacterial peritonitis (usually *E. coli*, now less often pneumococcal) in ascites
- Drugs:
  excess diuretics (hypokalaemia, hypomagnesaemia, or uraemia)
  sedatives
  opiates (including codeine, co-proxamol)
- Alcohol abuse
- Progression of underlying disease
- Excessive dietary protein (only in severe chronic liver disease)

• Hepatocellular carcinoma (p. 176)

Clinical features

Hepatocellular dysfunction
• Jaundice:
increasing
• Encephalopathy:
personality change, inability to draw a 5-pointed star
drowsiness, inappropriate behaviour
stuporous, inarticulate speech
coma
the changes are graded 1–4 (grade 5 means no response to
painful stimuli), but this is only clinically valuable in
fulminant hepatic failure (Table 1.6, p. 39)
• Hepatic fetor:
sweet, sickly smell
precedes coma
• Asterixis
arms outstretched, wrists hyperextended, fingers apart
slow (every second), flapping movements at the wrist
• Fever and other signs of infection may be absent

Portal hypertension
• Ascites—develops or increases (p. 149)
• Varices are not a sign of decompensation, but bleeding (p. 12)
often triggers acute-on-chronic hepatic failure
• Venous hum—heard as a buzzing over the liver. It is rare

Investigations
• Rectal examination for melaena
• Culture urine, blood and sputum if available
• Ascitic tap and urgent Gram stain on admission. Neutrophil
count in ascitic fluid >250/cm^3 is an indication for antibiotics,
even if no organisms are seen (p. 25)
• Electrolytes, urea, full blood count, coagulation studies
• α-fetoprotein
• Electroencephalography (EEG) is the most reliable method of
detecting encephalopathy and can be used for monitoring progress,
but repeated clinical examination is sufficient for most patients

Management

Acute episode
- Identify and treat the provoking factor, especially infection—intravenous cefotaxime 1 g twice daily is appropriate until the organism is identified
- Dietary protein and salt restriction
  protein <40–60 g/day (p. 389)
  no salt added to food
- Lactulose starting at 90 ml/day and increasing until mild diarrhoea develops (more effective than neomycin 4 g/day, which is now rarely used)
- Magnesium sulphate enema—if constipation is present when starting treatment
- Vitamin K 10 mg for 3 days should be given intravenously if the prothrombin time >22 sec (INR >1.5), although coagulation rarely returns completely to normal. Intramuscular injection is probably safe if the prothrombin time is <45 sec, but less pleasant for the patient
- Fresh frozen plasma is indicated if there is active bleeding (2–4 units rapidly, repeated after 8 h if bleeding continues)
- Intravenous saline must be avoided, especially in the presence of oedema or hyponatraemia due to liver disease, because salt (and water) are avidly retained due to secondary hyperaldosteronism. Added salt on food and sodium-containing drugs (many antacids, p. 77) should also be avoided
- B vitamins (intravenous Parentrovite HP 1 + 2 vials for 3 days) should be given to alcoholics, who often have dietary deficiency
- Ranitidine 50 mg intravenously three times daily (in 20 ml, slowly), or 150 mg orally twice daily, decreases the risk of stress-induced gastric erosions
- Monitor:
  clinical state (encephalopathy) daily
  daily weight (more practical than a fluid balance chart)
  daily electrolytes, urea and full blood count
  twice weekly bilirubin, AST, ALP, albumin and INR, or PT
- Patients aged <60 years with acute-on-chronic liver failure not due to alcohol may be suitable for a liver transplant, although this is best deferred until after recovery from the acute episode (p. 180 and Appendix 1)

After recovery
• Discharge the patient only when the weight, diuretic dose and mental state are stable
• Normal dietary protein intake can be resumed when the encephalopathy resolves. Protein restriction should be avoided if possible, because patients are protein-depleted and the diet is unpleasant
• Continue dietary salt restriction (no salt added to food or cooking) to decrease reaccumulation of ascites
• Lactulose can be decreased to 10–30 ml at night, before discharge and discontinued in outpatients
• In a few patients encephalopathy returns when dietary protein intake is normal. These will continue to need lactulose as well as continued protein restriction

5.3   Ascites
Ascites means free fluid in the peritoneal cavity. It is thought that peripheral vasodilatation is the initial event that decreases renal blood flow, which triggers salt and water retention. Portal hypertension is then the driving force that causes fluid to accumulate in the peritoneal cavity.

Causes
Most cases (90%) are due either to chronic liver disease or carcinomatosis with peritoneal seedlings (Table 5.5).

Table 5.5 Causes of ascites

Common	Less common	Rare
Cirrhosis	Nephrotic syndrome	Budd–Chiari syndrome
Carcinomatosis	Cardiac failure	Portal vein block
		Tuberculous peritonitis
		Chylous ascites
		Pancreatitis
		Urinary ascites
		Constrictive pericarditis
		Meig's syndrome
		Pseudomyxoma peritonei
		Peritoneal mesothelioma

5.3   Ascites

• Rapid onset of ascites is a feature of decompensated cirrhosis, malignancy (including hepatoma), portal or splenic vein thrombosis, or Budd–Chiari syndrome
• Ascites in an alcoholic cirrhotic with pancreatitis may be due to hepatic decompensation or pancreatitis. High ascitic amylase distinguishes pancreatic ascites, but needs discussion with the biochemist
• Severe right heart failure, constrictive pericarditis or Budd–Chiari syndrome can be confused with cirrhosis. The clinical signs (hepatomegaly, elevated jugular venous pressure and ascites) are the same, so a high index of suspicion and echocardiography are indicated if cirrhosis has not been proven by liver biopsy. Cirrhosis secondary to cardiac failure is extremely rare and if the two conditions coexist, alcohol is the likely cause. A large ovarian cyst can occasionally simulate ascites, but unlike ascites, the centre of the abdomen is dullest to percussion

Investigations
Examination of ascitic fluid is essential when ascites is first diagnosed, or if the clinical condition changes. The colour, protein content, results of microscopy and culture should be recorded on every sample; other tests are performed as indicated (Tables 5.6 and 5.7). Investigation of the underlying cause is then appropriate.
• Consider non-hepatic causes of ascites if liver enzymes and coagulation studies are normal. Pay particular attention to:
   serum albumin (consider intestinal loss, as well as urinary)
   urine protein (24-h collection)
   echocardiography (to exclude cardiac causes)

Management
The aim is a gradual, controlled loss of ascitic fluid. Diuretics are usually adequate, and the traditional measures of fluid restriction or a low-sodium diet merely make the patient's life miserable. There is a current debate about diuretics or paracentesis, but diuretic treatment remains the conventional approach and paracentesis is probably best reserved for refractory ascites.
   Fluid loss >500 ml (0.5 kg) each day exceeds the capacity of the peritoneum to absorb ascites and results in hypovolaemia, unless peripheral oedema is present. Other drugs should be reviewed and

5.3   Ascites

NSAIDS stopped because they cause fluid retention and deterioration in renal function.

Table 5.6 Ascitic fluid investigations

Condition	Investigation	Interpretation
All ascitic fluid	Colour	Table 5.7
	Protein*	<25 g/l, transudate (cirrhosis, or hypoalbuminaemia) >30 g/l, exudate (malignancy, or inflammation), but there is substantial overlap between the two groups
	Culture	Any growth is abnormal
Patient unwell	Gram stain	>1 bacterium/ml or >250 polymorphs/ml indicate bacterial peritonitis
	Ziehl–Nielsen	If tuberculosis is suspected
Malignancy	Cytology	Fresh specimen necessary Malignant cells are diagnostic
Pancreatitis	Amylase	Varies between laboratories
Milky (chylous) ascites	Triglyceride	>5 mmol/l is abnormal Normal in pseudochylous ascites
Ascites from a biliary leak	Bilirubin	Ascitic fluid/serum bilirubin ratio >1.0 is abnormal

* The serum–ascites protein gradient (serum albumin–ascitic albumin) is more accurate than the ascitic protein content alone for identifying the cause of ascites. An exudate (such as malignancy) has a protein gradient <11 g/l, and a transudate (such as portal hypertension) has a gradient >11 g/l.

Table 5.7 Colour of ascitic fluid

Pale straw	Haemorrhagic	Turbid	Milky
Cirrhosis Nephrotic Cardiac failure	Carcinomatosis Pancreatitis	Infection Pancreatitis Tuberculous	Chylous Pseudochylous

Small or moderate amounts of ascites
• Treated as an outpatient, starting with spironolactone 100 mg/day and no salt added to the food, rather than a low-sodium diet. Amiloride (5–15 mg/day) is an alternative if side effects of spironolactone are unacceptable

5.3   Ascites

• Review and weigh every week (aim for 2–4 kg/week) until ascites disappears
• Increase spironolactone by 100 mg/day every 3–5 days if ascites persists. The half-life of spironolactone is increased in liver disease; more frequent dose increases do not allow a steady state to be achieved
• Admit to hospital if spironolactone 200–300 mg/day at home is ineffective (Fig. 5.2)

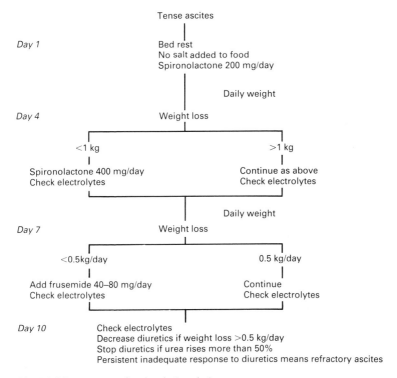

Fig. 5.2 Management of ascites in hospital.

Refractory ascites

Ascites that persists despite treatment as in Fig. 5.2, or ascites causing respiratory distress or pain, are indications for paracentesis.
• Ensure that all specimens (Table 5.6, p. 150) have been taken and that the cause of ascites has been established

• Start therapeutic paracentesis, with intravenous colloid replacement (10 g albumin/l of removal):
> remove up to 3000 ml ascites/day for 3 days
> replace with 30 g albumin, or 1000 ml synthetic colloid, to avoid hypotension and the hepatorenal syndrome
• Diuretic therapy may then prevent reaccumulation of ascites
• Paracentesis with colloid replacement is increasingly used as standard treatment of ascites, because it provides rapid relief. The risks of infection or rapid drainage causing renal impairment may be no greater than the hazards of high-dose diuretics, but this remains controversial
• Surgical insertion of a peritoneo-venous (LeVeen) shunt is only occasionally justified by the underlying condition—infection or blockage of the shunt are common

Malignant ascites
Repeated paracentesis is often necessary because the response to diuretics and salt restriction is poor. Instillation of cytotoxic drugs into the peritoneum occasionally helps, but specialist advice should be asked. A peritoneo-venous shunt may provide relief for several months before it blocks.

Chylous ascites
Chylous ascites is caused by lymphoma obstructing lymphatics, surgical transection of lymphatics during aortic aneurysmectomy, intestinal lymphangiectasia, or occasionally the nephrotic syndrome. Pseudochylous ascites, caused by malignancy or infection, looks the same but has a normal triglyceride content (Table 5.6, p. 150)

Treatment is with diuretics, salt restriction and dietary fat substitution with medium-chain triglycerides. Resection of a localized area of lymphangiectasia may be possible.

5.4   Portal hypertension
Portal hypertension usually arises from post-sinusoidal obliteration due to cirrhosis. Obstruction of the hepatic, portal or splenic veins (Fig. 5.3) may also raise portal pressure and cause collateral venous dilatation (varices).

5.4   Portal hypertension

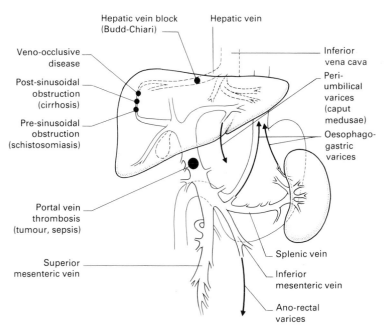

Fig. 5.3 Sites of obstruction causing portal hypertension and varices. (Adapted from Weatherall D.J. *et al.* (eds) (1987) *Oxford Textbook of Medicine,* 2nd edn. Oxford University Press, p. 12.24)

Causes

Three main groups exist: pre-sinusoidal, hepatic (sinusoidal) and venous outflow obstruction (post-sinusoidal) (Table 5.8). The distinction is practical because pre-sinusoidal causes have relatively normal hepatocellular function, which means that encephalopathy after a gastrointestinal bleed is less common and the results of surgical decompression are better. Hepatic causes are commonest in the West, but schistosomiasis is commonest worldwide.

Clinical features

The consequences of chronically raised portal venous pressure are varices, ascites, splenomegaly, hypersplenism, or portal hypertensive gastropathy.
• Varices—oesophageal varices are common, gastric and anorectal varices are less common. Umbilical varices (caput medusae) only occur if the umbilical vein remains patent after birth, and are very rare
• Ascites (p. 148)

5.4 Portal hypertension

Table 5.8 Causes of portal hypertension

Pre-sinusoidal:
Extrahepatic:
  portal vein thrombosis
  splenic vein thrombosis
Intrahepatic:
  schistosomiasis
  sarcoidosis
  myeloproliferative disease
  primary biliary cirrhosis*

Hepatic:
  cirrhosis*
  chronic active hepatitis
  congenital hepatic fibrosis

Venous outflow obstruction:
  Budd–Chiari syndrome
  veno-occlusive disease

* Portal hypertension in cirrhosis is complex and partly due to post-sinusoidal obliteration.

• Hypersplenism—recognized by splenomegaly, anaemia, thrombocytopenia and leucopenia. It indicates severe, long-standing portal hypertension and is a bad prognostic sign.
• Portal hypertensive gastropathy is an unusual cause of bleeding from the gastric mucosa. It may be becoming more common, due to variceal sclerotherapy

Investigations
The diagnosis is made by finding splenomegaly or varices in the presence of chronic liver disease.
• Liver biopsy—histological proof of chronic liver disease should always be established if possible
• Endoscopy is best for detecting oesophageal and gastric varices. Asymptomatic patients with cirrhosis need not be endoscoped, because the benefit of treating varices prophylactically is uncertain
    Difficulty arises when liver histology is apparently normal in the presence of varices and splenomegaly. This is an indication for:
• Ultrasound—with hepatic and portal vein Doppler studies if possible, looking for venous obstruction
• Portal, splenic and hepatic venography—best performed at a specialist referral centre, together with review of liver histology

Management

Treatment of portal hypertension is directed at the complications of bleeding varices (p. 12) or ascites (p. 150). Specific treatment of the underlying disease (such as abstinence in alcoholic cirrhosis, venesection in haemochromatosis, or anticoagulation in coagulopathies) is also appropriate.

Variceal prophylaxis
- Sclerotherapy (p. 14) is not indicated unless a bleed has occurred. It must be systematic and done repeatedly to be of value
- Varices recur after obliteration in about 40%
- Propranolol 20–40 mg three times daily to reduce resting pulse by 25% decreases the risk of bleeding, by reducing portal pressure, but does not alter mortality and is often poorly tolerated

Indications for surgical decompression
- Surgery (portal–systemic shunting, oesophageal stapling, or transection) should be considered if three episodes of bleeding varices occur despite sclerotherapy, and liver function is good (albumin normal, no encephalopathy during bleeding). This usually means patients with pre-sinusoidal portal hypertension

Portal or splenic vein thrombosis

Malignancy, pancreatitis, portal sepsis, or haematological disorders (below) can cause thrombosis of the portal or splenic veins. 50% are idiopathic. Rapid development of ascites without deteriorating hepatocellular function is the clue.

Treatment is directed at the ascites and underlying cause. Anticoagulants are not often indicated, because of the risk of variceal bleeding. Surgery is usually unsatisfactory because the veins used for grafting are blocked.

Budd–Chiari syndrome

Hepatic vein obstruction may be caused by haematological disorders (polycythaemia, protein C deficiency, antithrombin III deficiency, anticardiolipin antibody, paroxysmal nocturnal haemoglobinuria), malignancy, trauma, or oral contraceptives.

5.5 Hepatitis

Abdominal pain, tender hepatomegaly and ascites are variable it may present as a severe, acute condition, or as a mild, chronic illness. Liver biopsy is diagnostic. Ultrasound is helpful, especially with Doppler studies of portal venous flow. Preservation of Reidel's lobe on an isotope liver scan is characteristic but unusual. Treatment of the underlying disease, anticoagulation or surgical decisions (including transplantation) are best made at a referral centre.

Veno-occlusive disease
Non-thrombotic obliteration of intrahepatic venules is diagnosed by liver biopsy, but may be difficult to distinguish from Budd–Chiari syndrome. Pyrrolizidine alkaloids (*Senecio*, or comfrey herbal teas), irradiation and cytotoxic drugs are possible causes.

5.5 Hepatitis
Hepatitis involves inflammation of the whole liver. Most episodes are sub-clinical, detected (if at all) by abnormal liver enzymes, but the spectrum extends to subacute hepatic necrosis and fulminant failure. It may be caused by viral or bacterial infections, drugs, chemicals or toxins.

Causes
See Table 5.9

Table 5.9 Causes of hepatitis

Common	Uncommon	Rare
Hepatitis viruses	Hepatitis	Delta virus (Hepatitis D)*
A	C (parenteral non-A, non-B)	Cytomegalovirus
B	E (enteral non-A, non-B)	Herpes simplex
Alcohol	Epstein–Barr virus	Coxsackie A and B
	Drugs (p. 141)	Echovirus
		Measles
		Arenavirus (Lassa)
		Flavivirus (yellow fever)
		Leptospirosis
		Mycoplasma
		Rickettsia (typhus)
		Chemicals (iron, CCl_4)
		Toxins (mushrooms)

* Only with existing hepatitis B infection

5.5   Hepatitis

Clinical features

A high prevalence of asymptomatic hepatitis is suggested by the frequency of patients with antibodies to hepatitis A or B without recalling a specific illness.

History

- The incubation period (Table 5.10) varies widely
- Prodrome (2 days–2 weeks)—malaise, anorexia, distaste for cigarettes, nausea, myalgia, fever. These features are characteristic of viral hepatitis and less common in other causes of jaundice
- Jaundice:
  prodromal symptoms start to resolve
  itching is rare (except in alcoholic cholestatic hepatitis)
  dark urine and yellow (not clay-coloured) stools are common
- Associated symptoms can occur in acute hepatitis B, including arthralgia, arthritis and an urticarial rash
  The differences in incubation, people at risk and progression to chronic disease are shown in Table 5.10.

Table 5.10 Differences between types of viral hepatitis

	A	B	C	D	E
Incubation (weeks)	2–6	8–24	6–12	Uncertain	2–8
Transmission	Faeces Saliva	Blood Semen Saliva Perinatal	Blood	Blood ?Semen	Faeces Saliva
Epidemic	Yes	No	?Yes	No	Yes
Risk factors	Children Institutions Seafood Travel to Middle/ Far East Seasonal (winter) Homosexuals	Middle/ Far East Drug abuse Homosexuals Haemophiliacs Renal dialysis Neonates of HBV-positive mothers	Transfusion Haemophiliacs	Always with HBV Drug abuse Homosexuals	Travel to North India, Middle East, Mexico
Chronic disease	No	5–20%	20–50%	30–50%	?No
Prevention	Immunoglobulin Vaccination	Immunoglobulin Vaccination	Screen blood products	None	None
Carrier	No	Yes (10%)	Yes	?Yes	?No

5.5 Hepatitis

Examination
• Jaundice (anicteric cases are detected by liver enzyme tests)
• Tender hepatomegaly
• No signs of chronic liver disease (Table 5.2, p. 139) except in alcoholic hepatitis, when fever is also prominent
• Splenomegaly is commonly present in alcoholic hepatitis, infectious mononucleosis (Epstein–Barr virus), or rickettsial infections. It occurs in about 15% uncomplicated viral hepatitis

Outcome
• Complete recovery may take several weeks, or occasionally months. Lassitude and anorexia are commonly the most persistent symptoms
• Fulminant hepatic failure (p. 39) hardly ever occurs in hepatitis A, but develops in about 1% symptomatic hepatitis B infections, 2–5% hepatitis C (parenteral non-A, non-B) and is even more common in hepatitis D
• Chronic liver disease may follow acute viral hepatitis, but the risk depends on the virus (Table 5.10, p. 157). This includes chronic persistent (p. 162) or chronic active hepatitis (p. 164), cirrhosis (p. 170) and hepatocellular carcinoma (p. 176)
• Relapse, usually with a milder attack, occurs in 2–10%. Recovery may still be complete, or it may indicate progression to chronic liver disease
• Asymptomatic carriers (5–10% following hepatitis B) may have normal liver function or chronic liver disease

Investigations

Liver enzymes
• An AST more than 10 times the upper limit of normal is the hallmark of acute hepatitis (Table 5.3, p. 140). The pattern of change in relation to serological markers is shown in Fig. 5.4
• Predominant cholestasis is unusual in viral hepatitis, but more common in alcoholic hepatitis

Other blood tests
• Monospot or Paul–Bunnell test is advisable in young adults who are HAVIgM- and hepatitis B-negative. Epstein–Barr virus DNA or IgM can be measured if there is doubt about the diagnosis

5.5   Hepatitis

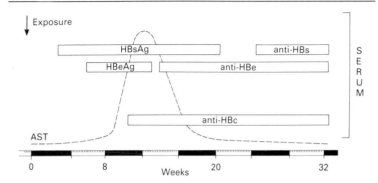

Fig. 5.4 Time course of enzyme and serological changes in acute hepatitis B. (Adapted from Weatherall D.J. *et al.* (eds) *Oxford Textbook of Medicine*, 2nd edn. Oxford University Press, p. 12.214.)

• Neutropenia is common in viral hepatitis before jaundice appears. Atypical monocytes are seen in infectious mononucleosis, and rarely in cytomegalovirus, or toxoplasmosis. Haemolytic anaemia is a rare complication of hepatitis B

Serology
• Hepatitis A IgM (anti-HAVIgM) and hepatitis B surface antigen (HBsAg) should always be checked
• Hepatitis B e antigen (HBeAg) should be checked if HBsAg-positive, to assess infectivity
• Delta antigen should be checked if the patient is HBsAg-positive and a drug abuser or unwell
• Tests for hepatitis C are not yet widely available, but are appropriate if anti-HAVIgM and HBsAg are negative

Meaning of markers
• Hepatitis A:
  anti-HAVIgM antibody indicates recent infection (within 8 weeks) and disappears soon after jaundice appears
  anti-HAVIgG antibody indicates immunity, appears within 2 weeks of infection and persists for years

Hepatitis B (Table 5.11)
• Occasionally infection without detectable HBsAg occurs, or anti-HBs can disappear on recovery
• Persistence of HBsAg for more than 6 months defines a carrier.

5.5   Hepatitis

Table 5.11 Serological markers in hepatitis B

Stage	HBsAg	HBeAg	Anti-HBs	Anti-HBe	Anti-HBc IgM	Anti-HBc IgG
Incubation	+	+	–	–	–	–
Acute hepatitis	+	+	–	–	+	+
Carrier	+	+ / –	–	– / +	+ / –	+
Convalescence	–	–	+	+	+ / –	+
Recovery	–	–	+	–	–	+
Vaccination	–	–	+	–	–	–

About 10% per year will subsequently develop antibodies
• The complete virus is called the Dane particle. Anti-HBc acts against the core, which is formed in the hepatocyte nucleus

Management

Acute attack
No specific treatment is available and most patients will settle with symptomatic treatment.
• Bed rest is unnecessary. Exercise has no effect on the severity of the attack or relapse rate, but most patients with hepatitis prefer to avoid exercise
• Careful hand washing and a high standard of personal hygiene are essential to prevent transmission. Cups, eating utensils and towels are traditionally not shared until the jaundice resolves, if the diagnosis is hepatitis A, but this is unnecessary
• Admission to hospital is only necessary for severe attacks or if the patient is unwell and lives alone. Isolation is unnecessary, but gloves should be worn when handling all excreta (urine, faeces, vomit) or when taking blood
• It is essential to withdraw drugs or alcohol whether or not these are the causative agent
• Patient preference is the best guide to diet. A low-fat diet is often preferred by patients, but otherwise no special diet is needed
• Every case of hepatitis must be notified to the Medical Officer for Environmental Health (p. 346)

Contacts
• It is usually too late to treat close contacts of hepatitis A (shared bathrooms or kitchens and physical contact) with human normal

immunoglobulin (5 ml intramuscular injection), but this should be discussed with a consultant in communicable diseases if more than one case occurs
• Sexual partners of hepatitis B patients should be tested for HBsAg and given recombinant vaccine if not immune (see below). Hyperimmune HBV immunoglobulin can be given as well if abstinence is impracticable whilst active immunity develops (2–4 weeks)

Follow-up
• Abstinence from alcohol is often recommended until liver function has returned to normal, but moderate drinking (4–8 units/ week) is not harmful. Total abstinence must be advised after alcoholic hepatitis
• Normal activity, including work, can be resumed as soon as the patient feels ready, but this often takes 2–6 weeks
• Liver enzymes should be checked after 6 weeks and again after 6 months if they have not returned to normal
• Abnormal liver enzymes elevated >2-fold after 6 months are an indication for further investigations, including liver biopsy. Minor abnormalities can be observed with repeat blood tests every few months, and only investigated if there is an increasing trend

Chronic hepatitis (see p. 162)

Immunization

Hepatitis A
• Passive immunization with intramuscular human normal immunoglobulin 5 ml is effective for 4 months. It is indicated for:
  travellers to highly endemic areas (Indian subcontinent, Middle East, South America, Mexico), who will not be staying in hotels
  it is cheaper to test travellers for antibodies to HAV rather than to give immunoglobulin indiscriminately
  close contacts (family, institutional members) of some patients with acute HAV (p. 157)
• Active immunization with live-attenuated, killed and recombinant vaccines are under trial

Hepatitis B
• Passive immunization with two doses of intramuscular

hyperimmune HBV immunoglobulin 500 IU, 1 month apart should be given to:

close contacts of patients with acute HBV

neonates born to HBV-positive mothers (200 IU within 12 h of birth and 0.5 ml (10 μg) recombinant HBV vaccine at separate sites. Second and third doses of recombinant vaccine at 1 and 6 months)

• Active immunization with recombinant HBV vaccine (three doses, 1 and 6 months apart) is indicated for:

HBsAg-negative close contacts of patients with acute HBV

haemophiliacs

renal dialysis patients

patients requiring repeated transfusion

staff of institutions for mentally retarded

laboratory staff

health care personnel (including doctors, dentists, nurses)

people working abroad in highly endemic areas

drug abusers, prostitutes and homosexuals are not readily vaccinated, but should be offered vaccination if the opportunity arises

• Booster doses are needed every 5–10 years at present

5.6 Progressive liver disease

Chronic hepatitis

Chronic hepatitis is defined as hepatic inflammation continuing for more than 6 months. Hepatitis B or C (parenteral non-A, non-B) are the usual causes, although autoimmune disease, drugs (p. 141), alcohol, or Wilson's disease may be implicated.

There are three types which are only reliably distinguished by liver biopsy. Liver biopsy is indicated if liver enzymes remain >2-fold elevated 6 months after acute hepatitis (p. 356). Biopsy is also indicated for patients with no history of acute hepatitis once other causes of abnormal liver enzymes have been excluded (Fig. 5.7, p. 181).

Chronic persistent hepatitis

• Asymptomatic with no physical signs. Non-specific symptoms ('post-viral malaise') cannot be attributed to chronic persistent hepatitis

5 Liver

5.6 Progressive liver disease

- Elevated AST (2–5 times normal). Bilirubin, ALP, coagulation and albumin are normal
- Histology shows mononuclear inflammatory cells within the limiting plate (Fig. 5.5)
- Treatment is not indicated
- Prognosis is good

Chronic lobular hepatitis
- Malaise and fluctuating jaundice are common
- AST is markedly elevated and other liver function tests are often abnormal
- Histology shows chronic inflammatory cells from portal tract to central area, and focal necrosis (Fig. 5.5)

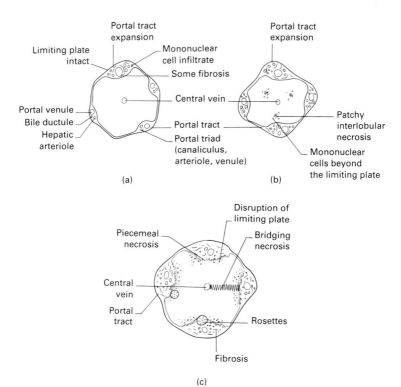

(a)

(b)

(c)

Fig. 5.5 Pathological features of chronic hepatitis. (a) Chronic persistent hepatitis. (b) Chronic lobular hepatitis. (c) Chronic active hepatitis. (Adapted from Sherlock, S. *Diseases of the Liver and Biliary System*, 7e, p. 281.)

- Treatment has not been evaluated. Steroids are reasonable for autoimmune disease (see below) but the usual cause is viral
- Prognosis is poor if the albumin is low. Rapid progression to cirrhosis may occur. Others improve spontaneously and the outlook for autoimmune disease is better than for viral causes

Chronic active hepatitis (CAH)

There are two main types (autoimmune and post-viral), and treatment differs. Alcohol, drugs, or Wilson's disease may cause similar histological patterns.

Autoimmune CAH
- Less common than post-viral CAH
- 75% women
- Malaise, arthralgia, or an urticarial rash sometimes precede jaundice by several months. 30% have associated autoimmune thyroiditis, diabetes, glomerulonephritis, ulcerative colitis or haemolytic anaemia
- Signs of chronic liver disease (Table 5.2, p. 139) are usual
- AST is elevated 2–20 times and the albumin is normal or low. Leucopenia and thrombocytopenia, due to hypersplenism, indicate severe disease. Serum IgG is usually elevated
- Anti-smooth muscle, or antinuclear antibody titres >1:40 are diagnostic. The term 'lupoid' hepatitis for antinuclear antibody-positive CAH should be avoided, because it is unrelated to systemic lupus erythematosus
- Histology shows a mononuclear infiltrate of the portal and periportal areas, piecemeal necrosis and fibrosis, or cirrhosis (Fig. 5.5, p. 163). Iron stains and copper analysis should be done, especially in young patients
- ERCP is indicated if the ALP is disproportionately elevated (>3-fold), because the histology of primary sclerosing cholangitis can occasionally be mistaken for chronic active hepatitis
- Treatment is with prednisolone 30 mg daily for one month, decreased by 5 mg daily each month, maintained on 5–10 mg daily, long term
- Steroids can sometimes be stopped after 2 years but active disease frequently recurs. Azathioprine 50–100 mg daily is an alternative if steroid side effects develop

- Repeat liver biopsy to assess progress is not usually justified if the clinical and biochemical response has been good

Post-viral CAH
- The clinical picture varies from mild non-specific symptoms to evidence of severe chronic liver disease. Arthralgia and an urticarial rash can occur, as in acute HBV infection
- The biochemical and histological features are the same as autoimmune CAH (p. 164). Autoantibody tests are negative, or present in low titre. Orcein stains of the liver biopsy will be positive in hepatitis B-associated CAH
- Treatment is controversial and still under evaluation. Intramuscular alpha interferon 5 MU three times weekly reduces the AST level and enhances development of antibodies in HBeAg-positive patients, but there is no evidence yet that it either prevents progression to cirrhosis or improves mortality. Steroids are contraindicated
- Prognosis is variable. Progression to cirrhosis or hepatocellular carcinoma is most rapid in HBeAg patients with continued viral replication (HBeAg-positive). Some patients do not develop cirrhosis after many years

Primary biliary cirrhosis (PBC)
The interlobular bile ducts are destroyed by chronic granulomatous inflammation of unknown cause. Increasing cholestasis leads to cirrhosis and the complications of portal hypertension.

Clinical features
- 90% women
- Age 40–60 years
- Incidental detection of an elevated ALP is now the commonest presentation. Most (80%) asymptomatic patients have progressive disease and will develop symptoms, although this may take years
- Pruritus almost always precedes jaundice by 6 months–2 years and lethargy is common
- Skin pigmentation, xanthelasma, xanthomata, hepatomegaly and a palpable spleen are characteristic signs. Malnutrition and ascites are very late signs because hepatocellular function is relatively preserved, although oesophageal varices are common

- Osteoporosis is common. Fat-soluble vitamin deficiency often causes bone pain (osteomalacia) and disordered coagulation in the later stages

Investigations
- Elevated ALP (5–20 times normal). This is initially the only biochemical abnormality and hepatic origin is confirmed by an elevated γ-glutamyl transferase. AST may be slightly elevated but albumin remains normal until late
- Antimitochondrial (M2) antibodies are present in high titre in 98%. These are specific to PBC, although M4 antimitochondrial antibodies may occur in autoimmune CAH
- Serum IgM and cholesterol are usually elevated
- Ultrasound (to exclude other causes of cholestasis, p. 193)
- Liver biopsy demonstrates chronic inflammation around the bile ducts, with granulomas and cirrhosis. Occasionally primary sclerosing cholangitis can cause diagnostic confusion

Management
The results of liver enzymes should be recorded at each outpatient visit. Treatment is initially symptomatic, although a minority will later need to be considered for hepatic transplantation.
- Pruritus—cholestyramine 4–12 g/day. Oxymetholone 100 mg/day is helpful in intractable pruritus
- Diarrhoea—codeine phosphate 30–60 mg/day or a low-fat diet, as tolerated (p. 388)
- Bone pain:
    1-α-cholecalciferol 1 μg daily
    effervescent calcium 1.5 g daily
- Fat-soluble vitamins—monthly intramuscular injections of vitamin A 100 000 U and vitamin K 10 mg are indicated for prophylaxis when jaundice develops. Acute vitamin deficiencies need higher doses (Table 13.14, p. 392)
- Ascites—diuretics (Fig. 5.2, p. 151)
- Varices—sclerotherapy if bleeding occurs (p. 14)
- Disease-modifying drugs continue under trial. Ursodeoxycholic acid 750 mg daily looks promising. Cyclosporin or colchicine are more controversial. Steroids and penicillamine are ineffective
- Hepatic transplantation is curative and should be considered for patients <60 years with deep jaundice (bilirubin >100 μmol/l), or

uncontrolled pruritus. The earlier the referral, the better the results of transplant, and when clotting is disordered or ascites develops, time is short (p. 182 and Appendix 1)

Prognosis
• Mean survival in asymptomatic patients is 12 years, but some patients have rapidly progressive disease
• Once jaundice develops, survival is <2 years
• 5-year survival following transplant is 75% and improving

Haemochromatosis
This autosomal recessive metabolic disorder causes inappropriate intestinal iron absorption and tissue damage from iron deposition ('bronze diabetes'). It is uncommon (3–8:10 000 population), but increasingly recognized and an iron stain should be performed on all liver biopsies that reveal chronic hepatitis or cirrhosis.

Clinical features
• Age 40–60 years, usually male, because menstrual loss protects premenopausal women
• Pigmentation—bronze to slate-grey
• Hepatomegaly—with signs of chronic liver disease (Table 5.2 p. 139). The liver may be tender. A bruit suggests a hepatoma, which develops in 10%
• Diabetes—70%, but exocrine pancreatic malfunction is rare
• Testicular atrophy, loss of libido, pubic and axillary hair are due to impaired pituitary function caused by iron deposition, as well as chronic liver disease affecting hormonal metabolism
• Arthritis—in metacarpophalangeal and larger joints. Chondrocalcinosis may be visible on X-rays
• Cardiac failure (dilated cardiomyopathy) occurs in 30% due to iron deposition

Investigations
• Abnormal liver enzymes depend on the amount of liver damage
• Serum iron is high and total iron binding capacity is low, with a high saturation (often >80%). Ferritin is markedly elevated when cirrhosis is present, but may only be at the upper limit of normal in earlier stages
• Liver biopsy is diagnostic. All biopsies should routinely be

stained for iron (Perl's stain). Alcohol, chronic haemolysis (with or without repeated transfusion), hepatic porphyria, or excess iron ingestion may cause hepatic siderosis to a lesser degree
• CT scan is not routine and magnetic resonance imaging (MRI) is under trial. Since hepatic density correlates with iron load, CT scans have been used as an alternative to repeated liver biopsy, but management is possible without repeated scans or biopsies

Management
• Venesection to a haematocrit <0.50 and total iron binding capacity >50 μmol/l (saturation <40%, or ferritin <100 μg/l) is the best treatment. This initially means twice-weekly venesection and is best arranged with the haematologists
• Outpatient checks:
  ask about fatigue, dyspnoea, arthritis and control of diabetes
  record liver and spleen size
  check liver enzymes, iron and iron binding capacity (if not being measured by the haematologists) and glycosylated haemoglobin (if diabetic)
  deterioration in liver enzymes despite normal iron studies suggests a hepatoma and α-fetoprotein should be checked
• Screen first-degree relatives by HLA typing. If the HLA type (usually A3) is the same as the index case, the risk of haemochromatosis is about 95%. Measuring total iron binding saturation is less sensitive, but substantial iron overload is likely if >60%
• Homozygote relatives should have a liver biopsy, then be followed up if there is no evidence of haemochromatosis, preferably at a specialist centre, with total iron binding saturation measurements every 6–12 months. Venesection is usually indicated if saturation >40%
• Heterozygote relatives should only have a liver biopsy if liver enzymes are abnormal or iron binding saturation is >40%. Follow-up is probably unnecessary if enzymes and saturation are normal
• Oral iron chelating agents are not yet available

Prognosis
• Liver histology may improve with effective venesection
• Cardiac failure is a poor sign

• Survival should be improved if the diagnosis is made before irreversible liver damage occurs

Wilson's disease

The metabolic defect of copper metabolism causing copper deposition in the liver and brain (hepatolenticular degeneration) remains unknown. The prevalence is probably 30/million population.

Features

• Neuropsychiatric features usually precede hepatic disease in young adults, although the converse is true in children
• Chronic active hepatitis, cirrhosis or, rarely, fulminant hepatic failure may be the presenting feature
• Kayser–Fleischer rings at the periphery of the cornea can only be detected by slit lamp examination, but may be absent in fulminant disease
• Haemolytic anaemia occasionally occurs

Management

• Diagnosis is established by the combination of low serum caeruloplasmin (<0.2 g/l) and low serum copper (reference range from the laboratory), increased urinary copper excretion (>1.0 μmol/24 h) and excess hepatic copper in a liver biopsy. All young patients with chronic active hepatitis should have these tests
• Penicillamine must be given for life. Referral to a specialist centre is advisable. There is a risk of fulminant failure if penicillamine is stopped suddenly. Trientine or tetrathiomolybdate are alternatives if the patient cannot tolerate penicillamine
• The family should be screened (serum caeruloplasmin, serum copper and 24-h urinary copper), but liver biopsy is not needed if these tests are negative. Genetic counselling should be offered to relatives

Hepatic granulomas

Granulomas on liver biopsy are usually an unexpected finding and often increase diagnostic confusion (Table 5.12). Granulomatous hepatitis is a misnomer, because neither the histological nor

Table 5.12 Causes of hepatic granulomas

Common	Uncommon	Rare
Sarcoidosis	Brucellosis	Histoplasmosis
Tuberculosis	Drugs:	Coccidioidomycosis
Primary biliary cirrhosis	hydralazine	Blastomycosis
Idiopathic (20–40%)	allopurinol	Berylliosis
	many others	Crohn's disease
	Q fever	Whipple's disease
		Hodgkin's disease
		Syphilis
		Leprosy
		Schistosomiasis
		Ascariasis

biochemical picture is that of hepatitis. Symptoms are those of the underlying disease.

• The usual dilemma is to distinguish sarcoidosis from tuberculosis, because steroids for the former would be totally wrong for the latter. Sarcoidosis is usually distinguished by chest X-ray (hilar lymphadenopathy, middle zone infiltrates), elevated serum angiotensin-converting enzyme, negative Mantoux and positive Kveim tests, but these do not always resolve the dilemma. A trial of antituberculous chemotherapy and re-biopsy is then the safest course of action

• Idiopathic hepatic granulomas have a good prognosis. Occasionally there is a prolonged febrile illness, sometimes with acute abdominal pain and arthritis. Prednisolone 30 mg/day is then indicated, but only after investigation has excluded other (particularly infective) causes

5.7 Cirrhosis

Cirrhosis means loss of normal hepatic architecture due to fibrosis, with nodular regeneration. It implies irreversible liver disease.

Causes
Most (70%) are due to alcohol, hepatitis B or hepatitis C (Table 5.13). Up to 20% are of unknown cause (cryptogenic).

Clinical features
Presentation varies from asymptomatic abnormal liver function tests to end-stage liver disease. A long period of compensated

5.7 Cirrhosis

Table 5.13 Causes of cirrhosis

Common	Uncommon	Rare
Alcohol	Primary biliary	Haemochromatosis
Hepatitis B	Autoimmune CAH	Wilson's disease
Hepatitis C		α_1-antitrypsin deficiency
(parenteral non-A, non-B)		Secondary biliary (strictures,
Cryptogenic		sclerosing cholangitis,
		atresia, cystic fibrosis)
		Cardiac (chronic right
		heart failure
		Budd–Chiari syndrome
		Drugs:
		methotrexate
		others

cirrhosis, when the patient feels well, is common. The equilibrium is easily upset as hepatic reserve dwindles, leading to:

• Hepatocellular failure (p. 146):
  encephalopathy
  bleeding disorder
  cutaneous signs (Table 5.2, p. 139)
  altered drug metabolism (p. 143)
  malnutrition (loss of muscle bulk)
• Ascites (p. 148)
• Portal hypertension (p. 152):
  splenomegaly
  hypersplenism
  bleeding varices
Other features include:
• Increased risk of hepatocellular carcinoma (p. 176)
• Tendency to infections (especially spontaneous peritonitis)
• Increased frequency of peptic ulceration
• Risk of renal failure following surgery (hepatorenal syndrome, p.198)

Diagnostic pitfalls
Some of the clinical features of cirrhosis may be simulated by portal or splenic vein thrombosis, Budd–Chiari syndrome, or constrictive pericarditis (p. 149).

Investigations
A clinical diagnosis should usually be confirmed by liver biopsy,

because biochemical tests correlate poorly with histological changes and treatable causes may be overlooked, even in alcoholics.

Blood tests

• Liver enzymes may be normal in the compensated phase. Marked elevation of the AST or ALP occur in alcoholic hepatitis or biliary cirrhosis, until the terminal stages when the levels fall (no functioning hepatocytes, no enzymes)
• HBsAg, antimitochondrial, antinuclear and anti-smooth muscle antibodies should be measured if the cause is not clearly alcohol-related. Elevated serum IgA, IgM, or IgG are common in alcoholic, primary biliary and autoimmune diseases respectively, but of no help in management
• Thrombocytopenia and leucopenia are features of hypersplenism. Clotting should be normal (INR <1.3), prothrombin time <22 sec) before percutaneous liver biopsy

Liver biopsy (p. 356)

• Biopsy can usually be delayed until after recovery from an acute presentation
• Ascites and disordered clotting should be treated before biopsy, because the risk of haemorrhage (normally <1:100) is increased. Fresh frozen plasma 2 units immediately before biopsy is more effective at correcting disordered coagulation than vitamin K
• Transjugular liver biopsy is safe in experienced hands for decompensated cirrhotics if the diagnosis needs to be established despite coagulation that cannot be corrected
• Histological features include fibrosis and nodular regeneration

Management

Cirrhosis need not be progressive, even if it is irreversible.

General measures

• Alcohol—complete abstinence is not necessary unless the aetiology is alcoholic, but restricted intake (<4 units/week) is sensible advice
• Nutrition—a normal diet is possible in compensated cirrhotics. During encephalopathy protein should be restricted (40 g/day and evenly distributed). Salt should not be added to food if ascites develops (p. 148)

- Drugs—NSAIDs, sedatives and opiates should be avoided (p. 143)
- Complications (portal hypertension, ascites) are treated in the standard way (pp. 150, 155), whatever the cause

Specific treatment
- Alcoholics—abstinence alters the prognosis from 30% to about 70% survival at 5 years
- Hepatitis B and C—interferon improves biochemical liver function, but has not yet been shown to improve mortality (p. 165). It should be considered for HBeAg-positive patients, at a referral centre
- Primary biliary cirrhosis—ursodeoxycholic acid may be of value (p. 166), pending a decision about transplantation
- Haemochromatosis—venesection may improve liver histology (p. 168), although established cirrhosis is irreversible
- Wilson's disease—penicillamine (p. 169)
- Surgery for extrahepatic biliary strictures or atresia

Alcohol and the liver
Four pathological types of alcoholic liver disease are recognized: fatty liver, acute hepatitis, chronic active hepatitis and cirrhosis. Why some (especially women, Indians and Afro-Caribbeans) are susceptible to liver disease and others develop cerebral, pancreatic, or cardiac disease remains unknown. The amount of alcohol consumed is not directly related to the degree of damage, but WHO recommendations are <21 units/week for men and <14 units/week for women. (1 unit is equivalent to one glass of wine, one (pub) measure of spirits, or half a pint of beer.) Alcohol abuse does not exclude less common causes of chronic liver disease, including autoimmune CAH or haemochromatosis.

Fatty liver
- The mechanism is complex. Ethanol oxidation to acetaldehyde increases reduced nicotinamide adenine dinucleotide (NADH), which favours triglyceride accumulation by decreasing fatty acid metabolism
- A palpable liver, increased MCV (>98 fl) and mildly disordered liver enzymes are usually the only features, but these may also be the only signs of established cirrhosis
- Fatty change is rapidly reversible upon abstinence from alcohol

• Liver biopsy is necessary to confirm the diagnosis and exclude irreversible disease. It may also reinforce the need for abstinence. It is reasonable to recheck liver enzymes after 2 months' complete abstinence in alcoholic patients without signs of chronic liver disease, and only to biopsy those whose enzymes remain abnormal
• Obesity, diabetes and parenteral nutrition are other causes of fatty liver

Acute hepatitis
• Jaundice, fever, signs of alcohol withdrawal (tremor, agitation, perspiration), tender hepatomegaly and biochemical changes of hepatitis (Table 5.3, p. 140) are characteristic. A cholestatic picture is more common than in viral hepatitis, as is a polymorphonuclear leucocytosis
• A heavy binge is usually the provoking factor, often on top of established liver disease. 30% die
• Fulminant hepatic failure is not uncommon and the risk is increased by even moderate doses of paracetamol

Chronic active hepatitis (CAH)
• The clinical and biochemical features are the same as in other types of CAH (p. 164), so other causes should be excluded, even in drinkers
• Progression to cirrhosis is almost certain without abstinence

Cirrhosis
• Telangiectases and Dupuytren's contracture are more common findings in alcoholic cirrhosis than in other types, but other clinical features are similar (Table 5.2, p. 139)
• A micronodular cirrhosis is usual
• Management is directed at complications (ascites, portal hypertension, encephalopathy). Abstinence may still alter the course of end-stage alcoholic cirrhosis; it is never too late to stop drinking
• The risk of hepatoma is increased

General points on management
• Detoxification is trying for everybody. A suggested protocol is shown in Fig. 5.6

5 Liver

5.7 Cirrhosis

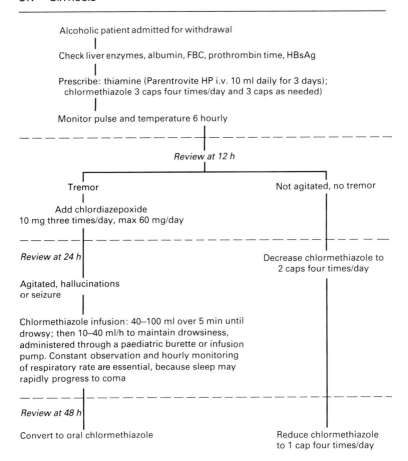

Alcoholic patient admitted for withdrawal
|
Check liver enzymes, albumin, FBC, prothrombin time, HBsAg
|
Prescribe: thiamine (Parentrovite HP i.v. 10 ml daily for 3 days);
chlormethiazole 3 caps four times/day and 3 caps as needed)
|
Monitor pulse and temperature 6 hourly

Review at 12 h

Tremor   Not agitated, no tremor
|
Add chlordiazepoxide
10 mg three times/day, max 60 mg/day

Review at 24 h   Decrease chlormethiazole to
| 2 caps four times/day
Agitated, hallucinations
or seizure
|
Chlormethiazole infusion: 40–100 ml over 5 min until
drowsy; then 10–40 ml/h to maintain drowsiness,
administered through a paediatric burette or infusion
pump. Constant observation and hourly monitoring
of respiratory rate are essential, because sleep may
rapidly progress to coma

Review at 48 h
Convert to oral chlormethiazole   Reduce chlormethiazole
                                         to 1 cap four times/day

Maximum duration of chlormethiazole should not exceed 9 days

Fig. 5.6 Detoxification of alcoholics.

- Vitamins A, C, B_1, folate are commonly deficient. Parentrovite HP 10 ml should be given intravenously over 2–3 min (intramuscular injection is painful), every day for 3 days to all alcoholic patients admitted to hospital
- Alcoholics with a high MCV (sometimes 115 fl) should still have folate, B_{12} and thyroid function checked
- Careful examination of peripheral nerves, coordination, eye movements, short-term memory and mental state is often

rewarding. Wernicke's encephalopathy (confusion, nystagmus, cranial (VI) nerve palsy, ataxia) is a medical emergency and reversible in the early stages with thiamine. The signs, or those of Korsakoff's psychosis (short-term memory loss and confabulation) can be overlooked by the unwary
• Counselling services and psychiatric intervention have variable results. They should be discussed with the patient and arranged if the patient is willing to cooperate (Appendix 1). Whilst there are some striking successes, there are more recidivists. Family involvement is as important as organized care

Prognosis
• 15% of alcoholics develop cirrhosis over 10 years
• Child's classification (A, B, C) of cirrhosis depends on jaundice, ascites, encephalopathy, albumin and nutrition. It is useful for comparing the outcome of variceal bleeding or surgery in groups of patients with cirrhosis, but not helpful for predicting the course in an individual
• 5-year survival in alcoholic cirrhotics is 50% overall, 30% for continued drinkers and 70% for abstainers

5.8 Tumours

Hepatoma
Primary hepatocellular carcinoma is the most common malignant tumour in the world, although rare in the West. 80% of all patients have pre-existing cirrhosis and all types of cirrhosis predispose to hepatoma, although hepatitis B is the commonest cause world-wide.

Causes
• Hepatitis B is strongly associated (100-fold increase in risk)
• Alcoholic cirrhosis is the commonest predisposing factor in Europe and North America

Clinical features
• Rapid development of ascites, increasing liver size or jaundice in a patient with known cirrhosis should always suggest a hepatoma
• Fever, weight loss and right upper quadrant pain are typical

- A hepatic arterial bruit or rub are highly suggestive but rare. A bruit can also sometimes be heard in acute alcoholic hepatitis

Investigations
- Elevated α-fetoprotein (>4 ng/ml) occurs in 80%. Other causes are rare, but include testicular, ovarian or pancreatic tumours, hydatidiform mole and pregnancy
- Ultrasound is as sensitive as CT scanning for detecting hepatic tumours and should be the first imaging technique. CT scanning should be performed if there is doubt, or if anatomical relations of the tumour are not clearly demonstrated by ultrasound
- Liver biopsy, if necessary under ultrasound control, is safe and a histological diagnosis should be obtained in all patients. A rare, fibrolamellar type of hepatoma occurs in non-cirrhotics and has a better prognosis
- Angiography is indicated if surgery is planned, or for therapeutic embolization, or intra-arterial chemotherapy. It is unnecessary for planning surgery if ultrasound demonstrates tumour in both lobes of the liver, because this means incurable disease

Management
- Surgical resection may be possible in 20–30%. Tumour must be confined to one lobe of the liver, without extra-hepatic spread. Referral to a specialist centre for preoperative assessment is recommended
- Transplant has an unacceptable recurrence rate, except in localized tumours of the fibrolamellar type. The occasional success in hepatocellular carcinoma, however, means that it is worth discussing exceptional cases (young patients, prepared to accept a <10% chance of cure) with a transplant centre
- Chemotherapy (mitozantrone, adriamycin, or multiple drugs) is unsatisfactory at present. 10% respond, but mean survival is only 9 months
- Angiographic tumour embolization and radiotherapy are palliative measures, but cannot be expected to offer a cure
- Prevention by hepatitis B vaccination is a hope for the future

Prognosis
- Median survival is 12 weeks after diagnosis. 5-year survival after lobectomy for resectable tumours is about 15%

Metastases

In Europe 90% of liver tumours are metastatic. Colorectal, breast, lung, gastric, or pancreatic cancers are the common primary sites. Metastases are said not to occur in cirrhotic livers. Median survival after diagnosis of hepatic metastases is 2–4 months. Earlier diagnosis by ultrasound is increasing this period (the 'lead time'), although prognosis remains unchanged.

Single hepatic metastases from colorectal cancer should be considered for resection at a specialist centre in patients age <50 years (p. 297). >2-year survival has been reported. Chemotherapy or arterial embolization offer no better results than for primary liver tumours.

Benign tumours

Haemangiomas are usually found incidentally on ultrasound or CT scanning. They may be confused with metastases (although the density is different) and present a hazard at liver biopsy, but are otherwise unimportant. Hepatic adenomas are very rarely associated with the oral contraceptive pill and these are best resected.

5.9   Abscesses

Hepatic abscess (often multiple) may be occult and surprisingly difficult to diagnose.

Pyogenic

• Cholangitis, diverticulitis, or following surgery are now the usual causes, as opposed to appendicitis, but often no cause can be found
• Fever (90%), weight loss and malaise are non-specific. Hepatomegaly and right upper quadrant pain occur in about 50%. Jaundice is a bad prognostic sign
• Blood cultures are negative in 50%. If *Streptococcus milleri* is grown, it is almost invariably due to a liver abscess
• Ultrasound of the liver is always indicated for patients with fever and mild derangement of liver enzymes. CT scanning is more sensitive for lesions near the diaphragm
• Needle aspiration under ultrasound or CT control identifies the organism in 90%. Mixed aerobes and anaerobes are usual

5.9   Abscesses

- Percutaneous drainage of a single abscess and the one or two largest cavities of multiple abscesses should be performed by a radiologist. Surgical drainage is now rarely indicated
- Intravenous metronidazole 500 mg, amoxycillin 500 mg and gentamicin 80 mg three times daily should be given for 2 weeks, followed by oral amoxycillin 500 mg and metronidazole 400 mg three times daily for 6 weeks

Amoebic
- Very rare in those living in Europe, but patients may present years after living in the tropics
- 80% are aged <40 years
- Pain is more common and systemic features less common than in pyogenic abscesses. Point tenderness is typical, but dysentery is unusual (p. 336)
- Ultrasound and markedly elevated serum antibodies to *Entamoeba histolytica* are diagnostic in >90%. Hot stools should be examined for trophozoites (p. 336), which are highly suggestive of the diagnosis. Aspiration of thick, pink-brown 'anchovy sauce' pus is characteristic, but not indicated unless the diagnosis cannot be confirmed in other ways
- Metronidazole 800 mg three times daily for 10 days is effective in most patients, but is best followed by diloxanide 500 mg three times daily for 10 days to prevent recurrent invasive disease. Drainage is needed only for impending rupture, indicated by severe pain, pleuritic pain or hiccups. Recurrent fever may be due to secondary bacterial infection

Hydatid cysts
Symptomless hepatomegaly in Eastern Mediterranean, South American or Welsh farmers is occasionally due to cysts of *Echinococcus granulosus*.

Liver function is usually normal, eosinophilia often absent and serological tests may be only weakly positive. Ultrasound presents a characteristic appearance of multiple 'daughter' cysts, with clearly defined walls. The walls calcify with time and may be visible on plain X-ray. Hydatid complement fixation test should be checked before aspiration of any hepatic cysts in patients from endemic areas.

Hydatid cysts are often best left alone. Albendazole may be effective and is available on a named-patient basis (from SmithKline Beecham) for symptomatic disease. Liver biopsy is contraindicated because of the risk of anaphylaxis and surgical removal is only necessary for increasing size, complications of local pressure, or secondary infection.

5.10 Clinical dilemmas
General advice is given in Appendix 5.

Asymptomatic abnormal liver function tests
Elevated liver enzymes or serum bilirubin are an increasingly common incidental finding due to automated biochemical tests. Normal ranges (Table 5.3, p. 140) represent the 95th centile of a selected healthy population. At best this leads to earlier diagnosis of treatable disease, but at worst it exposes the patient to the complications of ill-advised investigations. The following plan is recommended:
• Ask about:
  alcohol intake
  drug treatment or abuse
  previous jaundice
  family history of hepatic or chronic disease
  recent viral illness
• Examine for:
  hepatomegaly and splenomegaly
  signs of chronic liver disease (Table 5.2, p. 139)
  lymphadenopathy
  urticarial rash or arthritis (associated with chronic hepatitis)
• Then investigate as in Fig. 5.7

Liver transplantation
Indications for liver transplant are given in Table 5.15 and relative contraindications in Table 5.16. The timing of transplant in chronic liver disease is difficult, so early discussion with a referral centre (Appendix 1) is advisable.

The other side of the coin is that every hospital has a responsibility to face the difficult task of finding donors.

5.10 Clinical dilemmas

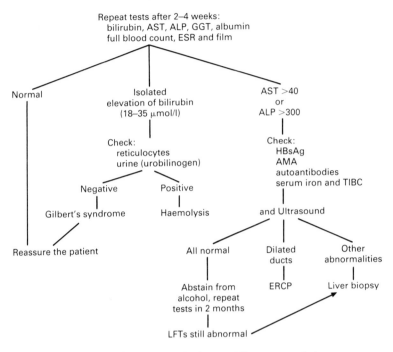

Fig. 5.7 Investigation of asymptomatic abnormal liver enzyme tests.

Table 5.14 Diseases potentially curable by transplant (adults)

Primary biliary cirrhosis (PBC)
Cryptogenic cirrhosis
Post-viral cirrhosis (except those still HBeAg-positive)
Autoimmune chronic active hepatitis
Primary sclerosing cholangitis (PSC)
Budd–Chiari syndrome
Fibrolamellar hepatoma
Fulminant hepatic failure (p. 39)
Metabolic disorders:
    Wilson's disease
    others (usually children)

5.10 Clinical dilemmas

Table 5.15 Relative contraindications to liver transplant

Alcoholic cirrhosis*
HBeAg-positive patients (but not HBsAg-positive alone)
Hepatocellular carcinoma
Previous upper abdominal surgery
Portal vein thrombosis
Extrahepatic malignant tumours
Cardiorenal disease
Age >60
Psychologically unable to cope with postoperative care

* Prognosis may be better than previously thought

Timing
• End-stage liver disease—histological evidence of irreversible liver damage (fibrosis), unremitting jaundice, ascites responding poorly to diuretics, incipient encephalopathy, or haemostatic disorder
• The timing is easier in PBC, because once the bilirubin is >100 μmol/l, the prognosis is usually less than 2 years
• The prognosis in the later stages of PSC or other types of cirrhosis is much more difficult to predict
• The patient and family should understand the irreversible nature of the disease, the likely delay of weeks (or months) whilst a matched donor is found, and the prognosis

Postoperative implications
• Hospital stay is usually 4 weeks
• Frequent blood tests are necessary (weekly for several months and then less frequently) to measure cyclosporin levels, biochemical and haematological tests, on top of outpatient visits
• Drug compliance must be good
• Graft rejection occurs in 25% and retransplant is necessary in 15%

Prognosis
• 75% 1-year survival in PBC, but results are constantly improving. After 1 year, the outlook is excellent. PBC has not been known to recur in the transplanted liver, although chronic rejection may look histologically similar
• 50% 5-year survival in PSC or cryptogenic cirrhosis

6 Gall Bladder and Biliary Tree

6.1 Clinical anatomy of the biliary tract

The biliary canaliculi adjacent to each hepatocyte drain into interlobular, then septal, bile ducts which combine to form intra-hepatic ducts visible on cholangiography. The right and left hepatic ducts join at the porta hepatis to form the common hepatic duct, which unites with the cystic duct from the gall bladder to form the common bile duct. This enters the duodenum through the head of the pancreas (Fig. 6.1).

Gall bladder contraction is stimulated by cholecystokinin (secretin) after meals. Biliary flow is controlled by a pressure gradient between the common bile duct and duodenum, as well as

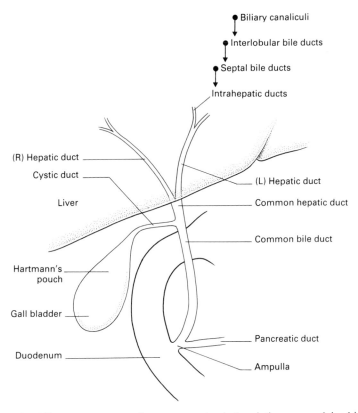

Fig. 6.1 Biliary tract anatomy. Important anatomical variations are explained in the text.

the peristaltic pump action of the sphincter of Oddi, which is also influenced by cholecystokinin.

Anatomical anomalies of pathological importance are:
• Separate exit points into the duodenum of the common bile duct and main pancreatic duct (endoscopic cannulation is difficult)
• Accessory artery superior to the ampulla of Vater in 1% (sphincterotomy can lead to major haemorrhage)
• Opening of the common bile duct onto a duodenal diverticulum (cannulation of the papilla is difficult and ERCP/sphincterotomy potentially dangerous, due to risk of perforation)
• Cystic duct fails to join the common hepatic duct in 20% (both the duct *and* its union must be identified before ligation at cholecystectomy)
• Cystic artery may arise from the left hepatic or gastroduodenal arteries, rather than the right hepatic artery

6.2   Gall stones

Bile is concentrated in the gall bladder, which acts as a reservoir between meals for bile acids (cholic and chenodeoxycholic acids), which are essential for emulsifying lipids prior to digestion and absorption. Bile acids form the outer, hydrophilic layer of micelles which contain lipid-soluble cholesterol in the centre. Phospholipids insert into the micellar wall to increase the micellar capacity for cholesterol.

Insufficient bile acids (caused by failure of enterohepatic recycling in terminal ileal disease, for example), or imbalance between cholesterol and phospholipid concentrations in bile, will lead to precipitation of cholesterol crystals from the supersaturated bile, which then form the nucleus for gall stone formation (lithogenic bile).

Pigment stones are caused by bilirubin forming insoluble calcium precipitates in bile. Black, brittle pure pigment stones account for 70% of radio-opaque gall stones. Brown pigment stones are soft, often intrahepatic and unusual (Fig. 6.2).

Prevalence

On ultrasound studies of a normal population, 10–15% people have gall stones, which become more common with age. Conditions predisposing to gall stones are shown in Table 6.1.

6 Gall Bladder and Biliary Tree

6.2 Gall stones

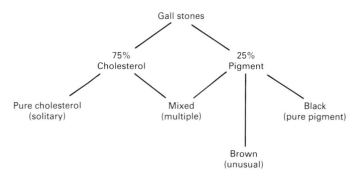

Fig. 6.2 Types of gall stones.

Table 6.1 Conditions predisposing to gall stones

Cholesterol	Black pigment	Brown pigment
Sex (2F:1M)	Chronic haemolysis:	Sclerosing cholangitis
Obesity	sickle cell	Oriental:
Diet (low fibre)	spherocytosis	biliary parasites
Race (Europe, USA,	prosthetic valve	
American Indians)	Cirrhosis	
Cirrhosis (30%)	Biliary infection:	
Terminal ileal:	*E. coli, Clostridium* sp.	
Crohn's		
resection		
Drugs:		
oral contraceptive		
clofibrate		

Symptoms
Most gall stones remain 'silent' in the fundus of the gall bladder. Migration to the cystic duct and impaction causes acute or chronic cholecystitis which resolves when disimpaction occurs, or progresses to complications (Fig. 6.3).
• Silent stones—15% develop symptoms over 15 years
• Acute cholecystitis—persistent, severe right upper quadrant pain, fever and leucocytosis (p. 22). Acalculous acute cholecystitis is rare and caused by bacterial infection, polyarteritis or trauma
• Chronic cholecystitis—recurrent biliary colic, dyspepsia, fat intolerance and non-specific features (p. 22)
• Common bile duct stones—jaundice, abdominal pain

6 Gall Bladder and Biliary Tree

6.2 Gall stones

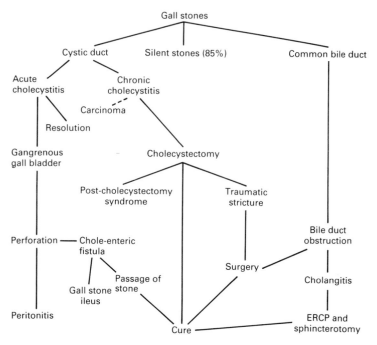

Fig. 6.3 Consequences of gall stones.

- Cholangitis—jaundice, fever, abdominal pain (p. 199), usually due to stones in the common bile duct
- Gangrenous gall bladder and empyema—septic and severe illness, with local peritonism
- Biliary fistula—from a chronically inflamed gall bladder into the small intestine or colon, resulting in air in the biliary tree and resolution of symptoms or, very rarely, impaction at the ileocaecal valve and gall stone ileus
- Perforation—local or diffuse peritonitis after acute cholecystitis
- Cholangiocarcinoma—jaundice, weight loss, pain (p. 201). More common in patients with gall stones, but does not justify prophylactic cholecystectomy

Investigations

Ultrasound
- Most effective non-invasive method of detecting stones, but often

finds incidental, silent stones. Stones may occasionally be missed even in experienced hands. In some patients the gall bladder cannot be identified, because of gas, fibrosis or unusual anatomy
• Also useful for diagnosing biliary obstruction, acute or chronic cholecystitis and for assessing gall bladder function when performed before and after a fatty meal (p. 361)
• CT scan is usually better for visualizing common bile duct stones

Blood tests
• All are normal in chronic cholecystitis or silent stones
• Elevated ALP or γGT suggests common duct stones. Leucocytosis occurs in acute cholecystitis or cholangitis
• Serum cholesterol is unrelated to biliary cholesterol, but is elevated in primary biliary cirrhosis

Other tests
• Plain abdominal X-ray—mandatory in acute abdominal pain. May show calcified stones, enlarged liver or air in the biliary tree (chole-enteric fistula, clostridial cholangitis, or post-intervention)
• Oral cholecystography—indicated for assessing gall bladder function before non-surgical treatment (p. 191)
• Isotope (HIDA) scanning—useful in acute cholecystitis (p. 23)
• ERCP—for diagnosis and treatment of biliary obstruction (p. 195)
• Percutaneous transhepatic cholangiogram (PTC)—indicated when dilated intrahepatic ducts are detected on ultrasound and ERCP is not readily available. Complementary to ERCP if proximal biliary anatomy needs clarifying (a cholangiocarcinoma may block the flow of contrast), or for stenting tortuous strictures (p. 195)
• Intravenous cholangiography and the bromsulphthalein (BSP) test for assessing biliary excretory function, are obsolete

Indications for surgery
Most decisions are straightforward. Difficulty arises in deciding whether gall stones in patients with non-specific symptoms are the cause or merely incidental (Table 6.2).
    Mini-laparotomy cholecystectomy (through a 5–10cm incision) or laparoscopic cholecystectomy (through a peri-umbilical incision and two upper quadrant punctures for instrument manipulation) are recently developed techniques. Advantages over standard

6.2   Gall stones

Table 6.2 Symptomatic or incidental stones?

	Symptomatic	Incidental
Pain	Acute episodes <60 sec Like labour pains 1–72-h duration	Constant dull ache or none Variable Most days
Pain-free interval	Several weeks/months	Rare
Fat intolerance	Common	Common
Flatulence	Common	Common
Bloating	Less common	Common
Physical signs	RUQ tenderness or none	RUQ tenderness or none
Ultrasound	Gall stone(s) Thickened wall	Gall stone(s) Normal gall bladder
Oral cholecystogram	Non-functioning	Functioning (may be poor in the elderly)

RUQ: right upper quadrant.

cholecystectomy are the short hospital stay (<48 h) and early return to work (<1 week), and unlike non-surgical options (dissolution or lithotripsy), there is no risk of stone recurrence. It is premature to recommend either technique as an alternative to standard cholecystectomy.

Absolute indications

• Acute cholecystitis—optimum treatment is surgery in the same admission, on the next available operating list (p. 23)
• Chronic cholecystitis—typical history of biliary colic and a contracted or non-functioning gall bladder shown by ultrasound or cholecystography after a fatty meal
• Common bile duct stones age <70 years—ERCP and sphincterotomy are unnecessary in patients who also need a cholecystectomy. In patients >70 years or those at poor operative risk, endoscopic sphincterotomy alone has a lower mortality, although the risk of recurrent stones remains
• Gangrenous gall bladder—emergency cholecystostomy is often safer than cholecystectomy. Later elective cholecystectomy or spontaneous closure are then possible
• Gall stone ileus—to relieve intestinal obstruction , with later cholecystectomy

6.2   Gall stones

• Elective cholecystectomy is indicated if gall stones are considered to be the cause of symptoms
• Irritable bowel syndrome, peptic ulcer, chronic pancreatitis, or renal tract disease may produce similar symptoms to chronic cholecystitis and should be excluded if doubt exists
• Post-cholecystectomy syndrome (p. 203) is more common in patients who present with non-specific symptoms (flatulent dyspepsia)

Non-surgical options
These options must be balanced against a safe operation (mortality 0.1% age <50 years, 0.5% >50 years) which removes all gall stones without recurrence, although retained stones occur in about 2% and other complications (including post-cholecystectomy syndrome) in 10%. Minimally invasive surgery (mini-laparotomy or endoscopic cholecystectomy) is being developed (p. 189).

Only 10–20% patients with symptomatic gall stones are suitable, and treatment is unsuccessful in up to a third. The risk of recurrent stones is the main drawback of all techniques that leave the gall bladder *in situ*. Technology is rapidly developing and indications are continuously being revised. Symptoms must be present before any treatment is contemplated.

Indications
• Patient declines surgery
• When the surgical risk is unacceptable
• Functioning gall bladder demonstrated by oral cholecystography or ultrasound before and after a fatty meal
• Non-calcified gall stones on abdominal X-ray or ultrasound. CT scan is needed to assess the degree of calcification
• Solitary stones must be <1 cm for reasonable success, although larger stones can be fragmented by lithotripsy
• Patient understands the risk of recurrence and need for long-term treatment

Ursodeoxycholic acid (UDCA)
8–12 mg/kg/day as a single dose for 4 months (50% dissolution rate) and continued for up to 2 years. Diarrhoea is the main side effect, but is less common than with chenodeoxycholic acid which it has largely superceded. Treatment (750 mg/day) for each year

costs over £500. Recurrence after successful treatment is 10%/year for 5 years, then plateaus (50% at 10 years), so maintenance treatment may be indicated, similar to lithotripsy.

External shock-wave lithotripsy (ESWL)
General, epidural, or spinal anaesthesia is needed, although immersion is no longer necessary. Transient biliary colic occurs in about 35% and 2% develop pancreatitis. UDCA (500–750 mg/day) is needed after ESWL and up to 90% are free of stones after 1 year, but recurrence without continued UDCA is 50% at 5 years.

Contact dissolution
Methyl-tert-butyl ether (MTBE) via percutaneous cholecystotomy remains experimental.

6.3   Cholestatic jaundice
Cholestatic jaundice is due to interuption of bile flow anywhere in the biliary tree. The site of obstruction is either extra-hepatic, when there is mechanical obstruction to the main bile ducts, or intra-hepatic when the obstructing lesion is usually not visible (except with intra-hepatic strictures, stones, or tumour). 'Obstructive jaundice' usually refers to extra-hepatic causes. About 20% patients with clinical or biochemical features of cholestasis have hepatocellular disease.

Causes

Extra-hepatic obstruction (Table 6.3)
About 70% cholestatic jaundice is due to extrahepatic obstruction. Dilated intra-hepatic ducts occur in high obstruction (at the porta hepatis), and extra-hepatic ducts dilate in distal obstruction, which is readily detected by ultrasound.

Intra-hepatic obstruction (Table 6.4)
• Benign recurrent cholestasis presents as recurrent cholestatic jaundice lasting for several weeks, for which no cause can be found
• Jaundice in Hodgkin's disease is usually extra-hepatic, due to lymph nodes obstructing the porta hepatis. Intra-hepatic cholestasis is usually pre-terminal

6.3 Cholestatic jaundice

- Septicaemia or total parenteral nutrition occasionally cause cholestatic jaundice, usually in a patient with multi-organ failure

Table 6.3 Causes of extra-hepatic cholestasis

Common	Uncommon	Rare
Common duct stones	Portal lymph nodes	Pseudocyst
Panceatic cancer	Pancreatitis:	Choledochal cyst
	acute	
	chronic	
	Post-traumatic stricture	
	Cholangiocarcinoma	
	Ampullary carcinoma	

Table 6.4 Causes of intra-hepatic cholestasis

Common	Uncommon	Rare
Drugs:	Viral hepatitis	Benign recurrent
phenothiazines	Alcoholic hepatitis	Hodgkin's disease
many others	Sclerosing cholangitis	Intra-hepatic stones
Primary biliary cirrhosis	(primary: PSC)	
(PBC)	Cirrhosis	
	Metastases	
	Septicaemia	
	Cholangiocarcinoma	

Clinical features
- Jaundice appears slowly, often preceded by pruritus
- Itching and pale stools are typical in both intra- and extra-hepatic cholestasis (Table 6.5)

Table 6.5 Physical signs in cholestatic jaundice

Pale stools
Dark orange urine
Scratch marks (excoriation)
Polished nails (itching)
Finger clubbing
Xanthelasma (eyelids)
Xanthomas (tendons, palmar creases)
Hepatomegaly
Palpable gall bladder (especially carcinoma)

• Dark urine also occurs in hepatocellular (but not pre-hepatic) jaundice, but urobilinogen is only absent in complete bile duct obstruction
• Extra-hepatic cholestasis may be associated with pain and fever, indicating cholangitis. Urgent blood culture, antibiotics and drainage are then indicated (p. 199). This is rare in intra-hepatic cholestasis

Investigations

Confirmation of cholestasis
• ALP is markedly elevated (>3 times, often 10 times, normal). Hepatic origin is confirmed by elevated γGT
• Bilirubin concentrations reflect the duration of cholestasis. The highest levels are reached in complete obstruction by carcinoma or end-stage intra-hepatic disease (such as primary biliary cirrhosis)
• An isolated high ALP without elevated bilirubin suggests intra-hepatic disease (PBC or PSC)—as long as Paget's disease is excluded!

Identifying the cause
The main aim is to distinguish intra- from extra-hepatic cholestasis. The sequence of investigations is shown in Fig. 6.4.

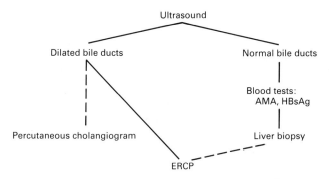

Fig. 6.4 Sequence of investigations in cholestatic jaundice.

• Ultrasound is not good at identifying common bile duct stones, although it will detect a dilated common bile duct (diameter >7 mm)

• Percutaneous transhepatic cholangiography (PTC) is indicated in preference to ERCP if:

ERCP is not readily available

ERCP does not opacify all of the biliary tree (cholangiocarcinoma can obstruct flow)

therapeutic stenting of a high, tortuous stricture is necessary (best performed from above, in conjunction with ERCP)

• A dilated common bile duct without an obstructing lesion occurs:

shortly after an obstructing stone has passed (air may also be seen in the biliary tree)

after cholecystectomy (for years, but rarely >9 mm diameter)

Indications for ERCP

Diagnostic

• Jaundice with dilated intrahepatic ducts
• Cholangitis (urgently, within 48 h)
• Jaundice or elevated ALP with normal-calibre intrahepatic ducts, when liver biopsy does not establish a diagnosis and especially if the patient has ulcerative colitis (high chance of PSC)
• Post-cholecystectomy pain (p. 203)
• Recurrent acute or chronic pancreatitis (Fig. 4.2, pp. 119 and 120)

Therapeutic

• Sphincterotomy for common bile duct stones (Fig. 6.5, p. 197)
• Stenting of malignant strictures (Fig. 6.5, p. 196)

Management

Once the site of obstruction has been determined by ERCP or PTC, the surgeons should be contacted and a joint decision made about endoscopic or surgical drainage for extra-hepatic obstruction

Common bile duct stones

• Patients >70 years:

endoscopic sphincterotomy (2–10 mm incision through the ampulla) allows the stones to pass, often with some further pain

subsequent cholecystectomy is not required in 90%

• Fit patients <70 years:

early cholecystectomy and exploration of the common duct is necessary, to remove the source of stones

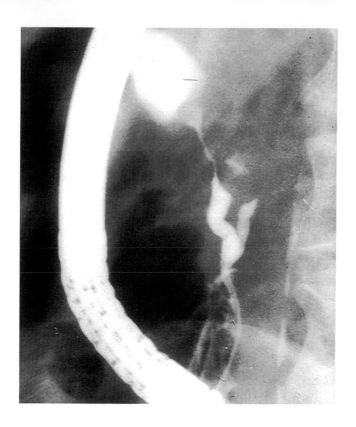

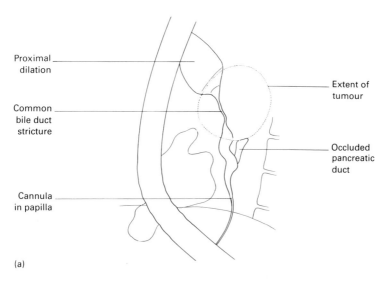

Proximal dilation

Common bile duct stricture

Cannula in papilla

Extent of tumour

Occluded pancreatic duct

(a)

Fig. 6.5 (a) ERCP demonstrating a blocked pancreatic duct due to a carcinoma which has caused stricturing of the common bile duct leading to dilatation of the proximal biliary tree.

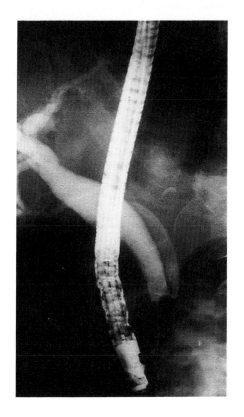

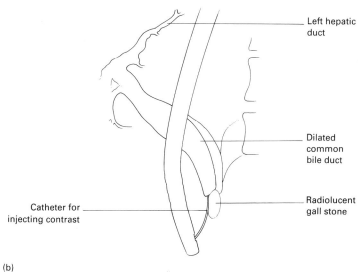

Left hepatic
duct

Dilated
common
bile duct

Radiolucent
gall stone

Catheter for
injecting contrast

(b)

Fig. 6.5 (*continued*) (b) ERCP in a patient with obstructive jaundice due to a gall stone impacted in the common bile duct. (Courtesy of Dr Roger Chapman.)

sphincterotomy is unnecessary and merely risks complications
- Retained stones after cholecystectomy:
  ERCP is diagnostic and therapeutic (sphincterotomy)
- Acute cholangitis or acute pancreatitis with common bile duct
stones at any age are indications for urgent sphincterotomy

Malignant strictures
- Endoscopic insertion of a stent is indicated if curative surgery is
not possible
- The success rate (85%) is similar to surgery, but complications
and hospital stay are appreciably reduced
- Duodenal obstruction by tumour following stent insertion (which
might otherwise have been avoided by surgery) is rare (<5%)
- Repeat ERCP for blocked stents is required in 20% with
malignant obstruction, after 3 months. Most stents block in time
- High or tortuous strictures are best stented by joint endoscopic
and percutaneous radiological manipulation. If this fails, jaundice
can sometimes be relieved by hepatic segment III biliary diversion
in expert hands

Benign strictures
- Single benign strictures (often post-traumatic) are best treated
surgically at a specialist referral centre, although balloon dilatation
at ERCP is occasionally possible

Surgery in cholestatic jaundice
- Mortality and complications are common—up to 50% if the
patient has underlying cirrhosis
- Contributing factors are the age of the patient (often elderly),
sepsis (especially cholangitis), cause of jaundice (cirrhosis or
malignancy) and prediposition to renal failure (hepatorenal
syndrome)

Hepatorenal syndrome

Features
- Renal failure in the presence of acute or chronic liver disease
(commonly, but not necessarily, cholestatic)
- Precipitated by hypotension during surgery, excessive diuretic
therapy or paracentesis, and aggravated by sepsis

• Hyponatraemia and a high urea are invariable. Urine sodium is low (<10 mmol/1), but there is little response to fluid challenge
• Renal tubular function is unusually preserved, so sodium is avidly reabsorbed, water retained and ascites becomes refractory
• Hyponatraemia, uraemia and hepatic failure contribute to terminal coma

Management
• Prevention is the key, because the prognosis is dismal once hepatorenal syndrome is established. The following decrease the risk:

> avoid hypotension, nephrotoxic drugs (aminoglycosides), and excessive diuretic therapy or paracentesis for ascites (p. 149)
> recognize and treat sepsis promptly
> 10% mannitol 20 ml/h intravenous infusion before and during surgery, to maintain a diuresis

• Hyponatraemia is extremely difficult to treat. It is exacerbated by diuretics for refractory ascites
• Fluid restriction (1000 ml/day), salt restriction (<50 mmol/day) and intravenous salt-poor albumin (100 ml 20% for 3 days) to expand the intravascular compartment are temporary measures
• Dialysis is ineffective
• Active measures are inappropriate if the underlying disease cannot be treated

6.4 Cholangitis

Bacterial cholangitis
Ascending infection in the biliary tree occurs when the main bile ducts are obstructed, usually by stones. Surgery or endoscopic procedures can introduce infection.

Features (Charcot's triad)
• Jaundice
• Pain—usually central, severe and colicky
• Fever—may be minimal in the elderly, those on steroids and the immunosuppressed

Management
• General—blood cultures, intravenous fluids, pethidine

6.4   Cholangitis

• Antibiotics—intravenous piperacillin 4 g four times daily is more effective than ampicillin and metronidazole
• Ultrasound—to look for a dilated common duct (>7 mm), although obstructing stones are rarely seen
• Drainage—urgent (<48 h) ERCP and sphincterotomy if common bile duct stones are present, whatever the age. Mortality is 5–10% emergency surgery and exploration of the common duct has a mortality of 30% in poor-risk patients

Sclerosing cholangitis

Primary sclerosing cholangitis (PSC)
All parts of the biliary tract may be involved in a fibrosing process that ultimately leads to biliary cirrhosis. The cause is unknown. 75% have associated ulcerative colitis.

Clinical features
• 70% are male
• Asymptomatic elevation of ALP in a patient with ulcerative colitis (rarely Crohn's disease) is highly suggestive. The activity of the colitis appears to be inversely related to the severity of PSC, although patients usually have a pancolitis
• Pruritus, jaundice, right upper quadrant pain and weight loss occur in the later stages
• Bacterial cholangitis and oesophageal varices due to portal hypertension occur less commonly than in other types of progressive liver disease
• Rapid deterioration may be due to a cholangiocarcinoma in later stages, which is more common in those with ulcerative colitis

Investigations
• ALP is elevated along with the GGT. Antimitochondrial antibodies are negative
• Ultrasound excludes other causes of cholestasis (gall stones are also more common in ulcerative colitis)
• ERCP is diagnostic. It demonstrates irregular stricturing and dilatation (beading) of intra-hepatic ducts. 30% have a stricture of an extra-hepatic bile duct. Diffuse cholangiocarcinoma can rarely cause this appearance

* Liver biopsy may be characteristic, but the diagnosis must be confirmed by ERCP. Histological appearances can be confused with chronic active hepatitis, but an unusually high ALP in these patients is an indication for ERCP (p. 164)
* Sigmoidoscopy and rectal biopsy should be performed in patients who have not previously been diagnosed as having ulcerative colitis

Management
* There is no specific treatment. Symptomatic treatment is the same as for primary biliary cirrhosis (PBC, p. 166)
* Colectomy does not alter the course of PSC in ulcerative colitis
* Hepatic transplantation should be considered in patients with end-stage disease (deep jaundice, ascites), although the timing is more difficult and the outcome less good than for PBC (p. 180)

Prognosis
* Mean duration from the onset of symptoms to death is 7 years, but the time is very variable
* 5-year survival after transplantation is 50%

Secondary sclerosing cholangitis
* Very rarely, an identical picture to PSC can be caused by long-standing biliary obstruction due to a benign stricture or common duct stones

6.5 Cholangiocarcinoma
Carcinoma may arise anywhere in the biliary tree. The site determines the presentation—distal tumours obstruct main ducts and present early; intrahepatic tumours present late and may be mistaken for hepatomas. There is a high prevalence in Thailand and the Far East, possibly due to liver fluke (*Clonorchis sinensis*) infection.

Clinical features
* Age >60 years
* Associated with:
  biliary cirrhosis (primary or secondary)
  PSC
  ulcerative colitis
* Jaundice, followed by pruritus (pruritus precedes jaundice in

PBC or PSC). Carcinoma of the pancreas or ampulla are more common causes. The jaundice occasionally fluctuates, which can be deceptive

- Pain—epigastric and mild
- Weight loss and diarrhoea, due to fat malabsorption
- Rapid deterioration in a patient with PBC or PSC
- Hepatomegaly or a palpable gall bladder are quite common, but splenomegaly and ascites are rare

Diagnosis
Investigations for cholestatic jaundice (ultrasound and ERCP or PTC, Fig. 6.4, p. 194) will suggest the diagnosis.

- Ultrasound may detect a tumour mass, as well as dilated ducts
- ERCP shows an abrupt or irregular obstruction to contrast, usually at the hilum. A percutaneous transhepatic cholangiogram is then indicated to define the extent, if intervention (relief of jaundice) is considered feasible
- Difficulties include:
  histological confirmation. Liver biopsy rarely shows tumour even in intra-hepatic lesions and brush or bile cytology obtained at ERCP is not easy to interpret
  distinguishing distal lesions from pancreatic cancer. CT scan may show the site of the main bulk of the tumour
  widespread intra-hepatic cholangiocarcinoma looks like PSC. The clinical course over a few weeks points to the diagnosis
- Blood tests show a cholestatic picture. α-fetoprotein is normal

Management
Cure is rarely possible unless a tumour is found incidentally at hepatic transplant for PBC or PSC. Surgery should be considered for distal, localized tumours in young patients that present with jaundice early. Referral to a specialist centre is advisable.
Symptomatic treatment includes:

- Endoscopic stenting of distal strictures to relieve jaundice and itching. This is difficult, because most tumours are at the porta hepatis (p. 195)
- Cholestyramine 4–12 g/day, or oxymetholone 100–150 mg/day, for pruritus
- Analgesics for pain
- Low-fat diet for diarrhoea

Prognosis
- The tumours are slow growing. Mean survival is 14 months, but may be up to 5 years

6.6   Clinical dilemma

Post-cholecystectomy symptoms

Recurrent symptoms occur in 15% patients who have an elective cholecystectomy. Most are attributed to ill-defined motility disorders, but there are other important causes.

Causes
- Retained common bile duct stone
- Duodenal or gastric ulcer
- Chronic pancreatitis
- Renal tract disease (including pelvi-ureteric junction obstruction)
- Irritable bowel syndrome
- Post-cholecystectomy syndrome
  Post-cholecystectomy syndrome describes recurrent colicky pain, fat intolerance, often with diarrhoea and dyspepsia, without a retained stone or other cause. Spasm of the sphincter of Oddi and a long cystic duct remnant have been implicated, but the irritable bowel syndrome is probably the cause.

Management
- Careful history—to identify differences from pre-cholecystectomy symptoms and associated features of other diseases
- Initial investigation:
  ALP, GGT (elevated in retained stones)
  full blood count
  urine for blood, protein, bilirubin and urobilinogen
  abdominal ultrasound (the common bile duct is usually slightly dilated after cholecystectomy, 7–9 mm)
- Subsequent investigations are indicated if severe symptoms persist, or if initial investigations are abnormal:
  upper gastrointestinal endoscopy
  ERCP—to exclude a retained stone and chronic pancreatitis.
  Sphincterotomy sometimes relieves the post-cholecystectomy syndrome, but a long cystic duct remnant is not an indication for surgery

6.6   Clinical dilemma

- Antispasmodics (mebeverine 135 mg three times daily) are occasionally helpful. The many alternatives (aluminium-containing antacids, cholestyramine, treatment for non-ulcer dyspepsia (p. 76), antidepressants, laxatives, exclusion diet) indicate how difficult it is to treat effectively

7 Small Intestine

7.1   Diarrhoea

Food, fluid and intestinal secretions amount to 7 l/day. Normally 5 l is absorbed by the small intestine and 1.5–2 l by the colon. The residual 100–200 ml (or 100–200 g when solid) is excreted as faeces. Consequently a 10% decrease in fluid absorbed by the colon will double the stool volume. There is, however, considerable reserve colonic absorptive capacity which compensates for increased ileal effluent volume in osmotic or secretory conditions (see below) until that capacity is exceeded, when diarrhoea develops.

Diarrhoea means increased stool water. Stool volume of >200 ml/day (weight >200 g/day) is a practical definition and usually results in an increased stool frequency. Patients may describe increased stool frequency alone, a single loose motion or even rectal discharge as diarrhoea. A careful history is essential and stool weight should be measured on a 24-h basis when the cause of diarrhoea is not apparent.

Causes
Common causes of recurrent or persistent diarrhoea are shown in Table 7.1. Classification into osmotic, secretory, motility and combined types (Table 7.2) helps when planning later investigations (see Fig. 7.2, p. 212), but diagnosis initially depends on excluding colonic causes and identifying common conditions.
• Persistent diarrhoea after acute gastroenteritis may be due to persistent infection (especially *Giardia lamblia*), acquired hypolactasia, hypogammaglobulinaemia, unrecognized disease (coeliac, ulcerative colitis), or post-dysenteric irritable bowel syndrome (p. 319), which is the commonest reason
• Common drug-induced causes include antibiotics, magnesium-containing antacids, beta blockers and NSAIDs, as well as alcohol

Osmotic diarrhoea
• Due to malabsorbed osmotically active substances (such as carbohydrate and peptides), which retain water in the intestinal lumen. Diarrhoea occurs when the extra ileal effluent exceeds colonic absorptive capacity, and may be intermittent (if the colon compensates for the fluid load), or only present when there is associated colonic disease (such as hypolactasia with Crohn's colitis)

207

7 Small Intestine

7.1 Diarrhoea

• Characterized by an osmotic gap; measured osmolality is 20% greater than the osmolality calculated from stool electrolytes (twice the sum of Na + K concentrations) in osmotic diarrhoea

Table 7.1 Causes of diarrhoea

Common	Uncommon	Rare

Gastroenteritis:
  viral (rota, echo)
  bacterial (*Salmonella,*
   Campylobacter sp.)
  parasitic (*G. lamblia*)
  toxin (*E. coli,*
   Shigella sp.)
Irritable bowel syndrome
Drugs (many, alcohol)
Colorectal carcinoma
Ulcerative colitis
	Crohn's disease
	Coeliac disease
	Hypogammaglobulinaemia
	Bacterial overgrowth
	Chronic pancreatitis
	Thyrotoxicosis
	Pseudomembranous colitis
	Laxative abuse
	Food allergy
	Ileal/gastric resection
	Hypolactasia
		Autonomic neuropathy
		Tropical sprue
		Ischaemic colitis
		Microscopic colitis
		Collagenous colitis
		Pellagra
		Addison's disease
		Hypoparathyroidism
		Amyloidosis
		Behçet's disease
		Polyarteritis nodosa
		Whipple's disease
		Mastocytosis
		Carcinoid
		VIPoma
		Gastrinoma
		Medullary thyroid
		  cancer
		Uraemic colitis
		Zinc deficiency

Secretory diarrhoea
• Secretion, stimulated by a toxin (such as cholera toxin) or peptide (such as vasoactive intestinal polypeptide, VIP), is mediated by cyclic nucleotides. 'Travellers' diarrhoea' is usually due to *E. coli* enterotoxin (Table 7.2)
• Characterized by a stool volume >400 ml during fasting (see Fig. 7.2, p. 212)

Table 7.2 Mechanisms of diarrhoea

Osmotic	Secretory	Motility	Combined

Hypolactasia
Drugs (lactulose,
  magnesium
  salts)
Malabsorption
	Toxins:
	  E. coli
	  Vibrio cholerae
	  Staphylococcus aureus
	  Cl. perfringens
	Peptides: VIP
		Irritable bowel
		Drugs (senna,
		  phenolphthalein)
			Ulcerative colitis
			Coeliac disease

7   Small Intestine

7.1   Diarrhoea

Combined mechanisms
- Diarrhoea is frequently due to multiple factors
- The diarrhoea of ulcerative colitis, for example, is caused by disordered motility, decreased sodium absorption by inflamed epithelial cells, altered mucosal permeability, prostaglandin or short-chain fatty acid-induced changes in ion transport, decreased capacity of the rectal reservoir and loss of blood or mucus into the lumen

Clinical features

History
- Duration >3 weeks (or less in the very young, very old, dehydrated, or debilitated) needs investigation
- Morning diarrhoea is a feature of alcohol abuse and irritable bowel syndrome, but may indicate more serious pathology (such as inflammatory bowel disease)
- Night-time diarrhoea or weight loss favour an organic cause
- Blood (altered or fresh) indicates a colonic cause
- Fat globules in the pan after flushing suggests steatorrhoea
- Recent travel abroad (including USA, USSR, or Europe) suggests giardiasis
- Weight loss despite a good appetite is typical of thyrotoxicosis
- Undigested food, odour, abdominal cramps, bloating, flatulence and audible borborygmi are non-specific
- Always ask about drugs, alcohol intake, contacts, family history, arthritis, iritis and skin rashes (erythema nodosum, dermatitis herpetiformis)

Examination
- Look for dehydration, weight loss, skin rashes and abdominal surgical scars. Clubbing sometimes occurs in active Crohn's disease
- Feel for an enlarged thyroid or an abdominal mass, which indicates colonic carcinoma or Crohn's disease
- Rectal examination and sigmoidoscopy are essential

Initial investigations
For all patients with recurrent or persistent diarrhoea (>3 weeks), or for diarrhoea in the very young, very old, dehydrated, or debilitated.

7.1 Diarrhoea

Stool sample
• Microscopy for *Giardia lamblia* (other parasites and ova when from abroad), and cysts of *Cryptosporidium* if immunodeficient
• Culture for *Salmonella, Shigella, Campylobacter, Yersinia* spp.
• *Cl. difficile* toxin assay when antibiotics have been recently taken
• Electron microscopy (for viruses) only in children, or an epidemic

Sigmoidoscopy
• Record the distance reached, stool and mucosal appearance
• Always take a biopsy of any identifiable lesion and a representative area, because 10–20% patients with Crohn's disease have microscopic changes even when the mucosa looks normal, microscopic colitis will otherwise be missed, and histology provides an independent record of the sigmoidoscopic findings

Blood tests
• Microcytic anaemia suggests a carcinoma or inflammatory bowel disease
• Macrocytosis may be due to coeliac disease, distal ileal Crohn's disease, or alcohol
• A high ESR points to active inflammatory bowel disease, carcinoma or occasionally infective causes. If the ESR is normal, the C-reactive protein (CRP) should be measured if possible, because this can be elevated independently of the ESR. Both Crohn's disease and carcinoma, however, can occur with a normal ESR and CRP
• Low potassium (<3.5 mmol/l) occurs in severe diarrhoea. Laxative abuse, colonic villous adenoma, or very rarely a VIPoma may be the cause
• Albumin, immunoglobulins and thyroid function tests are best checked at the first or second visit, so that they are not overlooked

Barium enema
• If age >40 years
• If <40 years, carcinoma is unlikely. Irritable bowel syndrome is the most likely diagnosis if other tests are normal and infective causes excluded, so review after treatment (p. 321) is better than a barium enema

7.1 Diarrhoea

• A barium enema is indicated at any age if diarrhoea is severe, if blood is present in the stools, or if histology or blood tests are abnormal

Subsequent investigations
The following plan is recommended if the results of initial investigations do not establish a diagnosis and symptoms justify invasive investigation (Fig. 7.1).

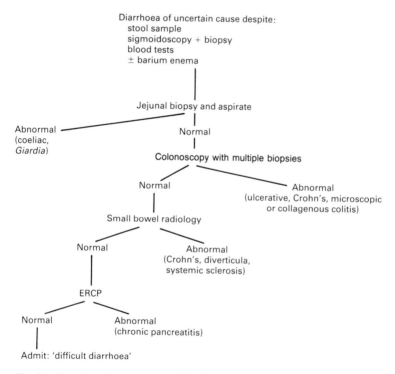

Fig. 7.1 Outpatient investigation of diarrhoea.

Difficult diarrhoea
If the cause of diarrhoea remains obscure after outpatient investigation (Fig. 7.1), then admission is usually necessary to distinguish between organic disease and a motility disorder (Fig. 7.2). Diarrhoea due to organic disease has a stool volume >200 ml/day,

which usually does not settle on admission. Functional diarrhoea (due to an irritable bowel) often disappears on admission and the stool weight is usually <200 g/day (volume <200 ml/day).

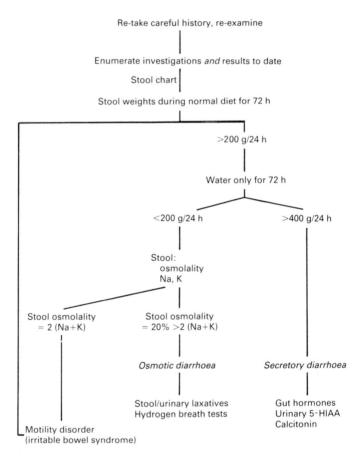

Fig. 7.2 Investigation of difficult diarrhoea.

General points
• Lactulose breath test is a non-invasive method of detecting bacterial overgrowth (p. 229). Breath hydrogen normally rises as the lactulose (or any carbohydrate load, including glucose) reaches the colon, but when lactulose is broken down by small intestinal bacteria this rise occurs <1 h after ingestion

• Lactose breath test is a non-invasive method of detecting lactase deficiency (p. 229). Hypolactasic subjects exhale more hydrogen than normal (>20 ppm) within 2 h of taking a lactose load. Subjects with normal lactase levels produce little or no hydrogen
• Xylose absorption is an unreliable screening test for carbohydrate malabsorption. Jejunal biopsy or double sugar tests (p. 365) are preferable
• Isotope scans (SeHCAT, p. 362) for bile salt malabsorption give less information about the terminal ileum than good small bowel radiology, or reflux of barium during a barium enema
• Stool should be examined for laxatives (addition of sodium hydroxide turns the stool red in the presence of phenolphthalein), and the urine for anthracene derivatives or senna alkaloids, if the diagnosis is obscure. Examination of the patient's bedside locker ('lockerotomy') is acceptable if laxative abuse is strongly suspected and there is no alternative

Management
The cause of diarrhoea should be identified and treated if possible.
• Oral rehydration solution (sodium chloride 3.5 g, sodium citrate 2.9 g, potassium chloride 1.5 g and glucose 20 g in 1 litre (WHO formula), or Dioralyte) is indicated for severe diarrhoea in the young or elderly
• Codeine phosphate 30–60 mg/day is the first choice when stool frequency needs to be controlled
• Loperamide 4 mg, then 2 mg after each loose stool can be used for acute gastroenteritis or motility disorders. Although drugs are best avoided if possible, there is no convincing evidence that clearance of intestinal pathogens is delayed. It should not be used in children, because fatal paralytic ileus has been reported
• Amitriptyline 25 mg at night is sometimes effective for motility disorders, because of anticholinergic effects
• Antibiotics are only indicated for a few, microbiologically confirmed, infections (*Giardia lamblia*, *Yersinia enterocolitica*, severe shigellosis, or bacterial overgrowth) (p. 327). Excretion of *Salmonella* sp. is prolonged by inappropriate antibiotics and increases the risk of a carrier state

Travellers' diarrhoea
Enterotoxigenic *E. coli* cause most acute, self-limiting episodes of diarrhoea in travellers (Table 7.3).

Table 7.3 Differential diagnosis of diarrhoea after foreign travel

Travellers' diarrhoea (enterotoxigenic *E. coli*)

*Giardia lamblia**

Infective diarrhoea:
  Salmonella sp.
  Shigella sp.[†]
  Campylobacter sp.[†]
  Yersinia enterocolitica
  E. coli 0157[†]
  rotavirus

Post-infective hypolactasia* (when drinking milk)

Latent disease revealed by infection*:
  ulcerative colitis[†]
  coeliac disease
  Crohn's disease
  ileocaecal tuberculosis

Other infections:
  *Strongyloides stercoralis**
  hepatitis A or B (community-acquired non-A, non-B)
  acute falciparum malaria
  Cryptosporidium sp.
  amoebic dysentery (*Entamoeba histolytica*)[†]
  fasciolopsiasis,* capillariasis,*
  Schistosomiasis,[†] enterobiasis,[†] trichuriasis[†]

Tropial sprue*

*Usually chronic diarrhoea.
[†] Often bloody diarrhoea.

- Incubation is 1–5 days
- Sudden onset of severe diarrhoea with abdominal pain is only serious in the young, debilitated, or elderly
- Resolution within 48–96 h is usual. <5% persist for more than 3 weeks and then need investigation to exclude underlying disease
- Symptomatic treatment (p. 213) is indicated and drugs avoided if possible. If the patient's job is affected and rapid control of symptoms needed, co-trimoxazole 2 tablets and loperamide 4 mg, taken once, followed by loperamide 2 mg after each loose motion, appears to be more effective than loperamide alone
- Preventive advice includes avoiding salads, uncooked vegetables, shellfish, ice cream and unsterilized water (including ice) in uncertain areas. Antibiotics are not recommended, although

sulphonamide combinations (co-trimoxazole 2 tablets twice daily) provide partial protection. Sulphonamides can produce sensitivity to sunlight
• Persistent diarrhoea may be due to post-dysenteric irritable bowel syndrome, persistent infection, hypolactasia or unmasked latent disease (Table 7.3), and is investigated in the same way as for other causes (p. 209 and Fig. 7.1, p. 211)

7.2   Malabsorption

Defective luminal digestion, mucosal disease or structural disorders are the mechanisms of malabsorption. Fat, carbohydrate, protein, vitamin or mineral malabsorption may predominate, but combined deficiency is usual except in metabolic defects.

Causes

Knowledge of the mechanism is more useful for deciding about investigations than for classifying causes (Table 7.4). More than one mechanism commonly operates; mucosal disease may be associated with defective digestion and sometimes with structural change as well.
• Hypoalbuminaemia and vitamin K or D deficiency in cirrhosis may be due to liver disease as well as malabsorption
• Crohn's disease may cause malabsorption from distal ileal disease (vitamin B_{12} and bile salts), mucosal disease, disaccharidase

Table 7.4 Causes of malabsorption

Common	Uncommon	Rare
Coeliac disease	Tropical sprue	Small bowel lymphoma
Chronic pancreatitis	Parasites (*Giardia lamblia*)	Lymphangiectasia
Cirrhosis	Bacterial overgrowth	Whipple's disease
Crohn's disease	Drugs	Thyrotoxicosis
Biliary obstruction	Short bowel	Zollinger–Ellison
Post-infective	Resection:	Metabolic defects
	gastric	Mesenteric ischaemia
	terminal ileal	Mastocytosis
	pancreatic	Amyloidosis
	Pancreatic cancer	HIV enteropathy
		α-chain disease
		Starvation

deficiency, enteroenteric fistulae, bacterial overgrowth, or a short bowel
- Other causes are discussed below

Clinical features

Diarrhoea
- Steatorrhoea is due to defective digestion of fat, resulting in malabsorption. Pancreatic exocrine insufficiency (p. 117) is the usual cause and severe steatorrhoea is rare in mucosal or structural disease. It is characterized by pale, bulky, malodorous motions, with oily globules in the pan after flushing
- Stool bulk is increased more than frequency, unlike the diarrhoea of colonic disease
- Malabsorption occasionally occurs without diarrhoea. Intestinal causes (coeliac disease, bacterial overgrowth) are then likely

Weight loss
- Weight loss occurs whatever the cause of malabsorption, but may be minimal during malabsorption of specific nutrients (such as vitamin B_{12} malabsorption from bacterial overgrowth)

General symptoms
- Lassitude, anorexia, abdominal bloating, discomfort and borborygmi may be inappropriately dismissed as an irritable bowel

Specific features (see Tables 13.2–13.4, pp. 373 and 374)
- Hypoalbuminaemia causes dependent oedema or, rarely, ascites
- Hypocalcaemia causes paraesthesiae and tetany if severe
- Vitamin deficiencies can cause cheilitis (riboflavin), glossitis (B_{12}), bruising (K), bone pain or myopathy (D), night blindness or xerophthalmia (A), dermatitis (niacin), neuropathy or psychological disturbance (thiamine or E)
- Mineral deficiencies can cause paraesthesiae or tetany (calcium), muscle weakness (calcium, magnesium), skin rashes, anaemia or leucopenia (zinc, copper). They are rare and often multiple

Investigations
Once malabsorption has been documented, the site and severity must be established.

7.2   Malabsorption

Documentation
• Stool sample for fat globules (rarely present except in
malabsorption), but often not detected
• 3-day faecal fat estimation is helpful if malabsorption cannot be
documented in other ways (>5 g/day (13 mmol/day) is abnormal
on a normal diet), although not popular with the laboratory. The
doctor must talk to the patient to ensure a proper collection.
Results are more accurate if expressed as a percentage of intake
over a 5-day collection (>7% of fat intake (>7 g on a 100-g fat diet)
is abnormal)
• ^{14}C triolein breath test (p. 368) is useful if available
• Full blood count, folate and vitamin B_{12} estimation (anaemia
and folate deficiency are common in mucosal disease and B_{12}
deficiency in terminal ileal disease or bacterial overgrowth)
• Prothrombin time or ratio (INR), may indicate vitamin K
deficiency and is also necessary before invasive tests (such as
jejunal biopsy)
• Albumin, calcium and alkaline phosphatase (hypoalbuminaemia
indicates severe malabsorption and osteomalacia causes
hypocalcaemia or an elevated ALP). Serum magnesium should be
measured if symptoms of hypocalcaemia respond slowly to
treatment, since it may be low (<0.7 mmol/1)
• The xylose test to assess carbohydrate absorption has a 25%
false-negative rate and is not recommended (p. 365). Enteric
protein loss can be documented by assessing faecal radioactivity
after intravenous ^{51}Cr-albumin injection. It is rarely necessary and
is best done at a specialist referral centre

Identify the site
Jejunal biopsy is the definitive investigation for mucosal lesions
and small bowel radiology for structural causes. Defective luminal
digestion may be confirmed by lactose breath test or mucosal
enzyme assay.
• Low duodenal biopsies at endoscopy are usually satisfactory for
detecting villous atrophy, but normal villi may appear flattened
over duodenal glands. Jejunal biopsy with a Crosby capsule,
steerable Meditech catheter, or multiple Quinton biopsy
instrument (p. 352), is indicated if endoscopic biopsies are not
definitive. Causes of villous atrophy are shown in Table 7.5
(p. 224)

• Aspiration of jejunal juice for *Giardia lamblia* and culture is advisable in any patient who has a jejunal biopsy. Swallowing a piece of string (whilst retaining the end!) and examination for parasites is not used in Britain, because jejunal biopsy is always necessary as well

• Small bowel radiology will usually identify distal ileal disease, diverticula, strictures, systemic sclerosis or tumours (Fig. 7.3). Small bowel enema demonstrates the mucosal pattern better than a barium meal and follow-through (p. 359). Flocculation, thickened folds and slight dilatation are all non-specific

• Lactose breath test is the most convenient non-invasive way of establishing hypolactasia, but it is usually simpler to document symptoms before and after stopping milk and milk products (p. 230) for a week. Enzyme assay is usually impracticable and unnecessary

• Ultrasound and then ERCP to detect chronic pancreatitis is indicated once mucosal and structural causes of malabsorption have been excluded

• Terminal ileal absorption can be assessed by ^{75}SeHCAT or $^{57/58}$CoB$_{12}$ isotope studies

Assess severity

• Document weight *and* height (Appendix 3) and laboratory evidence of malabsorption

• Other methods of nutritional assessment are rarely necessary in clinical practice (p. 371)

Coeliac disease

Coeliac disease (gluten-sensitive enteropathy) is defined as small intestinal villous atrophy (Fig. 7.4) which resolves when gluten is withdrawn from the diet. Gluten is a group of proteins derived from wheat, barley and rye but not oats, rice or maize; α-gliadin is the toxic moiety, but how it acts is unknown.

Distinguishing features

Coeliac disease may present at any age, but is most commonly diagnosed as failure to thrive in infancy, growth retardation in childhood, or nutritional deficiencies in adults.

• Symptoms of malabsorption may be provoked by infection, pregnancy or surgery

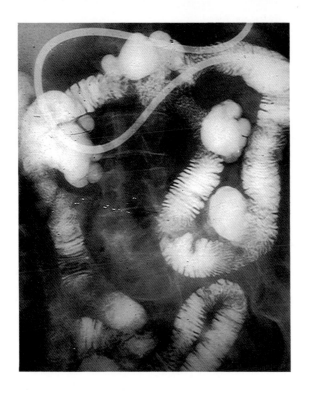

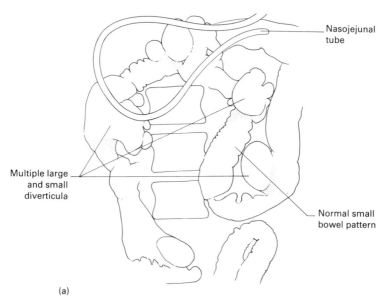

(a)

Nasojejunal
tube

Multiple large
and small
diverticula

Normal small
bowel pattern

Fig. 7.3 Small bowel radiology and malabsorption. (a) Small bowel enema showing multiple jejunal diverticula which caused malabsorption due to bacterial overgrowth.

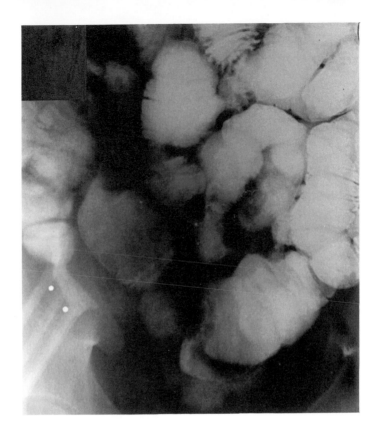

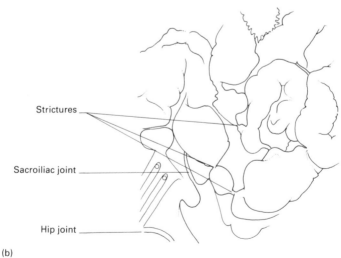

Strictures

Sacroiliac joint

Hip joint

(b)

Fig. 7.3 (*continued*) Small bowel radiology and malabsorption. (b) Small bowel study in a patient with malabsorption due to extensive Crohn's disease, causing multiple strictures.

7.2 Malabsorption

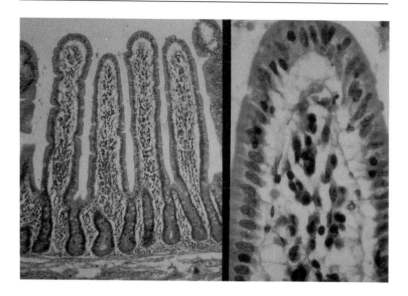

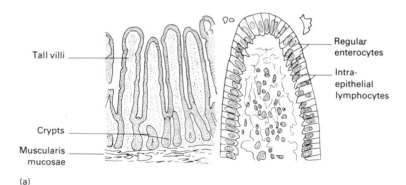

Tall villi

Crypts

Muscularis mucosae

Regular enterocytes

Intra-epithelial lymphocytes

(a)

Fig. 7.4 Histological features of coeliac disease. (a) Histological appearance of normal jejunal mucosa. Tall villi (left, × 70). The villus height : crypt depth ratio is at least 3:1. Tip of a villus showing a few intra-epithelial lymphocytes (right, × 320). H&E stain.

• Diarrhoea may be absent or intermittent and symptoms non-specific (lethargy, bloating, flatulence) for many years. Constipation may coexist with coeliac disease
• Aphthous ulcers are common, but clubbing is rare. Hyposplenism (Howell–Jolly bodies, target cells) may be detected on the blood film

221

7.2   Malabsorption

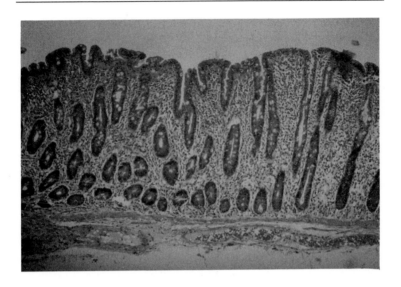

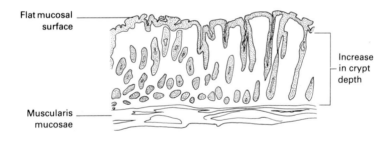

Flat mucosal surface

Increase in crypt depth

Muscularis mucosae

(b)

Fig. 7.4 (*continued*) Histological features of coeliac disease. (b) Subtotal villous atrophy showing total absence of villi and a corresponding increase in depth of the crypts, producing an apparently increased mucosal thickness. H&E stain, × 70.

- Refractory iron deficiency anaemia may be the only feature
- Isolated nutritional deficiencies (megaloblastic anaemia, myopathy and bone pain) may occur, especially in the elderly
- Examination may be normal (even well nourished), or reveal signs of nutritional deficiencies (p. 373) through to severe malabsorption

Associated disorders
• Dermatitis herpetiformis (intensely itchy vesicular papules on the elbows or buttocks)—up to 96% have villous atrophy and even those without villous atrophy respond to gluten withdrawal
• Autoimmune disease—diabetes, thyrotoxicosis, Addison's disease
• Arthritis—rheumatoid or seronegative arthritis are unusual associations
• Pericarditis, spinocerebellar degeneration, pancreatic insufficiency and liver disorders are very rare associations

Diagnosis in adults
• There is no alternative to jejunal biopsy and a second biopsy to document resolution of villous atrophy, after 3–6 months on a gluten-free diet. Clinical recovery after gluten withdrawal may be coincidental, if villous atrophy is due to a transient cause (such as *Giardia lamblia*, Table 7.5), and the implications of a lifetime gluten-free diet are considerable. Subsequent gluten challenge is unnecessary in adults
• Villous atrophy is occasionally patchy, which can cause diagnostic confusion, especially on low duodenal biopsies (p. 352)
• Immunoglobulins should be measured, since IgA deficiency (2%) predisposes to intestinal infections and hypogammaglobulinaemia itself can cause villous atrophy, which may respond to globulin infusion
• A high index of suspicion is justified for children of coeliac patients and other family members with gastrointestinal symptoms (5% risk of coeliac disease)

Other causes of villous atrophy
Subtotal villous atrophy is almost always due to coeliac disease in European adults. Partial villous atrophy has other (rare) causes (Table 7.5).

Complications
• Malignancy—small intestinal T-cell lymphoma develops in <5%. Other types of small intestinal lymphoma originate from B-cells. Small intestinal adenocarcinoma is also more common. Recrudescence of symptoms, abdominal pain or deterioration despite a gluten-free diet should suggest the diagnosis

7.2 Malabsorption

- Ulceration in the small intestine—rare, but may cause pain, persistent anaemia or bacterial overgrowth. A small bowel enema is diagnostic

Table 7.5 Other causes of villous atrophy

Giardia lamblia
Acute infectious enteritis:
viral
bacterial
Hypogammaglobulinaemia
Bacterial overgrowth
Tropical sprue
Cows' milk sensitivity
Soya protein sensitivity
Lymphoma
Whipple's disease
NSAIDs
Radiation
HIV enteropathy
Starvation

Management

- Gluten-free diet (p. 386) for life, with advice from a dietitian. There is now good evidence that this decreases the risk of small intestinal malignancy
- The Coeliac Society (Appendix 1) provides useful advice, food lists, recipe books, support and motivation for patients
- 85% respond, although histological resolution may take 3–12 months. It is advisable to repeat the jejunal biopsy after 3–6 months on a gluten-free diet, but a gluten challenge is not necessary in adults and rarely in children if symptoms resolve and growth recovers
- Iron and folate supplements are needed if anaemic, until recovery. Specific deficiencies may need treating (hypocalcaemia: effervescent calcium 6–12 tablets daily, but serum calcium must be checked monthly)
- Annual outpatient review is advisable when stable, to confirm adherence to the diet and detect complications. Relapse is most readily detected by full blood count and folate, if macrocytosis is present, followed by repeat jejunal biopsy

Poor responders

If there is no clinical or histological improvement after 3 months (less if the patient is unwell), the possibilities are:
- Failure to adhere meticulously to a gluten-free diet. This is also the most common cause of recurrent symptoms after an initial response
- Concomitant:
  hypolactasia (due to mucosal atrophy)
  infection (giardiasis, other parasites)
  endocrine disease (Addison's disease)
- Untreated nutritional deficiency:
  folate
  iron
  calcium
  magnesium
  others, less commonly
- Small intestinal lymphoma
- Ulcerative jejunitis
- Hypogammaglobulinaemia
- Reasons unknown

All, except poor dietary compliance, are unusual.

Management of poor responders
- Emphasize the importance of complete gluten exclusion and ask the dietitian to review dietary compliance carefully. Check that contact with the Coeliac Society has been established. Give support, encouragement and motivation
- Exclude dairy products (in case of secondary hypolactasia) and reassess in 4 weeks
- Check that *Giardia lamblia* has been looked for in jejunal juice, and that hypogammaglobulinaemia or nutritional deficiencies have been corrected. Give a single dose of tinidazole 2 g, even if *Giardia lamblia* has not been identified
- Arrange a small bowel enema to exclude Crohn's disease, diverticula, lymphoma or adenocarcinoma
- Start prednisolone 20 mg/day, but only after other causes of a poor response have been rigorously excluded
- Re-biopsy to assess response after 3 months on steroids. Some still do not respond and should be referred to a specialist centre

Prognosis
- Gluten sensitivity persists for life
- Childhood coeliacs often become quiescent as young adults, but symptoms or complications may develop later if the diet is not continued (p. 224)
- Life expectancy is normal on a gluten-free diet

Tropical sprue
Post-infective tropical malabsorption affects adults of any race who have lived in India, Asia, or Central America, but is rare in Africa. Tropical sprue is a disease of residents rather than visitors and seems to be increasingly uncommon. It usually follows an acute attack of diarrhoea. The cause of mucosal damage is uncertain (p. 332) although secondary bacterial overgrowth and hypolactasia commonly exacerbate the malabsorption.

Distinguishing features
- Malabsorption in a person who has recently lived in the tropics (rarely in the sub-tropics or several years previously)
- Persisting diarrhoea after an acute attack of gastroenteritis
- Typical features of malabsorption:
  steatorrhoea
  weight loss
  anorexia and lethargy
  oedema, anaemia, glossitis

Investigations
Diagnosis is established by a consistent history, macrocytic anaemia, partial villous atrophy and response to tetracycline. Other causes of tropical malabsorption should be considered (Table 7.6).
- Macrocytic anaemia is due to folate deficiency, although vitamin B_{12} may also be low due to bacterial colonization
- Hypoalbuminaemia is usual and occasionally the AST is elevated
- Jejunal biopsy usually reveals partial villous atrophy (total atrophy is rare), but unlike coeliac disease the changes are more severe in the terminal ileum. Jejunal juice should be examined for *Giardia lamblia*
- Stools should be examined for parasites

7.2 Malabsorption

- Small bowel radiology is non-specific, but helps exclude diseases such as tuberculosis. Xylose and Schilling tests are non-specific and unnecessary

Table 7.6 Differential diagnosis of malabsorption from abroad

Giardia lamblia
Tropical sprue
Hypolactasia
Small intestinal tuberculosis
Lymphoma (immunoproliferative small intestinal disease, IPSID)
Strongyloides stercoralis
Cryptosporidium sp.
Visceral leishmaniasis
Clonorchis sinensis cirrhosis
HIV enteropathy
Filariasis
Calcific chronic pancreatitis
Idiopathic

Management
- Tetracycline 250 mg four times daily for 4 weeks
- Folic acid 5 mg three times daily for 2 months
- Lactose-free diet (p. 387, for concomitant hypolactasia)

Giardiasis

The flagellated protozoan *Giardia lamblia* is a common cause of diarrhoea and malabsorption, which may be superimposed on coeliac disease, tropical sprue, or hypogammaglobulinaemia. Infection may also be asymptomatic.

Distinguishing features
- Incubation is 2–3 weeks
- Transmission is through contaminated water or faecal–oral route
- Travel abroad is *not* necessary to acquire infection, although it is more prevalent outside Britain, and in male homosexuals
- Persistent diarrhoea after an acute attack of 'gastroenteritis' may continue for months. Frank malabsorption is unusual unless there is an underlying cause (such as immunodeficiency)
- The diagnosis should always be suspected when a patient first presents with diarrhoea after travelling

Investigations
• Stool examination for cysts or trophozoites detects about 60%
• Jejunal aspiration and biopsy (to exclude other causes of persistent diarrhoea or malabsorption, Tables 7.1 and 7.6, pp. 208 and 227) is the most reliable method of diagnosis if no stool cysts are seen
• Measure immunoglobulins if *Giardia lamblia* is acquired in Britain, or if there is recurrent infection. Family and close contacts should also be checked for symptomatic or asymptomatic carriers
• Tinidazole (below) may be given before a jejunal biopsy if stool examination is negative, but only if the patient is going to be followed up and biopsy performed if there is an incomplete response

Management
• Tinidazole 2 g (single dose) is as effective as metronidazole 800 mg three times daily for 3 days
• Mepacrine 100 mg three times daily for 1 week is an alternative for the rare problem of resistant giardiasis. Re-infection or an underlying disease is a more common cause of persistent symptoms after treatment

Bacterial overgrowth
Bacterial contamination of the small intestine results in diarrhoea or typical features of malabsorption. An underlying cause (Table 7.7) is almost always present. Bacterial (anaerobes, *E. coli*

Table 7.7 Causes of bacterial overgrowth

Duodenojejunal diverticula
Post-surgical loops ('blind loop')
Obstruction:
Crohn's disease
tumour
radiation stricture
pseudo-obstruction
Fistulae
Hypogammaglobulinaemia
Tropical sprue
Systemic sclerosis
Autonomic neuropathy (diabetes, amyloid)
Anacidity (autoimmune, vagotomy, old age, drugs)

and *Klebsiella* sp.) deconjugate bile salts, metabolize vitamin B_{12} and carbohydrate, but folate and fat-soluble vitamins are not malabsorbed. Normal jejunal juice contains $<10^4$ Gram-positive organisms/ml.

Distinguishing features
• Diarrhoea or malabsorption in patients with a structural small intestinal abnormality, or when immunocompromised
• Onset of diarrhoea in patients with otherwise stable chronic disease (diabetes, systemic sclerosis, Crohn's disease)
• Malabsorption with a low vitamin B_{12} and normal (or elevated) folate

Investigations
• Small bowel radiology is the first investigation when the diagnosis is suspected, to look for diverticula or strictures (Fig. 7.3, p. 219)
• Hydrogen breath test after lactulose is non-invasive. Breath hydrogen >20 ppm in <2 h indicates bacterial overgrowth (p. 367). Urinary indican measurements are too unreliable to be useful
• Jejunal aspiration is convenient if a biopsy is being performed to exclude other causes of malabsorption (after normal small bowel radiology), but air insufflation may destroy anaerobes

Management
• Tetracycline 250 mg four times daily for 4 weeks, with metronidazole 400 mg three times daily for 2 weeks. Either drug is probably inadequate alone
• Replacement vitamin B_{12} (1000 µg intramuscularly for 5 days)
• Vancomycin 125 mg four times daily for 1 week is second-line therapy if tetracycline is ineffective
• Recurrent courses when symptoms relapse, or maintenance tetracyline 250 mg daily (not vancomycin, because of potential ototoxicity) are often necessary, because surgical correction of the cause is rarely possible

Disaccharidase deficiency

Hypolactasia
Hypolactasia is the only common small intestinal enzyme

deficiency. Alactasia is rare and presents in neonates. Hypolactasia is usually primary, because the enzyme disappears after weaning in most races except North Europeans. Secondary causes include any cause of mucosal damage (viral gastroenteritis, coeliac disease, giardiasis, Crohn's disease) and is reversible once the disease is treated. Cows' milk protein intolerance occurs in children (and may cause villous atrophy), but probably not in adults.

The clinical problem is milk intolerance, which may not be recognized by the patient. Lactose is normally split into galactose and glucose which are rapidly absorbed. Undigested lactose causes an osmotic diarrhoea and excessive flatulence from fermentation. The colon adapts to absorb excess intestinal fluid, so diarrhoea is variable. Diagnosis is confirmed by a 50 g lactose–hydrogen breath test; a rise of >20 ppm H_2 in <2 h is abnormal (p. 367).

Avoiding milk and liquid milk products (yoghurt) is effective (p. 387). Butter and hard cheese contain little lactose, so intake is not restricted.

Other deficiencies

Sucrase–isomaltase deficiency is a rare disorder of childhood and trehalase deficiency results in mushroom intolerance.

Adverse reactions to food

It is important to distinguish between food allergy, sensitivity, intolerance and preference.

Food allergy is immunological (IgE-mediated type I hypersensitivity) and uncommon. *Food sensitivity* best applies to an identifiable non-immunological effect in susceptible individuals, be it pharmacological (tyramine in cheese) or due to enzyme deficiency (hypolactasia). *Food intolerance* applies to reproducible effects of certain foods for undefined reasons (some patients with irritable bowel syndrome, p. 322). *Food preference* or fads are psychological and not a reproducible cause of symptoms on blind testing.

Very few patients who believe food to be the cause of their symptoms have true food allergy. Many apparently have food sensitivity, for reasons that cannot be defined scientifically at present. Psychological aversion to certain foods is the most common reason for symptoms.

Distinguishing features
• Acute hypersensitivity reactions are usually caused by egg, shellfish, nuts, tomatoes or food additives (commonly tartrazine or monosodium glutamate). Labial or pharyngeal oedema, urticaria, wheeze or anaphylaxis occur rapidly and the relationship is readily recognized by the patient
• Chronic reactions to cows' milk or soya protein are rare in adults, but may cause diarrhoea, vomiting, abdominal pain or steatorrhoea due to villous atrophy. The immunological mechanism is uncertain
• Associated atopy (eczema, hay fever, asthma) or drug allergy are clues to the diagnosis of food allergy
• Reproducible food sensitivity or intolerance are recognized by testing with an exclusion diet with the help of a dietitian (p. 390). Lack of reproducibility either means that food is not the cause of symptoms, or indicates a food fad

Investigations
• Document the relationship between exposure to the specific food and symptoms; a food diary (diet on one page, symptoms opposite) is helpful for chronic symptoms
• An exclusion diet of low allergenicity (p. 390) with planned reintroduction of common food allergens (dairy products, egg, fish, nuts, additives and colouring agents) is then appropriate
• Challenge tests, skin tests and radioallergosorbent tests (RAST) are of little value unless done by specialists
• Invasive investigation to exclude other causes of symptoms (small bowel radiology or jejunal biopsy) is only indicated if clinical suspicion of an organic cause is very strong. Partial villous atrophy is almost never due to protein sensitivity in adults

Management
• The specific food should be avoided, but subsequent intolerances are common. Foods to which there has been intolerance can often be gradually reintroduced after a few months, for reasons that are obscure
• Mebeverine 135 mg three times daily may help abdominal pain, or codeine phosphate 15–30 mg as needed can be prescribed for diarrhoea

Short bowel syndrome
Massive intestinal resection to <1 m of remaining small intestine

231

may be due to Crohn's disease, mesenteric infarction, trauma, or radiation injury. The result is diarrhoea and malnutrition, due to loss of fluid, electrolytes, fat, bile acids, vitamin B_{12} or other nutrients. In the acute phase, loss of fluid and electrolytes are most important (up to 6 l/day), but adaptation occurs over 2 years. Management of the chronic phase is shown in Table 7.8.

Preservation of the ileocaecal valve, some terminal ileum and some jejunum have the greatest beneficial effect on subsequent symptoms; some patients remain well on 30 cm total (18 cm jejunum, 12 cm terminal ileum).

• Chronic vitamin and trace element deficiency can develop insidiously. Unexplained skin rashes or non-specific symptoms (malaise, weakness, paraesthesiae) are very suggestive

• Parenteral Addamel (trace elements), Vitlipid N (fat-soluble vitamins) and Parentrovite (water-soluble vitamins) are then best given together (Tables 13.14 and 13.15, p. 392) because laboratory measurements are inexact and deficiencies usually multiple

Table 7.8 Management of chronic short bowel syndrome

Problem	Mechanism	Management
Diarrhoea	Bile salts decrease colonic Na/H_2O absorption	Cholestyramine 4–12 g daily
	Lack of absorptive capacity	Small frequent meals
	Hyperosmolar luminal contents	Avoid milk and sweet drinks
	Rapid transit	Anticholinergic (Lomotil 2–6 tablets/day)
	Fatty acids stimulate H_2O secretion	Low-fat diet
Malnutrition	Steatorrhoea (calorie wastage)	Low-fat diet
	Reduced absorptive capacity	Check folate, Zn, Ca Mg, every 3 months Medium chain triglyceride diet* Home parenteral feed*
	Terminal ileal resection	Vitamin B_{12} 1 mg injection every 3 months
Gallstones	Bile acid depletion	Cholecystectomy*
Renal stones	Chronic dehydration	3 l fluid/day
	Chronic salt depletion	Dioralyte 1 l/day*
	Hyperoxaluria	Low oxalate diet $CaCO_3$ 7.5 g/day*

* When other measures fail.

Other causes of malabsorption
- Post-infective malabsorption may occur after gastroenteritis from any cause—bacterial, viral, toxin (travellers' diarrhoea), or parasitic (*Giardia lamblia*). Hypolactasia is the usual reason
- Drug-induced causes include:
  neomycin
  cholestyramine
  liquid paraffin and irritant purgative abuse
  antacids (interfere with iron, antibiotic, or antimalarial
     absorption)
  alcohol
- Lymphangiectasia may be primary, or secondary to lymphoma, tuberculosis, severe right heart failure or filariasis. Protein leaks into the lumen ('protein-losing enteropathy') and chylous ascites (p. 152) may develop
- Whipple's disease is a rare condition, usually in middle-aged men, with malabsorption, arthritis, pigmentation and occasional neurological features. It is diagnosed by jejunal biopsy and cured by tetracycline for 1 year. Patients are best referred to a specialist centre
- Metabolic defects, except hypolactasia, are not acquired by adults. Aminoacidurias (cystinuria, Hartnup disease), chloridorrhoea and acrodermatitis enteropathica (zinc deficiency) occur in children
- HIV enteropathy is characterized by diarrhoea and partial villous atrophy without an identifiable cause (p. 343)
- Starvation causes partial villous atrophy, defective intestinal immunity and possibly calcific pancreatitis. Susceptibility to enteric infection is increased. Impaired digestion of nutrients influences refeeding (calorie intake should be increased gradually, with replacement of vitamins and minerals). Chronic illness and postoperative complications are the commonest cause of starvation in adults in Britain (p. 371)
- Small intestinal lymphoma, and IPSID or α-chain disease are discussed on p. 238

7.3 Diverticulosis
Small intestinal diverticula are asymptomatic, or result in stasis of intestinal contents, bacterial overgrowth and malabsorption (p. 228). Perforation, inflammation and haemorrhage are much less common than in colonic diverticula.

Duodenal diverticulum
• A single diverticulum is usually an incidental finding on a barium meal (about 2%), adjacent to or involving the papilla, and associated with gall stones. It is then a hazard to ERCP examination
• A diverticulum in the duodenal cap rarely follows ulceration
• Treatment is unnecessary unless complications occur. Surgery is appropriate for perforation, haemorrhage, or contamination due to stasis, but these are very unusual

Meckel's diverticulum
2% of the population have this embryological remnant in the terminal ileum, but <5% cause symptoms.

Haemorrhage
• More common than in other small intestinal diverticula, because 20% have heterotopic gastric or pancreatic tissue which can become inflamed
• Occult or frank rectal bleeding may occur, especially in the young (p. 19)
• Small bowel enema will show a diverticulum more reliably than a ^{99m}Tc pertechnate isotope scan, which detects heterotopic gastric mucosa, but still sometimes with difficulty

Diverticulitis and perforation
• Cannot be distinguished clinically from appendicitis. Immediate management is similar (p. 235), but the surgeon must look carefully for a Meckel's diverticulum if the appendix is normal

Other
• Bacterial overgrowth, intussusception and herniation (Littré's) are all very unusual

Multiple diverticula
• Jejunal diverticula are usually multiple, on the mesenteric margin
• Diarrhoea due to bacterial overgrowth is the commonest presentation (p. 228), but most are asymptomatic
• Small bowel radiology is diagnostic (Fig. 7.3(a), p. 219)

• Maintenance antibiotics (p. 229), or repeat courses when symptoms recur are indicated once bacterial overgrowth has occurred
• Angiography is necessary for obscure gastrointestinal bleeding in a patient with multiple diverticula, prior to surgery, but such patients are best referred to a specialist centre

7.4 Appendicitis

Appendicitis is usually due to obstruction and invasion by *E. coli* or anaerobes. Caecal carcinoma in the elderly, Crohn's disease, *Yersinia enterocolitica*, tuberculosis, carcinoid tumour, or *Enterobius vermicularis* infestation are other rare causes.

Clinical features

• Occurs at any age, but most commonly diagnosed in the young. Mortality is 25% when age >70 years
• The pattern of central abdominal pain, shifting to the right iliac fossa, with anorexia and vomiting is most common in adolescents
• Abdominal rigidity may be absent when the appendix is retrocaecal or pelvic, and in obese or elderly patients
• Rectal examination is essential in all cases of abdominal pain
• The pain is higher and more lateral in pregnancy, with a higher incidence of peritonitis
• Subacute obstruction may occur in the elderly
• An appendix mass may be confused with a caecal carcinoma, Crohn's disease, tuberculosis, or an ovarian tumour
• Clues to the differential diagnosis (Table 1.3, p. 19) include:
  recent sore throat (mesenteric adenitis)
  previous episode (Crohn's disease)
  weight loss (Crohn's disease, caecal carcinoma)
  dyspepsia (cholecystitis, perforated ulcer)
  arthralgia (*Yersinia enterocolitica*, Crohn's disease)
  vaginal discharge (salpingitis)
  mid-menstrual cycle (ruptured follicular cyst)
  frequency (urinary tract infection)
  preserved appetite (non-specific, or gynaecological)
  Asian origin (ileocaecal tuberculosis)

Management
• Metronidazole 1 g suppository, oral clear fluids and observation
for 8 h is reasonable if peritonism is absent and the diagnosis
uncertain
• Surgery is needed for acute abdominal pain with peritonism
• Metronidazole 1 g suppository should be given 1 h before and
8 h after operation
• A normal appendix is found in up to 30%. Mesenteric adenitis,
Yersinia enterocolitica ileitis, Crohn's disease, Meckel's
diverticulitis, tubo-ovarian and 'non-specific' causes (p. 31) should
then be considered

Conservative management
• Indicated for an appendix mass, or when the risk of operation is
too great (such as in a ship at sea)
• Intravenous fluids, metronidazole 500 mg, ampicillin 500 mg
and gentamicin 80 mg are given 8-hourly
• 30 ml water can be allowed every hour
• Careful charts of pulse and temperature, as well as regular
re-examination determine progress
• Surgery must be performed if peritonitis develops

Appendix mass and abscess
• A tender right iliac fossa mass may be palpable after 5 days'
untreated appendicitis. Pain and pyrexia resolve with bed rest
• Interval appendicectomy is indicated after 3 months. A small
bowel enema to exclude Crohn's disease is necessary before
operation, if the history is atypical in any way
• An appendix abscess is distinguished by a swinging pyrexia and
point tenderness on rectal examination. Ultrasound will identify
the site and surgical drainage is indicated forthwith

'Grumbling appendix'
Recurrent right iliac fossa pain has often been attributed to a
'grumbling appendix'. The diagnosis is doubtful. Repeated attacks
of appendicitis may occur, but the patient is well in between.
    Chronic pain with evidence of organic disease (weight loss,
elevated ESR) is usually due to Crohn's disease at any age, caecal
carcinoma in the elderly, or rarely lymphoma or tuberculosis.

Pain without signs or abnormal investigations is likely to be due to irritable bowel syndrome (p. 319), but a small bowel enema is still warranted if pain persists, to exclude more unusual causes.

7.5   Tumours

Polyps

Single

Isolated small intestinal polyps are rare and suggest malignancy (Table 7.9), although they may be benign. Secondaries from melanoma or lung should be considered. Symptoms are unusual, but bleeding or intussusception can occur. Surgical resection is indicated to establish the nature of a polyp if one is detected by small bowel radiology, but localization at operation is difficult without per-operative endoscopy.

Polyposis

Multiple polyps are more common (Table 7.9) than single polyps. They are usually lymphoid (nodular lymphoid hyperplasia, in the ileum or rectum of children, or associated with hypogammaglobulinaemia), non-neoplastic hamartomas (Peutz–Jegher's syndrome, associated with buccal or labial pigmentation and intussusception) and rarely adenomatous (Cronkite–Canada syndrome, associated with alopecia and nail dystrophy).

Table 7.9 Causes of small intestinal polyps

Single	Multiple
Adenocarcinoma	Nodular lymphoid hyperplasia
Carcinoid	Peutz–Jeghers syndrome (hamartomas)
Secondary deposit	Lymphomatous polyposis
Benign adenoma	Endometriosis
Lipoma	Cronkite–Canada syndrome (adenoma)
Leiomyoma	

Associated features are usually sufficient for diagnosis, although jejunal biopsy or laparotomy may be necessary to exclude lymphoma.

Lymphoma

Intestinal lymphoma is rare, but after the stomach (p. 95) is the most common extranodal origin of lymphoma. Mediterranean lymphoma (IPSID, or α-heavy chain disease) is discussed below.

Features

• Present with obstruction (70%), haemorrhage (50%), or perforation
• Associated with coeliac disease (<5% coeliacs, usually >50 years and following dietary non-compliance, pp. 223 and 225). These are T-cell lymphomas, as opposed to the more usual B-cell lymphomas
• Weight loss, non-specific symptoms or failure to respond to gluten withdrawal in coeliac disease are common. A mass may be palpable

Management

• Diagnosis is established by small bowel radiology (Fig. 7.5), followed by laparotomy. Lesions may be annular, ulcerating, multiple, or occasionally diffuse, or missed by contrast radiology. Lymphoma may occur anywhere in the bowel
• Staging (Table 3.3, p. 96) is performed by thoraco-abdominal CT scan, bone marrow and frozen-section biopsies at laparotomy
• Resection of annular lesions is often possible, but lymphoma in coeliac disease has a bad prognosis
• Postoperative chemotherapy is usually indicated and should be discussed with an oncologist
• Annual follow-up after treatment should include abdominal examination for a mass, blood count, ESR and small bowel radiology if intestinal symptoms recur

Immunoproliferative small intestinal disease (IPSID)

• IPSID is common in the Middle East (especially Iraq), but important to recognize in Europe because the early stage can be cured by antibiotics
• Mediterrranean lymphoma or α-heavy chain disease are synonyms. Only 70% excrete α-chains in the urine and IPSID has been reported in indigenous Europeans. Hypogammaglobulinaemia is commonly associated and nodular lymphoid hyperplasia in adults may be premalignant

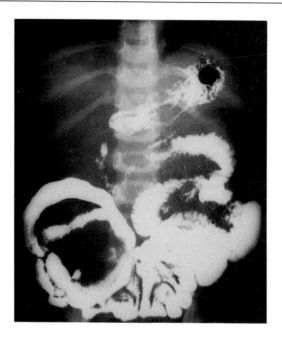

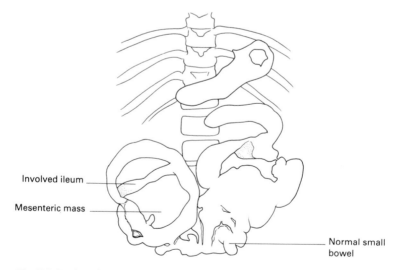

Fig. 7.5 Radiological features of small intestinal lymphoma. Small bowel lymphoma in a patient with coeliac disease giving rise to a large mesenteric mass in the right iliac fossa. This is displacing and compressing several ileal loops which show effacement of the fold pattern and nodular irregularity, indicating mucosal invasion.

- Lymphomatous polyposis, which is definitely malignant, is distinguished from IPSID histologically by normal intestinal mucosa between areas of lymphoid infiltration
- Diarrhoea, malabsorption, finger clubbing and weight loss in a young Middle Eastern adult are characteristic. Urine for α-chains, small bowel radiology and jejunal biopsy establish the diagnosis. Tetracycline 500 mg four times daily for 6 months is effective before extraintestinal spread occurs, but prognosis is poor after dissemination

Carcinoma

Small intestinal carcinoma is rare and usually of unknown cause. It is occasionally associated with coeliac disease, familial adenomatous polyposis (Gardener's syndrome), or Cronkite–Canada syndrome (p. 237).

- Obstruction or chronic blood loss are the usual presenting features. Other causes of a small intestinal stricture are shown in Table 7.10.

Table 7.10 Causes of small intestinal strictures

Crohn's disease
Adenocarcinoma
Lymphoma
Tuberculosis
Vasculitis
Secondary deposit
NSAIDs
Radiation
Surgical anastomosis
Yersinia enterocolitica

- Laparotomy is necessary, after small bowel radiology (Fig. 7.3(b), p. 219), for histological diagnosis and resection. Duodenal carcinomas are treated by pancreatoduodenectomy (Whipple's procedure).

8 Inflammatory Bowel Disease

8.1   Crohn's disease

Crohn's disease is characterized by chronic transmural granulomatous inflammation, with a tendency to form fistulae or strictures. It may affect any part of the gastrointestinal tract, often in discontinuity. The cause remains unknown.

General information

A few facts are helpful when explaining the disease to the patient:
- First recognized in 1932, but described earlier (1913, Dalziel)
- Affects 30–50 per 100 000 population
- 5 new cases/100 000/year in northern Europe, USA and Australia, but appears uncommon in other areas of the world
- Incidence has doubled since 1950, but may now be declining. It does not differ markedly between race, sex or social class in the UK
- Presents at any age, but usually 15–40 years. The site of disease and pattern of onset are unrelated to age
- 15% have a relative with Crohn's disease or ulcerative colitis (the same risk to children of an affected parent). Twins often have Crohn's disease together
- 4 times more common in smokers than non-smokers and possibly associated with oral contraceptive use
- Diet (high refined sugar), infective agents (atypical mycobacteria), mucins and altered cell-mediated immunity are postulated causes, but none explain disease discontinuity. Microvascular changes are probably secondary to inflammation
- At least half the patients have periods of remission lasting 5 years

Clinical features

The site of disease influences the presentation. Exacerbations of existing disease produce similar features that may be due to active inflammation, infection, or other complication.

The commonest site at presentation is the terminal ileum and proximal colon (40%), and equal numbers of the remainder have either small intestinal or colonic disease alone.

All sites

- Three symptoms occur in most patients: diarrhoea, abdominal pain and weight loss

---

• Acute abdominal pain may be confused initially with appendicitis
or yersinial ileitis (Table 1.3, p. 19), but a careful history usually
detects previous episodes that have not been recognized
• Fever, malaise, anorexia and lassitude are usual in active disease
• Weight loss alone, without diarrhoea or pain, may be the
presenting feature and may be confused with anorexia nervosa in
adolescents

Small intestinal disease
• Aphthous ulcers are common with active disease, but true
oropharyngeal Crohn's ulcers are rare
• Duodenal ulcers that are postbulbar, difficult to heal, or
associated with a high ESR may be due to Crohn's disease,
although they are exceptionally rare
• Colicky abdominal pain without systemic illness or local
tenderness suggests a fibrotic stricture
• Abdominal pain may also be due to biliary colic or renal calculi
• Malnutrition is usually due to anorexia
• Malabsorption is rare except in extensive small intestinal disease,
or after resection. More than 80 cm distal ileum must be diseased
or resected before vitamin B_{12} malabsorption occurs
• An abdominal mass is frequently palpable in small intestinal
disease, often in the right iliac fossa, but can be anywhere

Colonic disease (Crohn's colitis)
• Severe diarrhoea is more common than in small intestinal disease
• The rectum is usually spared, although perianal disease is
common and can be very difficult to treat (p. 261)
• Extraintestinal manifestations (Table 8.1) are more common than
in small intestinal disease
• Rectal bleeding is uncommon compared to ulcerative colitis, but
profuse haemorrhage is a very rare complication. Bleeding may
indicate a colonic carcinoma in chronic Crohn's colitis, but this is
rare
• Toxic dilatation is also much less common than in ulcerative
colitis, but may be the presenting feature (p. 36)

Perianal disease
• Associated with ileocolonic disease, less common in isolated
small intestinal involvement

8.1   Crohn's disease

• Recurrent abscesses, fistulae and violaceous fleshy skin tags, with or without ulceration, are characteristic. Pain and systemic illness are surprisingly rare
• Anal or rectal stenosis may cause constipation and spurious diarrhoea

Extra-intestinal manifestations

Occur in about 15%, but up to 30% in colonic disease. Some are markers of active disease and respond to treatment, others are unrelated to disease activity (Table 8.1). Differences from ulcerative colitis are discussed on p. 265 (Table 8.7).
• Sacroiliitis is unrelated to HLA B27, unlike ankylosing spondylitis
• Fatty liver is common in sick patients and non-specific
• Renal calculi are more commonly due to chronic dehydration and salt depletion than hyperoxaluria
• Nutritional deficiencies may account for obscure symptoms (p. 391), including weakness (vitamin D, potassium, magnesium), lassitude (iron, vitamin B_{12}, folate), rashes (niacin, zinc), or altered

Table 8.1 Extra-intestinal manifestations of Crohn's disease

	Common (5–20%)	Unusual (<5%)

Related to activity	Aphthous ulcers
	Erythema nodosum
	Finger clubbing
	Ocular:
	  conjuctivitis
	  episcleritis
	  iritis
	Arthritis (large joint)
		Pyoderma gangrenosum

Unrelated to activity	Gall stones
	Sacroiliitis
		Liver disease:
		  fatty
		  primary sclerosing
		  cholangitis
		Ankylosing spondylitis
		Renal:
		  stones
		  ureteric stricture
		  right hydronephrosis
		  nephropathy (oxalate, amyloid)
		Osteomalacia
		Nutritional deficiency
		Systemic amyloidosis

taste (zinc), but only occur in very extensive disease or after major resection

Investigations
Diagnosis depends on clinical and radiological features, but should if possible be confirmed by biopsy, since there is no specific diagnostic test. All patients should have the tests listed below, even if the diagnosis seems certain.

Establishing the diagnosis
- Sigmoidoscopy and rectal biopsy:
  even when the mucosa is macroscopically normal (up to 20% have microscopic granulomas)
- Small bowel radiology (p. 359):
  performed first if diarrhoea, pain and weight loss are the presenting features. A barium enema should subsequently be arranged to exclude Crohn's colitis (Fig. 8.1, Table 8.2).
- Barium enema:
  colonoscopy is preferable if there is rectal bleeding, but a barium enema is usually more readily available and may be combined with flexible sigmoidoscopy. Complete small bowel radiology is then advisable, even if the terminal ileum has been demonstrated by reflux of barium
- Blood tests:
  anaemia is common, usually due to iron deficiency rather than vitamin B_{12} or folate deficiency
  elevated ESR or platelet count and a low albumin in a patient with recurrent abdominal pain and weight loss is usually due to Crohn's disease

Table 8.2 Summary of radiological features of Crohn's disease

General	Structural	Mucosal
Rectal sparing	Strictures	Aphthoid ulcers
Discontinuity	Fistula	Rose-thorn ulcers
	Asymmetrical disease	Linear ulcers
	Dilatation	Thickened valvulae
	Pseudodiverticula	Cobblestoning
	Caecal distortion	Pseudopolyps
	Mass effect	

8.1 Crohn's disease

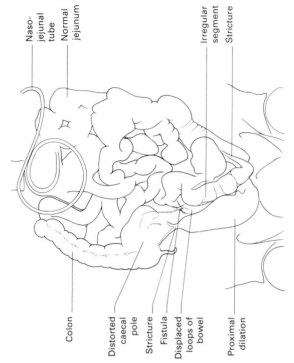

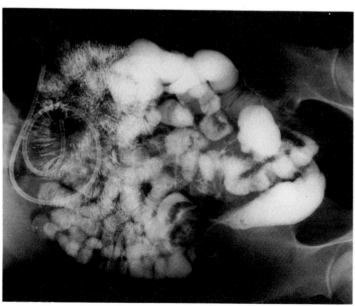

(a)

Fig. 8.1 Radiological appearance of Crohn's disease (*continued overleaf*). (a) Small bowel enema in distal ileal Crohn's disease, showing dilatation of the ileum proximal to a stricture, displaced loops of bowel due to a mass, a distorted caecum and a fistula.

Labels: Naso-jejunal tube, Normal jejunum, Irregular segment, Stricture, Colon, Distorted caecal pole, Stricture, Fistula, Displaced loops of bowel, Proximal dilation

8.1   Crohn's disease

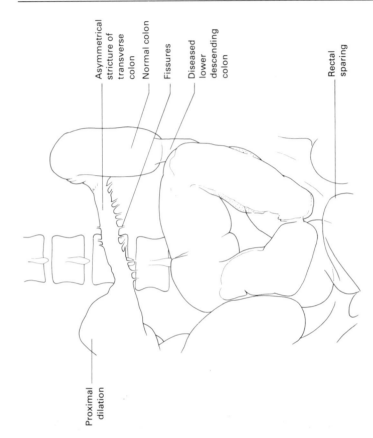

Asymmetrical stricture of transverse colon

Normal colon

Fissures

Diseased lower descending colon

Rectal sparing

Proximal dilation

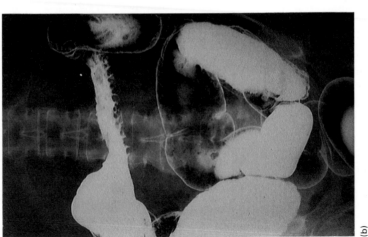

(b)

Fig. 8.1 (*continued*) Radiological appearance of Crohn's disease. (b) Barium enema in Crohn's colitis showing disease in two sites and rectal sparing.

antibodies to *Yersinia enterocolitica* are indicated when terminal
ileal disease is diagnosed at laparotomy for suspected
appendicitis
* Stool:
examination for pathogens and *Cl. difficile* toxin assay if
diarrhoea is severe
* Biopsy:
any inflamed tissue, or rectum even if uninflamed. Granulomata
are characteristic, but a chronic inflammatory infiltrate is more
common. Goblet cells are usually preserved (Table 8.10, p. 269)
* Colonoscopy with multiple biopsies is indicated if the barium
enema is equivocal, to assess strictures, colonic polyps and to
biopsy the terminal ileum if possible
* Laparotomy is occasionally necessary to distinguish Crohn's
disease from other causes of a small bowel stricture (Table 7.10,
p. 240), including malignancy. Resection or stricture plasty will also
be therapeutic

Assessing activity
Once the diagnosis has been made it is necessary to establish
whether symptoms are due to active disease or complications.
Assessment of disease activity is often difficult, because symptoms
(such as diarrhoea or abdominal pain) may be due to conditions
other than active disease (Table 8.5, p. 260). A combination of
clinical, blood and imaging tests is needed, as no one test is sufficient.
* Clinical:
anorexia, malaise, fever, tachycardia and weight loss indicate
active disease
severe disease may be present without all these features and
superimposed infection can mimic any of them
* Blood tests:
low serum albumin or anaemia, a high ESR, C-reactive protein
(CRP) or platelet count all indicate active disease
* Radiology:
ulcers (aphthous, rose-thorn, or linear), fistulae, or disease at a
new site, on small or large bowel radiology, suggest activity
* Endoscopy:
visible ulcers or histological evidence of acute inflammation on
biopsies are specific indicators of activity, but the site of active
disease (small intestine) may be inaccessible
* Ultrasound of the abdomen is valuable in experienced hands. It

can demonstrate thickened bowel loops, an inflammatory mass or an abscess
* ^{111}In-labelled leucocyte scanning helps differentiate active disease from a fibrotic stricture and may locate an abscess, but may not be available locally
* Crohn's Disease Activity Index, or the Dutch Activity Index, are useful for coordinating clinical trials, but of less value for assessing individual patients

Investigation of recurrent symptoms
Recurrent symptoms may have to be investigated as above, to detect active disease or disease at a new site, but the reasons for re-investigation must be clearly formulated. They should be relevant to subsequent therapeutic strategies, rather than to document the extent of disease for its own sake. Crohn's disease is a chronic condition and therefore patients will have numerous investigations over the years.

Contrast radiology should be limited to investigation of symptoms of subacute intestinal obstruction that do not resolve rapidly with treatment, or of complications (fistulae), when surgery may be indicated. Endoscopy is appropriate for colonic or upper gastrointestinal symptoms.

If symptoms do not follow the previous pattern of disease, consider other causes and arrange:
* MSU—for ureteric or renal involvement
* Plain abdominal X-ray—for subacute obstruction or stones
* Ultrasound—for gall stones, nephrolithiasis or hydronephrosis
* Lactulose–hydrogen breath test—for bacterial overgrowth (p. 229)

Differential diagnosis
As much care must be taken not to label a patient inappropriately as having Crohn's disease, as not to overlook the diagnosis in the first place. Features are diverse and the clinical alternatives are many, but only a few cause real difficulty (Table 8.3). Do not forget that other diseases can also develop after a diagnosis of Crohn's disease has been made.

Weight loss as the sole symptom
* May be inappropriately attributed to anorexia nervosa in an adolescent. Anaemia, a high ESR or platelet count strongly suggest Crohn's disease

8.1 Crohn's disease

Table 8.3 Differential diagnosis of Crohn's disease: site of disease

Site	Condition	Differentiating features
Duodenal	Tuberculosis	Biopsy persistent ulcers, chest X-ray
	Sarcoidosis	Chest X-ray, serum ACE*, Kveim test
Jejuno-ileal	Tuberculosis	Asian/African patients, Mantoux test Laparotomy
	Lymphoma	Smooth stricture(s). Laparotomy
	Adenocarcinoma	Single or multiple strictures (p. 240)
	Yersinia enterocolitica	Acute ileitis. Yersinial antibodies
	Behçet's disease	Aphthous ileal and orogenital ulcers
	Coeliac disease	Ulcerative jejunitis may occur (p. 225)
	NSAID stricture	History of slow-release NSAID ingestion, with no systemic illness
Colonic	Ulcerative colitis	(Table 8.10, p. 269)
	Ischaemic colitis	(Table 9.4, p. 309)
	Carcinoma	Shouldered stricture(s). Biopsy
	Infective colitis	Stool samples, biopsy (p.269)
	Schistosomiasis	Japanese/Middle Eastern patients. Cyst excretion, biopsy
	Radiation	History of pelvic malignancy, biopsy
	Solitary rectal ulcer	Constipation, anterior position, biopsy, no systemic illness

*ACE: angiotensin-converting enzyme.

• In older patients, gastrointestinal malignancy (pancreas, gastric carcinoma, or lymphoma) must be considered. Gastroscopy and ultrasound are indicated before small bowel radiology
• Diabetes can cause weight loss and recurrent perianal sepsis

Abdominal pain
• Symptoms resembling the irritable bowel syndrome (p. 319) with weight loss or anaemia are indications for further investigation
• Gall stones may coexist with Crohn's disease

Diarrhoea
• Ulcerative colitis, pseudomembranous, infective or ischaemic colitis (Table 9.4, p. 309) are distinguished by biopsy and stool culture, which must be repeated in cases of doubt
• Isolated diarrhoea that remains undiagnosed after colonic investigation is an indication for small bowel radiology, then jejunal biopsy and aspirate (Fig. 7.1, p. 211)

Right iliac fossa mass
- Caecal carcinoma is more common than Crohn's in the elderly
- Appendix abscess or ileocaecal tuberculosis occur at any age. Tuberculosis, amoeboma, or actinomycosis should be considered in Asian, African or South American patients. Ultrasound and serology help, but laparotomy may be necessary. The surgeon needs as much information as possible before operating

Rectal and perianal ulceration
- Carcinoma, lymphogranuloma venereum, syphilis, Behçet's disease, herpes simplex, cytomegalovirus or tuberculosis are less common causes than Crohn's disease. Biopsy and serology are usually diagnostic

Disease at other sites
Radiology resolves most of the dilemmas, but other conditions occasionally mimic the radiological appearances of Crohn's disease (Table 8.3, p. 251).

Management principles

General
- A confident and consistent approach, attention to nutrition, medical treatment of active disease and surgical management of complications are the principles of management
- Close liaison between medical and surgical teams is essential for optimal management of functional and structural problems (Table 8.4)
- Crohn's disease is only treated if there are symptoms; treat the patient, not the X-ray

Approach
- Explain that although the cause is unknown, inflammation and infection can be treated effectively. General information (p. 243) is often helpful for the patient
- Availability to deal with recurrent problems is reassuring. The patient should have a telephone number to call, either the medical secretary for an appointment, or an experienced nurse
- Patients should be seen and followed up by an experienced gastroenterologist, who can avoid unnecessary investigations and provide continuity

8 Inflammatory Bowel Disease

8.1 Crohn's disease

- Cautious optimism is advisable
- Patients may benefit from contact with the National Association for Colitis and Crohn's Disease (NACC, Appendix 1). Useful information leaflets are also available from the British Digestive Foundation (Appendix 1)

Nutrition

Most patients can eat anything. Patients should avoid foods that upset them and try to eat a balanced diet. A special diet is occasionally needed (Table 8.4). Many patients find that avoiding vegetables and other foods high in fibre mitigates abdominal pain during an acute episode, especially if there is small intestinal disease.
- Nutrition is especially important in children and adolescents, to maintain adequate growth
- Parenteral feeding or an elemental diet might be beneficial in active disease, but are not a substitute for steroids
- There is no evidence that decreasing sugar intake alters the pattern of disease, although a high sugar intake has been implicated in the aetiology (p. 243)

Table 8.4 Indications for special diets in Crohn's disease

Situation	Diet
Small intestinal stricture	Low-residue diet (p. 387)
Persistent diarrhoea without active disease	Try a lactose-free diet (p. 387), but see also p. 260
Malnourishment: during active disease perioperatively jejunoileostomy short (<100 cm) bowel	Enteral supplements (p. 376) Parenteral nutrition, central, or peripheral (p. 379) Dioralyte for excess fluid loss (p. 213) Enteral or parenteral nutrition (p. 231)
Steatorrhoea	Low-fat diet (p. 388)
Active disease unresponsive to steroids	Elemental diet (p. 377), but see also p. 256
Specific deficiencies	Iron, folate, fat-soluble vitamins, zinc (Table 13.14, p. 392)

Medical management

Severity can be difficult to assess. All symptoms should be taken seriously. The differentiation between severe and mild attacks is not as clear as in ulcerative colitis (p. 264).

8.1   Crohn's disease

Basic investigations for any acute episode include a full blood count, ESR, CRP (if available), albumin, electrolytes and stool sample for pathogens (p. 249). A plain abdominal X-ray is also indicated in severe attacks (to look for large or small bowel dilatation) and contrast radiology is advisable before surgical intervention.

Severe attacks
• Patients look ill, with severe symptoms, vomiting, fever >38 °C, tachycardia >90 bpm, or laboratory evidence (albumin <35 g/dl, high ESR, leucocytosis) of inflammation or infection. These features are indications for admission to hospital
• Intravenous fluids and replacement of electrolytes (especially potassium) are important. The patient may be dehydrated
• Intravenous hydrocortisone 100 mg four times daily is started
• Metronidazole 500 mg three times daily, orally if possible, can be useful, because there is often associated infection which may be impossible to distinguish from inflammation. It may also have a specific effect
• Blood transfusion may be needed to bring the haemoglobin up to 10 g/dl
• Fluids are allowed by mouth, but no food. It is uncertain whether avoiding food is of specific value, but patients are often anorexic and symptoms may be exacerbated by food
• Intravenous hydrocortisone and fluids are continued for 5 days, then feeding restarted, with oral prednisolone 40 mg/day
• Response should be monitored by symptoms (bowel frequency, pain, anorexia), examination (abdominal tenderness, fever, tachycardia) and blood tests (daily full blood count, ESR, CRP, albumin, electrolytes)
• Deterioration during intravenous treatment suggests a complication, or disease that is not going to respond to medical treatment, and is usually an indication for surgery (p. 256). Deterioration once feeding is restarted has similar implications
• Further investigations (p. 254) can be arranged when the patient is stable
• Once appetite returns and abdominal tenderness resolves, the patient can be discharged home, with an outpatient appointment for 2 weeks' time. The weight on discharge should be recorded
• Prednisolone is decreased to 20 mg/day over 2 weeks, then continued at 20 mg for 1 month, before decreasing by

5 mg/2–4 weeks. More rapid reduction can provoke early relapse, but the aim must always be to stop steroids during remission. Some patients are very sensitive to minor changes in steroid dosage and the minimum dose needed to control symptoms in these patients should be established

Mild attacks

• Patients are symptomatic and uncomfortable, often with abdominal tenderness and an elevated ESR or CRP. Vomiting, fever or a low albumin usually indicate a severe attack (p. 254)
• Outpatient treatment is reasonable
• Prescribe prednisolone 30 mg/day for a week, then 20 mg/day for 1 month. A low-residue diet is advisable if colicky pain is persistent
• Prednisolone can then be decreased slowly if symptoms have resolved, by 5 mg/2–4 weeks
• Response should be regularly assessed in outpatients (every 2–4 weeks, or less during the early stages). Symptoms, examination and blood tests (full blood count, ESR, CRP, albumin) are the guide. It is usually unwise to stop steroids until all have returned to normal
• Maintenance therapy is not indicated, but there is a group of patients in whom complete steroid withdrawal is difficult (p. 261)

Alternatives to steroids

• Sulphasalazine 2 g/day should be tried with steroids for Crohn's colitis, but the response is variable. Maintenance sulphasalazine might be beneficial and does no harm if tolerated. There is no evidence that it benefits small intestinal disease
• Mesalazine 1200 mg/day, or olsalazine 1000 mg/day may be alternatives to sulphasalazine, but the results of trials of these newer drugs (in active small and large bowel Crohn's disease) are awaited and their precise role is still being evaluated
• Azathioprine (2–2.5 mg/kg/day) is indicated as a steroid-sparing agent for patients with side effects from steroids, or for those who relapse rapidly when steroids are reduced. It is ineffective alone for active disease and takes about 1 month to have an effect. Duration of treatment is empirical; if there is a response then it should probably be continued for several months and full blood count monitored every 4–6 weeks

• Metronidazole 400 mg three times daily is indicated with steroids for perianal disease, or when infection coexists with active disease (see below). Ciprofloxacin 500 mg twice daily may give additional benefit

• Cyclosporin (5–10 mg/kg/day) is under trial, but recent reports are not very encouraging. It should not be used outside specialist centres

• An elemental diet (p. 377) can be used as an adjunct to steroids for extensive small intestinal, perianal, or steroid-resistant disease. The solution is often poorly tolerated because it is unpalatable, but it can be infused through a fine bore nasogastric tube. Whilst it may relieve pain from intestinal strictures, surgery is usually indicated

Outpatient review in Crohn's disease
Routine follow-up of patients (every 3–6 months) aims to detect early recurrence or complications and to monitor long-term therapy.

Documentation that is needed for each patient is most helpfully recorded on a special card at the front of the notes (Appendix 4):
• Date of onset of symptoms
• Site and extent of disease
• Presence or absence of positive histology
• Date of last small bowel/colonic examination
• Chronology of operations and complications
At each review:
• Ask about present symptoms and extra-intestinal manifestations
• Record weight and abdominal signs
• Check full blood count and liver function every 6 months, even if asymptomatic, to detect subclinical nutritional deficiency
• Explain the importance of early review if symptoms recur

Indications for surgery
70–80% of patients have an operation at some stage. The decision to operate depends on the degree of disability caused by the symptoms.

Major indications
• Symptomatic disease despite medical therapy

- Intestinal obstruction (subacute or acute) from strictures
- Local complications:
fistulae
abscess
perforation

Principles
- Limited resection of the most diseased area by an experienced surgeon
- Avoid bypass surgery; recurrence is common. End-to-end anastomosis is always preferable
- Staged procedures for sick patients with colonic disease (ileostomy, then resection of the diseased area, then restoration of continuity for example) are now performed less commonly because of better supportive care, including parenteral nutrition
- Perioperative corticosteroids are indicated for all patients, including elective procedures during remission, to reduce postoperative relapse. Give intravenous hydrocortisone 100 mg twice daily whilst nil by mouth, then prednisolone 20 mg/day decreasing by 5 mg/week

Special situations
- Strictureplasty is preferable for small intestinal strictures, since it avoids resection and anastomosis
- Limited resection (rather than a right hemicolectomy) is appropriate for ascending colonic or terminal ileal disease
- Localized transverse or distal colonic disease with a stricture or fistula may first be resected, but the relapse rate is fairly high and more extensive disease that needs surgery is best treated by proctocolectomy, which has a lower relapse rate. Pouch formation is absolutely contraindicated
- Split ileostomy and hydrocortisone 100 mg in 100 ml instilled into the distal limb daily may heal resistant colonic or perianal disease. Continuity can be restored after 18 months and a permanent ileostomy avoided
- Local surgery should be avoided for perianal fistulae, ulcers or haemorrhoids, because symptoms are usually few and recurrence common

Complications

Small intestinal obstruction
Diagnostic investigations: plain abdominal X-ray, markers of activity and cautious small bowel radiology.
• Usually due to active disease, but may be caused by bolus obstruction at a fibrotic stricture
• Chronic symptoms with few signs of active disease suggest fibrosis
• Radiographic intestinal diameter correlates poorly with symptoms

Toxic dilatation (p. 36)
Diagnostic investigations: temperature >38°C, colonic diameter >6.0 cm on plain X-ray (Fig. 1.3, p. 37, repeated daily), stool culture for pathogens and *Cl. difficile* toxin and blood cultures
• Much less common than in ulcerative colitis

Abdominal, pelvic or ischiorectal abscess
Diagnostic investigations: temperature chart, white cell count, ultrasound and culture of pus after aspiration. ^{111}In-labelled leucocyte scan or gallium scan are sometimes helpful, but may not be locally available
• Surgery is necessary to drain the abscess before antibiotics (intravenous cefuroxime 750 mg and metronidazole 500 mg three times daily for 1 week) can be effective. Steroids are also indicated (oral for ischiorectal, intravenous for abdominal abscesses) to suppress active Crohn's disease

Fistulae
Diagnostic investigation: contrast radiology, preferably when disease is quiescent.
• Perianal fistulae produce a discharge and may interfere with anal sphincter function (faecal soiling) or produce a stricture (palpable on rectal examination). Treatment is only indicated for symptoms (p. 261). A sinogram is not indicated unless surgery is considered
• Vesicocolic or vaginal fistulae (causing pneumaturia or faecal vaginal discharge) usually connect with the terminal ileum. Small bowel radiology is indicated before surgery. Rectovaginal fistulae often heal spontaneously

---

• Enterocutaneous fistulae follow surgery. Antibiotics, steroids and nutritional supplements allow a minority to heal spontaneously, but surgical resection of the fistulous track and connecting bowel is usually needed. The anatomy must be clearly defined by sinograms, small and large bowel radiology before surgery
• Enterocolic or entero-enteric fistulae cause profound weight loss, often, but not always, with diarrhoea. Steroids (prednisolone 40 mg/day), metronidazole 400 mg three times daily and an elemental diet or parenteral nutrition should be tried for 1 month or more, before considering surgery

Perforation
Diagnostic investigations: plain abdominal and erect chest X-rays
• Rarely presents acutely because an abscess cavity often forms, although features may be suppressed by steroids
• Surgery is indicated if perforation is detected

Massive rectal bleeding
Diagnostic investigations: clinical evidence, full blood count, prothrombin time.
• Rare in colonic disease (1%) and very rare in terminal ileal disease
• Transfusion alone is almost always sufficient. Colonoscopy is indicated after the bleeding stops
• Surgery for persistent bleeding (>8 units transfused) may be preceded by angiography if the distribution of colonic disease is unknown

Carcinoma
Diagnostic investigations: colonoscopy, biopsy
• Occurs in <5% patients with colonic disease. Diagnosis is often too late for a curative colectomy
• New symptoms, such as rectal bleeding without signs of active disease, are an indication for colonoscopy
• Small intestinal carcinoma is very rarely associated (p. 240)

Extra-intestinal complications (see Table 8.1, p. 245)

Management problems
Recurrent symptoms are not always due to active disease. The ESR, CRP and platelet count are usually elevated and the albumin

low ('inflammatory markers') when inflammation or infection are present.

Persistent abdominal pain (Table 8.5)
• Urine examination is always necessary, to look for haematuria (calculi), proteinuria (infection or inflammation) and for culture
• A plain abdominal film may show fluid levels, dilated bowel, loops separated by a mass, or calcified calculi
• Ultrasound of a mass, to look for an abscess cavity, inflammatory mass, thickened bowel loops or calculi is advisable before repeat small bowel radiology, because it is less invasive. Intestinal gas may obscure views

Table 8.5 Causes of abdominal pain in Crohn's disease

Inflammatory markers present	Inflammatory markers absent
Active Crohn's disease:	Stricture:
small intestinal	small intestinal
colonic	colonic
Abscess	Biliary colic
Pyelonephritis	Renal colic
Cholecystitis	Adhesions
	Steroid-induced peptic ulcers
	Other disease—ovarian, pelvic

Persistent diarrhoea
• Diarrhoea due to distal ileal disease or resection responds to cholestyramine 4 g 1–3 times daily
• Avoiding milk helps patients with hypolactasia
• Small bowel bacterial overgrowth is diagnosed by a lactulose–hydrogen breath test (p. 229), except after ileocolonic resection or entero-enteric fistula, when jejunal aspiration is more reliable. It is treated with tetracycline 250 mg four times daily for 4 weeks and metronidazole 400 mg three times daily for 2 weeks (p. 229). Recurrent courses every few months may be necessary
• Symptomatic control with codeine phosphate (up to 180 mg/day) or loperamide (up to 12 mg/day) is appropriate if other measures fail

8   Inflammatory Bowel Disease

8.1 Crohn's disease

Rapid relapse upon steroid withdrawal
Patients who relapse when steroids are reduced below 10 mg, or within 2 weeks of complete withdrawal, are best treated by:
• Prednisolone 30 mg daily to induce remission again, with azathioprine 2–2.5 mg/kg/day (usually 100–150 mg/day)
• Decrease prednisolone to 20 mg/day upon remission, then by 5 mg every month to 5 mg/day, then 5 mg on alternate days for 1 month. It may still not be possible either to withdraw steroids or to control symptoms completely, and a compromise may have to be struck between symptom control and steroid dosage
• Continue azathioprine until steroids are withdrawn and stop azathioprine after 6 months in remission. A full blood count every 1–2 months, or during any acute infection, is advisable to detect the rare complication of aplasia. More than 2 years' continuous treatment is not recommended, because of the theoretical risk of lymphoma
• Sulphasalazine 2 g/day (olsalazine 1 g/day, or mesalazine 1.2 g/day if not tolerated) should probably be given to any patient with colonic disease

Perianal disease
• Treatment is only necessary for symptoms, which are frequently trivial compared to the often horrific appearance
• Resolution is often independent of disease activity elsewhere
• Metronidazole 400 mg three times daily and topical steroid enemas twice daily are indicated for symptomatic disease, with sulphasalazine 1 g twice daily for associated colonic disease
• Spreading fistulation is an indication for oral steroids (prednisolone 30 mg daily) with metronidazole 400 mg three times daily. Azathioprine offers no specific advantage. An elemental diet, or adding ciprofloxacin 500 mg twice daily, sometimes help
• Surgery is only indicated for drainage of an abscess (acute local pain and tenderness) or complicated fistulae that fail to respond to intensive medical treatment. These are best treated at a specialist centre
• Pads are helpful for discharging sinuses

Ileostomy dysfunction (p. 277)

Crohn's disease in pregnancy
Advise patients to avoid conception until disease is inactive. There is then little risk to the pregnancy or the course of Crohn's disease.

Active disease during pregnancy is often relatively resistant to treatment, but sometimes remits spontaneously. Steroids, sulphasalazine and even azathioprine are used in the normal way (p. 255). The risks of active disease are greater than drug side effects.

Crohn's disease in adolescence

Retardation of growth and puberty, as well as loss of schooling, are additional problems, although the course of disease and treatment principles are the same as in adults.

Nutritional assessment and support are essential. Height and weight must be recorded on a centile chart at each visit. Falling below centile lines for height or weight is an indication for blood tests to assess activity and nutritional status (full blood count, folate, vitamin B_{12}, iron studies, calcium). Nutritional supplements (enteral sip feeds, p. 377) are usually tolerated, but if not, continuous and nocturnal enteral feeding are alternatives.

Active disease is treated as in adults, with prednisolone (starting at 0.75 mg/kg daily). Once symptoms are relieved, steroids may be prescribed as a double dose on alternate days, to decrease adverse effects. Rapid control of disease activity with adequate steroids, whilst providing nutritional supplements, also minimizes the adverse effects of steroids. Surgical resection of the most diseased area should be considered if the response is slow.

Prognosis

It is impossible to predict the course of Crohn's disease in an individual patient. Most patients have a good prognosis, although morbidity may be considerable for short periods.

Risk of relapse

- Crohn's disease cannot be cured
- About 10% relapse/year
- Patients with jejunoileal disease relapse more commonly than those with Crohn's colitis

Need for surgery

- 40% of patients have an operation within 10 years of the onset of symptoms and 80% after 20 years
- Half the operations are emergencies

• About 10% with colonic disease have a permanent ileostomy after 10 years

Recurrence after surgery
• 30% relapse within 5 years and 50% within 10 years, but only half of these need further surgery
• Recurrence is less common in colonic disease and the elderly, but more common in children

Mortality
• Overall mortality is twice that of the population
• Patients diagnosed before age 20 years have more than a 10-fold increase in mortality

8.2 Ulcerative colitis
Ulcerative colitis is an inflammatory disorder of the colonic mucosa characterized by relapses and remissions. The cause remains unknown.

General information
A few facts are helpful when explaining the disease to the patients:
• Affects 80/100 000 population (twice as common as Crohn's)
• 10 new cases/100 000/year, with no apparent increase in incidence recently. Race, sex and social class are not associated, although it is uncommon outside Western societies
• Most patients present aged 15–30 years, with a second peak at age 55–70 years, although no age is exempt. Proctitis is more common than total colitis, especially in the elderly
• 15% have a member of the family with ulcerative colitis or Crohn's disease. Ulcerative colitis in monozygotic twins affects both twins about half the time, but concordance in twins with Crohn's disease is more common
• Twice as common in non-smokers
• The cause is unknown, but cell wall-deficient bacteria, diet (low fibre, milk) and deficient immunoregulation have been implicated. Stress may exacerbate existing symptoms, but not cause the disease
• The pattern is usually intermittent. Chronic continuous symptoms with varying severity are less common. Single attacks with no recurrence are rare, and probably not true ulcerative colitis but caused by infection

8.2 Ulcerative colitis

Clinical features

General
• Bloody diarrhoea is the hallmark, usually with mucus
• Onset is usually gradual but can be abrupt, and there may sometimes be a previous history of episodic diarrhoea. Infection may trigger an abrupt onset or toxic dilatation
• Bowel frequency is broadly related to the severity of disease
• Crampy abdominal discomfort is common, but severe persistent pain suggests a complication or different diagnosis
• Systemic features (anorexia, malaise, fever) are common during an acute attack, except in ulcerative proctitis
• Signs (tachycardia, fever, abdominal tenderness or distension) are important when assessing severity (Table 8.6)

Table 8.6 Assessing the severity of ulcerative colitis

Feature	Mild	Moderate	Severe
Motions/day	≤4	4–6	≥6
Rectal bleeding	Small	Moderate	Large amounts
Temperature	Apyrexial	Intermediate	>37.8°C on 2 days out of 4
Pulse rate	Normal	Intermediate	>90 bpm
Haemoglobin	>11 g/dl	Intermediate	<10.5 g/dl
ESR	<30 mm/h	Intermediate	>30 mm/h

• Other features that help distinguish severe attacks are systemic upset (anorexia, malaise, weight loss), tender colon (but often notable by its absence), leucocytosis and hypoalbuminaemia
• Steroids can mask clinical features of severity
• Young patients with severe disease may appear misleadingly well

Extra-intestinal manifestations
10–20% are affected, especially those with pancolitis. Similar to those in Crohn's disease (Table 8.1, p. 245), with some important exceptions (Table 8.7)

Investigations
The aim is to confirm the diagnosis, assess the severity and extent of disease, and to detect complications.

8.2   Ulcerative colitis

Table 8.7 Distinctions between extra-intestinal manifestations of ulcerative colitis (UC) and Crohn's disease

Extra-intestinal feature	Comment
Primary sclerosing cholangitis (PSC, p. 200)	Affects 2–3% 80% with PSC have UC Less common in Crohn's disease
Cholangiocarcinoma (p. 201)	Usually complicates PSC, but very rare in Crohn's disease
Skin lesions	Consider drug-induced lesions, such as sulphasalazine, especially in UC
Large-joint arthritis	Possibly becoming less common in UC due to maintenance sulphasalazine
All extra-intestinal manifestations	Relieved by proctocolectomy in UC, except ankylosing spondylitis and hepatobiliary disease, but not in Crohn's disease

Establish the diagnosis
Sigmoidoscopy and biopsy:
• Diffuse mucosal changes in the rectum are invariable during active disease
• Infective colitis and occasionally Crohn's disease or ischaemia can look similar
• Characteristic microscopic features are an inflammatory infiltrate, goblet cell depletion, glandular distortion and crypt abscesses (Table 8.10, p. 269)
Air contrast barium enema:
• Shows symmetrical and confluent changes (Table 8.8,Fig. 8.2)
• Also establishes the extent of disease after an acute attack

Table 8.8 Summary of radiological features of ulcerative colitis

Acute (approximate order of severity)	Chronic
Normal (proctitis)	Increased retrorectal space
Granular mucosa	Granular mucosa
Absent faecal shadows*	Loss of haustra
Punctate ulcers	Tubular colon
Collar-stud ulcers	Pseudopolyps
Mucosal islands*	Backwash ileitis (pancolitis)
Toxic dilatation (>6.0 cm)*	Carcinoma

* Visible on plain abdominal X-ray.

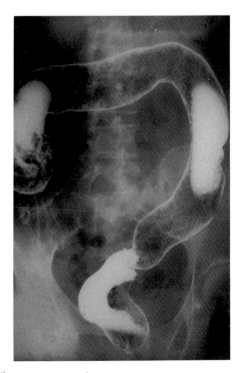

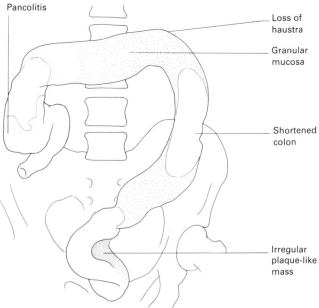

Pancolitis

Loss of
haustra

Granular
mucosa

Shortened
colon

Irregular
plaque-like
mass

Fig. 8.2 Radiological features of ulcerative colitis. Barium enema showing
carcinoma in long-standing ulcerative colitis, presenting as an infiltrative plaque.

• Should not be performed during severe disease unless major doubt exists about the diagnosis. An unprepared, single contrast 'instant enema' is appropriate if immediate management will be altered, but is not good for estimating the true extent of disease
Stool examination:
• Always necessary to exclude pathogens (*Salmonella* sp., *Shigella* sp., *Campylobacter* sp.) and *Cl. difficile* toxin

Establish the severity
• Clinical criteria (Table 8.6, p. 264)
• Sigmoidoscopy (Table 8.9), but mucosal changes may have been ameliorated by local steroids
• Blood tests:
anaemia (Hb <10.5 g/dl) and an ESR >30 mm/h indicate severe disease
leucocytosis, hypoalbuminaemia (<35 g/l) and hypokalaemia are also common in severe disease. If the ESR is normal, a CRP >10 mg/l has the same significance

Table 8.9 Sigmoidoscopic appearances in ulcerative colitis

Mild	Moderate	Severe
Diffuse erythema	Granular mucosa	Intense inflammation
Loss of vascular pattern	Petechial haemorrhages	Purulent exudate
	Contact bleeding	Spontaneous bleeding
	Discrete ulcers	

Establish the extent of disease
• Proctitis means that normal mucosa (pale, with a normal vascular pattern) is visible beyond the upper limit of inflammation at sigmoidoscopy
• Distribution of faecal shadows on a plain abdominal X-ray during an acute attack is a useful guide to the extent of disease; faecal shadows are absent from bowel with active mucosal inflammation. It can be misleading, however, in those with proximal constipation
• Barium enema documents the extent of macroscopic disease
• Colonoscopy and serial biopsy almost always show that disease is more extensive than appears on barium enema, because of microscopic changes. Prognostic factors (for carcinoma, or risk of a severe attack) are based on the extent of macroscopic disease, and the implications of microscopic changes are not clear

Investigation of relapse
- Sigmoidoscopy and biopsy are necessary to assess the severity (Table 8.9, p. 267), in association with the clinical features
- Stool for culture and *Cl. difficile* toxin must be taken
- Full blood count, ESR, electrolytes and albumin should be measured. The CRP may be elevated when the ESR is normal and has the same significance as a high ESR
- A plain abdominal X-ray is necessary in severe disease to look for signs of toxic dilatation or mucosal islands (Fig. 1.3, p. 37). When a moderate relapse is slow to settle, proximal constipation may be visible (p. 276)
- A repeat barium enema is unnecessary unless the extent of the disease is thought to have changed (such as after a severe attack in a patient with previous proctitis)

Outpatient follow-up in remission
- Duration and extent of disease should always be documented, preferably on a summary card at the front of the notes (p. 256 and Appendix 4)
- Sigmoidoscopy is only necessary if a relapse occurs
- Rectal biopsy is recommended at every sigmoidoscopy, because it provides an independent record of the macroscopic appearances, consolidates the diagnosis and, rarely, detects dysplasia
- Surveillance colonoscopy and multiple biopsy (see Fig. 8.3, p. 274) is indicated for total colitis after symptoms for 10 years. It is not necessary for left-sided disease
- Annual full blood count and liver function tests are recommended. Macrocytosis can be due to sulphasalazine, but other causes (alcohol, vitamin B_{12} or folate deficiency, myxoedema or haemolysis) should not be overlooked
- A mildly elevated AST is an indication for complete abstinence from alcohol for 4–8 weeks before repeating the test. Drug-induced liver damage should be considered (p. 141) and if the AST continues to rise, all drugs should be stopped if possible. A liver biopsy is indicated if >2-fold elevation persists for 3 months
- Persistently (>3 months), or >3-fold elevation in ALP, are indications for ultrasound to exclude gall stones, before ERCP to look for primary sclerosing cholangitis

8.2 Ulcerative colitis

Differential diagnosis
There are many causes of bloody diarrhoea, but only a few cause diffuse rectal changes visible on sigmoidoscopy. The main problems are differentiating ulcerative colitis from infective colitis or Crohn's colitis (Table 8.10).

Table 8.10 Differentiation of ulcerative from Crohn's colitis

	Ulcerative colitis	Crohn's colitis
Clinical:		
Bloody diarrhoea	90–100%	50%
Abdominal mass	Very rare	Common
Perianal disease	Very uncommon	30–50%
Sigmoidoscopy:		
Rectal sparing	Never	50%
Histology:		
Distribution	Mucosal	Transmural
Cellular infiltrate	Polymorphs	Lymphocytes
Glands	Distorted	Normal
Goblet cell depletion	Common when active	Absent
Granulomata	Absent	Diagnostic
Radiology:		
Distribution	Continuous	Discontinuous
Symmetry	Symmetrical	Asymmetrical
Mucosa	Shallow ulcers	Deep ulcers
Strictures	Very rare	Common
Fistulae	Never	Common

Infective colitis
- Identification of *Salmonella* sp., *Shigella* sp., *Campylobacter* sp., *Entamoeba histolytica*, or *Cl. difficile* in the stool do not exclude ulcerative colitis
- Infective colitis causes macroscopic and microscopic inflammation, but unlike ulcerative colitis, does not usually distort microscopic glandular architecture
- Repeat sigmoidoscopy and biopsy after the acute episode has settled is always advisable if doubt exists. The patient can be reassured if the second biopsy is normal, but follow-up is necessary if inflammation persists

Crohn's colitis
A definitive diagnosis is not initially possible in 15% and many of these turn out on long-term follow-up to have Crohn's colitis. This is one reason for repeat rectal biopsies (p. 268)

Other possibilities
• Ischaemic colitis—clinical features can be identical. Rectal sparing, 'thumb-printing' on plain abdominal X-ray and an 'instant' barium enema establish the diagnosis (see Table 9.4, p. 309)
• Radiation colitis—history of pelvic or abdominal node irradiation, with mucosal telangiectasia
• Microscopic colitis—no bleeding and macroscopically normal mucosa (p. 279)
• Pseudomembranous colitis (p. 280)
• Diverticular disease, polyps and colorectal carcinoma are readily distinguished as the cause of bloody diarrhoea, by barium enema
• Irritable bowel syndrome may coexist with ulcerative colitis (p. 324)

Management
Prompt treatment of acute attacks, maintenance therapy to reduce the relapse rate, selection of patients for colectomy and early detection of colorectal carcinoma are the principles of management. Patient education is essential to ensure early presentation during relapse.

Treatment of an acute attack involving any site other than proctitis depends on the severity (Table 8.6, p. 264). Proctitis is a special case because proximal progression is rare (<10%). The term 'fulminant attack' is best avoided, because treatment is no different from that for a severe attack.

Mild attacks
Prompt and decisive treatment brings rapid relief to the patient and reduces the risk of complications, so oral steroids are recommended, although they may initially appear unnecessary for mild symptoms.
• Oral prednisolone 20 mg/day for 1 month, then reduce by 5 mg/week
• Steroid retention enemas twice daily
• Sulphasalazine 1 g twice daily (mesalazine or olsalazine for intolerance)

• Failure to improve after 2 weeks is an indication for treatment as a moderate attack. Deterioration is an indication for admission

Moderate attacks

• Prednisolone 40 mg/day for 1 week, then 30 mg/day for 1 week, then 20 mg/day for 1 month, before decreasing by 5 mg/day
• Steroid enemas morning and night
• Sulphasalazine 1 g twice daily (mesalazine or olsalazine for intolerance). A higher dose (up to 4 g/day) may be more effective, but cannot usually be tolerated
• Admission is not essential unless symptoms fail to improve within 2 weeks, although for some patients (especially the elderly), bed rest and enemas in hospital are more comfortable

Severe attacks

Immediate admission is necessary when clinical features of a severe attack are present (Table 8.6, p. 264). Surgical colleagues should be informed. A severe attack may occur without colonic dilatation ('toxic dilatation') although this may subsequently develop.
• A plain abdominal X-ray and blood tests are taken on the way to the ward. Daily abdominal X-rays are then needed to detect mucosal islands, dilatation (Fig. 1.3, p. 37) or perforation, until fever, abdominal tenderness and tachycardia resolve
• Intravenous hydrocortisone 100 mg four times daily is given for 5 days
• Rectal steroids should also be given twice daily. Hydrocortisone 100 mg in 100 ml 0.9% saline, dripped through an intravenous giving set into the rectum, is often more comfortable for the patient than proprietary enemas
• Sips of fluid only by mouth; although the benefit of withdrawing food has not been proven, patients are usually anorexic and the response to reintroduction of food may help decide whether colectomy is indicated in difficult cases (p. 272). Parenteral nutrition is needed for malnourished patients or those who come to colectomy. Peripheral intravenous feeds (p. 381) are a useful temporary measure
• Intravenous fluids are needed to correct dehydration and maintain serum potassium at 4.0–4.5 mmol/l
• Blood transfusion is advisable if Hb<10 g/dl. Serum should be grouped and saved for possible surgery

- Daily (or twice daily in very sick patients) re-examination is essential, looking for a rise in pulse or temperature, increasing abdominal girth or tenderness
- Daily full blood count, ESR and electrolytes should be checked
- Failure to respond after 5 days, or deterioration at any stage, is an indication for colectomy. Delay increases the mortality
- 60% are in remission after 5 days, and 25% deteriorate and have a colectomy. A small group (15%) improve but continue to need careful observation. Relapse on reintroducing food and changing to oral steroids usually means that colectomy is required
- For those who improve, oral prednisolone 40 mg/day can be started after 5 days and decreased after 1 week to 30 mg/day for 1 week, then to 20 mg/day for 1 month. It can then be decreased by 5 mg/week unless relapse occurs (p. 276)
- Sulphasalazine may be poorly tolerated in severely ill patients, but should be reintroduced with oral steroids
- Antibiotics, including metronidazole, offer no benefit

Indications for emergency surgery
- Toxic dilatation (p. 36)
- Perforation
- Massive haemorrhage
- Failure of a severe attack to respond to intravenous steroids within 5 days. The decision and timing can be difficult, and should be made jointly by a senior physician and surgeon. Whilst some prefer to continue steroids for longer periods, the operative morbidity (and mortality) increases if surgery is inappropriately delayed
- Mucosal islands on a plain abdominal X-ray, or a sustained fever >38°C and stool frequency >8/day after 24-h treatment, predict a high probability that colectomy will be needed. Several gas-filled loops of small bowel on plain X-ray are also associated with the need for emergency colectomy
- A small proportion of patients with a severe attack show a moderate but incomplete response to intravenous steroids after 5 days. Deterioration when food is reintroduced is usually an indication for surgery

Proctitis
Local steroids and oral sulphasalazine are often sufficient, but proctitis can be very refractory, even to oral steroids

8.2   Ulcerative colitis

---

* Steroid retention enemas morning and night, then only at night when bowel frequency returns to normal, until 1 week after bleeding stops
* Some patients find foam enemas or suppositories easier to retain than fluid enemas. It is a matter for personal choice, although. suppositories may be useful for very localized disease
* Sulphasalazine 1 g twice daily (mesalazine or olsalazine for intolerance)
* Failure to control symptoms within 2 weeks is an indication for prednisolone 20 mg/day, reducing by 5 mg/week after 1 month.
* Refractory proctitis is discussed on p. 276

Maintenance treatment

* All 5-aminosalicylic acid compounds (sulphasalazine, mesalazine, olsalazine) reduce the relapse rate by about 4-fold, from 80% to 20% at 1 year
* Maintenance treatment should be continued for life, because the benefit is sustained
* Sulphasalazine 1 g twice daily remains the first choice, because it is cheap and well established. Higher doses (up to 4 g/day) are more effective and may be tried if relapse occurs whilst taking a lower dose, but are often poorly tolerated. Enteric-coated sulphasalazine may help
* Nausea or abdominal discomfort occur in 10% taking sulphasalazine, but more specific side effects (rash, haemolysis) are rare. Reversible oligospermia is frequent, so potential fathers should be changed to olsalazine or mesalazine
* Mesalazine (400–500 mg three times daily) or olsalazine (500 mg twice daily), are indicated for sulphasalazine intolerance
* Steroids have no effect on relapse rate and should be stopped once remission occurs
* Patients often benefit from contact with the National Association for Colitis and Crohn's Disease (NACC), even if symptoms are mild (Appendix 1). A booklet on ulcerative colitis is also available from the Digestive Diseases Foundation (Appendix 1).

Detection of colonic carcinoma

The risk of cancer increases with the extent and duration of disease (p. 279). It may be unrelated to age of onset, but is more prevalent in patients whose symptoms run a chronic continuous course.

8.2   Ulcerative colitis

Colitis distal to the splenic flexure does not justify surveillance. There is no evidence that maintenance sulphasalazine decreases the risk of cancer in ulcerative colitis. A register and recall system for patients with total colitis is advisable. The best surveillance programme has not been established, but Fig. 8.3 shows a plan.

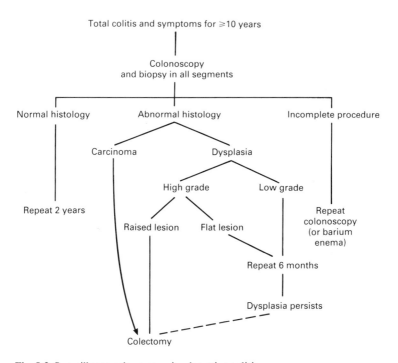

Fig. 8.3 Surveillance colonoscopy in ulcerative colitis.

Indications for surgery
Colectomy is the only cure for ulcerative colitis, although it does not affect some of the extra-intestinal manifestations (Table 8.7, p. 265). Colectomy with a temporary ileostomy and later ileoanal pouch construction is now popular, but proctocolectomy and permanent ileostomy retains a definite place.

Indications for elective surgery
Disease is usually extensive, but colectomy is occasionally needed

for distal colitis. The patient should talk to an ileostomist of the same sex and similar age before surgery.
- Continuous symptoms (often with general ill health and anaemia) despite treatment
- Frequent relapses unresponsive to medical treatment that materially affect the patient's life
- High-grade dysplasia, or frank malignancy

Indications for emergency surgery (p. 272)

Type of operation
- Proctocolectomy with a permanent ileostomy remains the standard procedure for elective surgery. Mortality is 2%, but ileostomy dysfunction occurs in about 15% (see Table 8.11, p. 277)
- Colectomy and later formation of an ileoanal pouch ('restorative proctocolectomy', J, W, or S pouches) is now popular because there is no permanent ileostomy. Good results (continence and 5 or fewer bowel actions/day) are obtained in two-thirds or more in experienced hands, but some need revision to a permanent ileostomy
- One-stage proctocolectomy is safer than sub-total colectomy and ileostomy for emergencies, in experienced hands. For patients who may subsequently have an ileoanal pouch, then sub-total colectomy is appropriate, leaving the rectal stump in place

Complications

Toxic dilatation
Clinical features of severe disease with mucosal islands and a colonic diameter of >6.0 cm on plain X-ray are diagnostic (Fig. 1.3, p. 37).

Perforation
- Diagnosed by free gas on plain X-ray, usually complicating toxic dilatation when surgery has been delayed too long, or colonoscopy during a severe attack
- Common signs (pain and peritonism) are often few and masked by steroids
- Colectomy after fluid, blood and electrolyte replacement is vital

8.2   Ulcerative colitis

Massive haemorrhage
* Diagnosis is not difficult except at presentation, when the mucosal pattern may be obscured by blood
* Clotting should be checked and corrected with fresh frozen plasma if the INR is >1.5 (prothrombin time >22 sec)
* As the underlying disease is likely to recur, colectomy is usually indicated if bleeding has not stopped after transfusing 4 units

Carcinoma (see p. 273)

Management problems

Refractory distal colitis, or proctitis
Distal colitis is resistant to treatment in a minority, but surgery is better avoided for limited disease. The therapeutic options below also apply to patients who relapse rapidly after a course of steroids, or who appear to be dependent on steroids.
* Relieve proximal constipation, visible on plain X-ray, by sodium picosulphate and magnesium citrate (Picolax) 1 sachet orally, or lactulose 30–60 ml/day
* Azathioprine 2–2.5 mg/kg/day in addition to prednisolone, until remission. A full blood count should be performed every 1–2 months, or if unwell, to detect the unusual complications of agranulocytosis or aplasia
* Mesalazine or sulphasalazine enemas twice daily, in addition to steroid enemas, are often helpful, but some patients find them difficult to retain
* Avoiding milk relieves diarrhoea in a minority, but does not affect disease activity
* Colectomy may be needed if there is still no response, but patients are best referred to a specialist centre; cyclosporin enemas and methotrexate are under trial, but should not be used except by specialists

Pregnancy
* Pregnancy has no consistent effect on colitis
* Relapse during pregnancy is treated in the standard way

Chronic continuous symptoms
* Usually an indication for colectomy if the disease is extensive

Stomas and pouches (Table 8.11)
Ileostomists and patients with pouches produce 500 ml effluent/day, which is largely fluid and high in sodium. Urine volume is decreased to compensate. Ileal adaptation develops over 12 months and volume decreases. Nutrient absorption is normal except when there is coexistent small intestinal disease or terminal ileal resection.

Table 8.11 Complications of ileostomies

Early	Late
Ischaemia	Dysfunction (fluid loss >1000 ml/day)
Wound infection	Small bowel obstruction
Small bowel obstruction	Parastomal herniation
Delayed perineal healing	Stenosis
	Retraction
	Local dermatitis
	Psychosexual
	Gall stones
	Renal calculi

Ileostomy dysfunction
• Loss of fluid and electrolytes causes lassitude, postural hypotension and dehydration
• Partial obstruction, recurrent disease (in Crohn's disease) or infection may be the cause, but often no reason is apparent
• Culture of effluent, plain abdominal X-ray and serum electrolytes are necessary. Small bowel radiology, if there is abdominal pain, and urinary and ileal effluent electrolytes guide replacement in severe cases
• Admission and intravenous fluids are indicated if there is clinical evidence of dehydration or postural hypotension
• Loperamide, up to 12 mg/day, decreases moderately increased fluid loss
• Oral electrolyte solutions (Dioralyte, p. 213) are indicated for chronic losses. The amount depends on electrolyte loss, but is often 2000–3000 ml/day

Subacute small bowel obstruction
• Adhesions, twisted ileal loops, stenosis, recurrent Crohn's disease, or parastomal herniation may be the cause

- Examination with a fibreoptic sigmoidoscope is advisable, but is often limited even in normal ileostomies
- Most settle spontaneously with intravenous fluids, nasogastric suction if there is vomiting, and intramuscular pethidine 50–100 mg for pain

Stenosis or retraction

- Digital examination of the ileostomy spout will detect stenosis and is advisable at outpatient visits during the first 6 months and if obstruction or bleeding occurs
- Retraction of the spout causes maceration of the skin and difficulties with bag adhesion. Surgical revision is necessary

Practical problems

- A specialist nurse (stoma therapist) is invaluable before elective procedures (to help plan the site or relieve anxiety) and after a stoma has been formed
- A badly sited stoma is rapidly recognized by the patient. Revision may be necessary if the stoma substantially interferes with daily activities (including sitting, if at an abdominal crease)
- Odour may be reduced by odour-proof bags or dietary changes (eggs, onions and beans are common culprits)
- Local dermatitis may be due to an allergy to the adhesive, or leaking effluent. Changing the type of appliance and an effective seal are the solutions
- Psychosocial difficulties may be helped through patient support groups (Ileostomy Association, National Association for Colitis and Crohn's Disease, Appendix 1), although patients without problems benefit as well

Pouches

All the problems of ileostomists may occur with ileoanal pouches. Pouchitis is an additional problem in 10–20%. Infection must be excluded. Pouchitis causes frequency, bleeding and an inflamed pouch mucosa and probably does not occur in pouches for familial adenomatous polyposis. Sulphasalazine 1 g twice daily, metronidazole 400 mg three times daily, or prednisolone 20 mg/day should be tried, in that order.

Prognosis
• About 25% have proctitis, 50% left-sided disease and 25% total colitis at presentation. Proximal progression in proctitis is rare (<10%), but occurs in about 25% with left-sided disease
• 80% on maintenance treatment with sulphasalazine, mesalazine or olsalazine have no relapse for 1 year
• About one relapse can be expected every 5 years, and only 4% remain symptom free after 15 years
• About 25% come to surgery
• There appears to be a substantial difference in mortality during a severe attack between those managed in specialist centres (<1%, including operative mortality) and those managed elsewhere (5%)
• Mortality is otherwise similar to that of the general population
• About 12–15% with pancolitis for 20 years develop colonic carcinoma (p. 273). The risk of carcinoma in colitis distal to the splenic flexure is probably no higher than in the general population

8.3 Non-specific colitis

General
If a definitive diagnosis of the type of colitis cannot be made after histological and radiological examination, this should be stated in the notes. This is an indication for regular follow-up, repeated sigmoidoscopy and biopsy, until a diagnosis is established.
  Differentiation between post-infective, ulcerative and diffuse Crohn's colitis is the usual problem (Table 8.10, p. 269). Small bowel radiology is essential if doubt about the diagnosis persists, because typical lesions of Crohn's disease may be asymptomatic.

Microscopic colitis

Features
• Watery diarrhoea
• Often female, aged >60 years
• Macroscopically normal mucosa on sigmoidoscopy and colonoscopy
• Serial biopsies show microscopic inflammation and lymphocytic infiltration (the term 'lymphocytic colitis' is also used)
• Other causes of diarrhoea (Table 7.1, p. 208), including coeliac disease, should be excluded

___

Treatment
- No treatment has been definitely established, but it is probably best to start with sulphasalazine 2 g/day. About 50% respond
- Prednisolone 20 mg/day until diarrhoea stops, then decreased slowly (5 mg/month) if there is no response to sulphasalazine
- Metronidazole 400 mg three times daily helps a proportion, but this is empirical
- Long-term results remain unknown

Pseudomembranous colitis

Pseudomembranous colitis is caused by *Cl. difficile* and usually follows prolonged or multiple antibiotics, especially ampicillin, clindamycin or lincomycin. It is diagnosed by sigmoidoscopy (punctate, adherent yellow-white plaques on an inflamed rectal mucosa) and detecting *Cl. difficile* toxin in stool. Histology may be diagnostic if a plaque ('summit lesion') is included in the biopsy, but may be difficult to distinguish from ulcerative colitis (although crypt abscesses are rare) or ischaemic colitis (Table 9.4, p. 309).

  Cl. difficile causes about 4% acute gastroenteritis in adults (p. 327) and pseudomembranous colitis represents the severe end of the spectrum.

  It can be difficult to distinguish pseudomembranous colitis from acute ulcerative colitis provoked by *Cl. difficile*. Treatment with both metronidazole (below) and steroids (p. 270) is advisable if doubt exists, and follow-up sigmoidoscopy and biopsy arranged once symptoms resolve (p. 269).

  Treatment with oral metronidazole 400 mg three times daily for 1 week is recommended. Relapse may occur (up to 30%) and should be treated with vancomycin 125–250 mg four times daily for 1 week or longer (several weeks, decreasing the dose gradually). Recurrent infection is rare and patients are best referred to a specialist centre.

Ischaemic colitis (see p. 307)

Collagenous colitis

A rare disorder, characterized by a sub-epithelial band of collagen on colonic biopsies. It may be associated with microscopic colitis,

8 Inflammatory Bowel Disease

8.3 Non-specific colitis

but is unrelated to connective tissue diseases. Treatment with steroids or sulphasalazine is empirical.

Diversion colitis

Inflammation in the defunctioned loop of a colostomy, causing a mucous discharge, appears to respond to sodium butyrate enemas.

9 Large Intestine

9.1   Constipation

Constipation means the passage of hard faeces infrequently, often with straining and discomfort. Patient reporting of constipation depends on early training, preoccupation with the bowel and expectations (p. 288). Some make exacting demands.

Causes

Diet or faulty bowel habit cause the vast majority, but less common, treatable causes should not be overlooked (Table 9.1).

Table 9.1 Causes of constipation

Common	Uncommon	Rare
Diet:	Anorectal disease:	Metabolic/endocrine:
inadequate fibre	fissure	myxoedema
Motility disorders:	stricture	hypercalcaemia
irritable bowel	mucosal prolapse	hypoka laemia
Age	Drugs:	porphyria
Pregnancy	opiates	lead poisoning
	aluminium antacids	Idiopathic slow transit
	anticholinergics	Neurological disorders:
	iron	cerebral disease
	cathartic colon	spinal cord lesions
	Intestinal obstruction:	aganglionosis
	carcinoma	
	pseudo-obstruction	

• Dietary causes are common in the elderly or depressed, although tricyclic antidepressants and pseudo-obstruction are additional causes in these groups
• Faecal impaction in the elderly or mentally impaired may cause spurious diarrhoea, urinary retention or irritability
• Chronic stimulant laxative use causes cathartic megacolon, hypokalaemia, or melanosis coli
• Idiopathic slow transit constipation is discussed on p. 288
• Neurological disorders may cause constipation due to inactivity or failure of rectal sensation and rectal reflexes. Constipation is a key feature of spinal cord lesions (such as transection, transverse myelitis, or cauda equina tumours). Drugs often contribute to constipation in Parkinson's or cerebrovascular disease
• Aganglionosis (due to Hirschsprung's or Chagas' disease) very rarely presents in adults, with constipation and megacolon

Investigation

General
The history must determine the frequency, nature and consistency of stool, so as to establish whether the patient really is constipated. Questions about diet and drugs, as well as rectal examination, sigmoidoscopy and proctoscopy are essential. Investigation is only indicated if there has been a recent change in bowel habit (<6 months), especially if age >40 years, or if there are associated features (rectal bleeding, weight loss).

Initial investigations
• Blood tests—a full blood count, electrolytes, calcium and thyroid function tests will identify most organic and treatable causes
• Sigmoidoscopy is always indicated. Melanosis due to chronic use of anthraquinone laxatives (such as senna) may be visible
• Barium enema is indicated if an organic lesion is suspected, especially if the change in bowel habit is recent

Special investigations
• Transit studies are useful to document slow intestinal transit when the bowel frequency is less than once a week. Fybogel 3 sachets/day is given for 2 weeks (to eliminate dietary causes of slow transit), then 20 oral radio-opaque markers are taken at once. Plain abdominal X-rays at 2 and 5 days normally show >75% excretion of markers by day 5
• Anorectal manometry (p. 366) is rarely indicated in adults, unless there is megacolon or megarectum (to exclude aganglionosis, when the rectosphincteric reflex is absent), a defaecation disorder (p. 289) is suspected, or if there is faecal incontinence. Defaecography at a specialist centre may demonstrate anterior mucosal prolapse or a rectocele. Perineal descent is often visible on careful clinical examination, when the patient strains

Management
Constipation due to colonic, anorectal or systemic disease must be identified and treated appropriately. The patient's idea of a normal bowel habit should be discussed. A reasonable aim is a soft motion every 1 or 2 days. The call to stool should not be ignored.

9 Large Intestine

9.1 Constipation

Diet
- Increased fibre intake is the key, but is not always well tolerated. There is no universal dose, but it must be accompanied by adequate fluids (about 1500 ml/day), which the elderly are sometimes reluctant to increase
- 100% wholemeal bread, leguminous vegetables (peas, beans and lentils) and fruit are simple dietary changes (p. 385)
- A tablespoon of bran (added to breakfast cereal, yoghurt or soup) may be necessary, but it should be of the coarse-milled variety
- Flatulence or abdominal distension may be increased on a high-fibre diet, and the elderly may develop faecal soiling if the softer stool cannot be controlled. A gradual increase in fibre intake is wise
- Constipation due to colonic strictures or spinal cord lesions may be exacerbated by increased dietary fibre

Laxatives
Laxatives are indicated to alleviate painful defaecation, when straining will exacerbate a condition (such as a hernia), for drug-induced constipation, before surgery or colonic examination. There are four groups of laxatives and 60 preparations, but bran and an osmotic laxative, with only an occasional stimulant, work for most. The diagnosis should be reassessed if two sorts of laxative are ineffective. The ultimate sanction for simple constipation is magnesium sulphate. Any laxative is dangerous in obstruction.

Bulk-forming laxatives
- For dietary constipation and painful anorectal conditions, with extra fluid
- Ispaghula husk (Fybogel), or sterculia (Normacol) are more palatable than coarse bran (1–2 tbsp/day), but more expensive

Osmotic laxatives
- Indicated when bulk-forming laxatives are ineffective, for proximal constipation in ulcerative colitis or hepatic encephalopathy
- The dose of lactulose (30–100 ml/day) is easier to regulate, but more expensive, than magnesium sulphate (10–20 ml of crystals in water 2-hourly, until effective)
- Sodium picosulphate with magnesium citrate (Picolax 1–2 sachets) works for proximal constipation in ulcerative colitis, but has some stimulant action

Stimulant laxatives
• For bowel clearance, neurological disorders, or temporary use in stubborn constipation
• Colic may be exacerbated and long-term use should be avoided (p. 285)
• Bisacodyl suppositories (1–2) act within 1 hour, senna tablets (2–4 at night) act the following morning
Faecal softeners
• Occasionally indicated for faecal impaction
• Arachis oil enema, or glycerine suppositories are useful and a disposable enema (such as Relaxit) is good for stubborn cases
• Liquid paraffin can cause granulomas or lipoid pneumonia, and is not recommended

General advice on constipation
Re-education is an important part of improving bowel habit.
• Do not ignore the call to stool
• Develop a regular time for defaecation each day
• Avoid excessive straining—this makes defaecation disorders worse
• Avoid prolonged sitting
• Aim for a soft, easily passed motion every day or two

Slow transit constipation
Young women (exceptionally men) occasionally present with gross constipation (bowel frequency once or twice a fortnight), abdominal discomfort and painful defaecation, but are otherwise in good health. No cause can be found and the diagnosis is confirmed by transit studies (p. 286). Barium enema is usually normal, but may show faecal loading in a dilated colon—idiopathic megacolon

Osmotic laxatives in sufficient doses soften the stool, but stimulant laxatives are often required on alternate days to increase stool frequency. Bulking agents may make abdominal discomfort worse. Cisapride 10–20 mg three times daily may be beneficial. Colectomy and ileorectal anastomosis are the last resort for disabling symptoms.

Megacolon
Megacolon or megarectum in adults is usually idiopathic. A long history of constipation is usual, although it may be intermittent and interspersed with episodes of faecal impaction with spurious

diarrhoea. A barium enema is diagnostic. Aganglionosis must be excluded by anorectal manometry (p. 366). Full-thickness rectal biopsy and silver stain to show the myenteric plexus is only justified if manometry shows inhibition of sphincteric relaxation. Idiopathic megacolon is treated in the same way as slow transit constipation, but referral to a specialist centre is necessary for manometry and makes subsequent management easier. Laxatives must be continued for life, to avoid episodes of faecal impaction, and this should be made clear to the patient and the general practitioner.

Defaecation disorders
Obstructed defaecation causes a sensation of incomplete evacuation (tenesmus). A local cause (tumour, rectal ulcer, mucosal prolapse) must be excluded by rectal examination, proctoscopy and sigmoidoscopy. The patient must strain during proctoscopy for mucosal prolapse to be seen. The descending perineum syndrome, with or without mucosal prolapse and ulceration, should be considered. Tenesmus is likely to be a feature of the irritable bowel syndrome (p. 320) if a cause is not visible on rectal examination and proctosigmoidoscopy.

Descending perineum syndrome
Women are most commonly affected, sometimes as a sequel to pudendal nerve damage during childbirth. Marked perineal descent during excessive straining at stool causes a sensation of incomplete evacuation and further straining. This results in rectal mucosal prolapse, ulceration and bleeding. Incontinence may develop. Diagnosis is made by careful inspection of the perineum during straining; >1 cm descent, which can be measured at a specialist centre, is abnormal.

Solitary rectal ulcer
Constipation with excessive straining at stool may be associated with an anterior rectal ulcer, rectal bleeding and a sensation of incomplete evacuation. Sigmoidoscopy shows a single (sometimes circumferential) ulcer; biopsies are essential to exclude Crohn's disease, carcinoma, or other causes of rectal ulcers (p. 252). Some are caused by insertion of a finger or foreign body, in a desperate attempt to initiate defaecation by severely constipated patients

Management of defaecation disorders

Treatment of constipation, advice to avoid straining and excluding serious disease are the principles of management. Mucosal prolapse is treated by submucosal injection of a sclerosant (such as phenol). Local steroids may relieve bleeding from mucosal ulceration. Barium enema, follow-up and repeat biopsies are indicated if rectal biopsies are equivocal, to exclude Crohn's disease and other pathology.

Should symptoms persist, referral to a specialist centre is advised, for anorectal studies, pelvic nerve conduction studies and defaecography, before surgery in selected cases. Anal dilatation for constipation in inappropriate cases (such as descending perineum syndrome with a lax anal sphincter) can provoke faecal incontinence.

9.2 Colonic polyps

Adenomatous polyps precede colorectal cancer, which can be prevented by the early recognition and treatment of polyps. Not all polyps are premalignant.

Classification

Polyps are mucosal projections into the lumen and may be sessile or pedunculated. There are four types, which cannot be reliably distinguished macroscopically, so polypectomy and histology are always indicated.

Metaplastic

• Commonest type—75% of all rectal polyps in adults >40 years; often multiple, usually flat, shiny and <5 mm in diameter
• No malignant potential

Adenomas

• Also common—50% of colonic polyps in patients >55 years
• A third of older Western patients have 1–2 colonic adenomas, but only 3% develop colorectal cancer
• Malignant potential is related to size (>1 cm), type (villous > tubulovillous > tubular) and histology (poorly > well differentiated)
• 25% are multiple
• Villous adenomas tend to recur locally after removal

9.2 Colonic polyps

Inflammatory
- Pseudopolyps after severe colitis of any cause
- Not neoplastic

Hamartomatous
- Juvenile polyps are developmental malformations, often large, pedunculated and vascular, but usually solitary. Very rarely there are multiple (>5) polyps—juvenile polyposis
- Peutz–Jeghers syndrome of buccal pigmentation and multiple intestinal hamartomas affects the colon in over 50% (p. 237)
- No malignant potential, but occasional foci of dysplasia in solitary polyps cause sporadic small or large bowel cancer in Peutz–Jeghers syndrome and juvenile polyposis

Other
- Nodular lymphoid hyperplasia in the rectum or terminal ileum is a normal variant in young people and recognized histologically, although radiological features may resemble Crohn's disease or polyposis.

Clinical features
Most colonic polyps are asymptomatic and detected on barium enema or endoscopy for unrelated gastrointestinal symptoms. Some present with rectal bleeding at any age, but diarrhoea (sometimes with profuse mucus and hypokalaemia) is a rare presentation of a villous adenoma.

Management
- Polyps identified on barium enema or sigmoidoscopy are an indication for total colonoscopy and polypectomy; small polyps other than those detected radiologically may be present
- Repeat colonoscopy 1 year after successful polypectomy is recommended, and then at 3-year intervals, if this is normal, until age 75 years
- A good way of permanently marking the site of suspicious or partially removed polyps, for follow-up or surgical identification, is by 'tattooing', with 1 ml intra-mucosal Indian ink
- All polyps must be examined histologically and the pathologist should say whether polypectomy has been complete. Incomplete

polypectomy is an indication for repeat colonoscopy within 3–6 months
• High-grade dysplasia or submucosal infiltration by carcinoma in a sessile polyp is usually an indication for colectomy; in a pedunculated polyp, a specialist pathologist may judge removal to be complete. Repeat colonoscopy after 3–6 months is recommended when excision is thought to have been complete
• Complications of polypectomy include immediate or delayed (up to 2 weeks) bleeding. Perforation is rare

Familial adenomatous polyposis
Multiple (>100) colonic polyps invariably progress to colorectal cancer in this autosomal dominant condition, unless colectomy is performed. Sporadic cases occur. Polyps may occur in childhood, but the increased cancer risk starts in teenagers. Gastric cancer and small intestinal adenocarcinoma are also more common and Gardner's syndrome (colonic polyposis and osteomas) is a variant. Other rare associations are tumours of the central nervous system, retinal pigment hypertrophy and large intra-abdominal desmoid tumours.

Management
• Proctocolectomy with an ileoanal pouch should be performed if adenomas are identified. Pouchitis probably does not occur (p. 278)
• Screening of all first-degree relatives is mandatory, probably best by fibreoptic sigmoidoscopy after age 15 years, every 2 years for life
• Some patients do not develop polyps until older than 35 years
• Genetic counselling is essential. The gene has been identified on chromosome 5, so genetic screening will be possible in the future

Cancer family syndrome (Lynch syndrome)
Rare families have a high incidence of colorectal cancer without polyposis (although adenomas may occur), especially at a young age (<45 years) and in the proximal colon. The inheritance is dominant. Family members may be at risk from other primary tumours (breast, ovary, endometrium) and benefit from colonoscopic screening every 5 years and annual pelvic ultrasound after age 25 years. Only a thorough family history identifies those at risk. Referral to a specialist centre may be advisable (Appendix 1).

Screening for colorectal cancer is also recommended if a first-degree relative (parent, sibling, or child) has developed colorectal cancer aged <45 years, or if two first-degree relatives have had colorectal carcinoma at any age (p. 297).

Pneumatosis coli

A rare condition with gas-filled submucosal cysts that look like polyps at colonoscopy, but which collapse on needle aspiration. A plain X-ray or barium enema shows multiple radiolucencies along the wall of the bowel, or throughout the abdomen if the small intestine is involved. It may be misdiagnosed as multiple polyps, colitis, or carcinoma if the radiolucencies are not recognized. There are often no symptoms, but diarrhoea with mucus, abdominal pain or rectal bleeding may occur.

No cause can usually be found, although it may be associated with emphysema. Treatment is only necessary for symptoms. 70% inspired oxygen through nasal cannulae for 5 days usually gives relief for long periods, but should be used with care if the patient has emphysema. Anticholinergic drugs (such as dicyclomine 10–20 mg three times daily) have been advocated, but are not often helpful.

9.3 Colorectal cancer

Adenocarcinoma of the colon is the commonest malignancy in Britain (lifetime incidence 3–5%) after lung cancer. It is potentially curable and preventable.

Causes

Adenocarcinomas almost always arise from pre-existing adenomatous polyps (except rarely after ulcerative, or perhaps Crohn's colitis).
• Environmental—lack of dietary fibre causing slow transit and increased exposure to toxic bacterial products of digestion, may explain the prevalence in Western communities. Colonic cancer is rare in the Far East and Africa, but the incidence is increasing
• Genetic—about 1% of all colorectal cancers are due to familial adenomatous polyposis, and another 5% occur in cancer family syndromes. The remainder are sporadic, but 10–15% of first-degree relatives will develop the disease
• Ulcerative and Crohn's colitis (pp. 259 and 273)

• Suggested associations with Barrett's oesophagus, cholecystectomy, coffee drinking or cholesterol are unproven

Clinical features

Features vary with the site of the tumour. Most colorectal cancers are left-sided, but a third are proximal to the splenic flexure. Inflammatory bowel disease-associated cancers are evenly distributed.
• Bleeding—less than half have visible rectal bleeding. Fresh blood on the outside of faeces does not exclude a tumour, which may coexist with haemorrhoids
• Change in bowel habit—more common in distal tumours. Tenesmus is common in rectal cancer
• Abdominal pain—is non-specific. It may be due to spasm, partial obstruction in distal lesions or local invasion in caecal tumours
• Anorexia, weight loss or an abdominal mass (especially caecal) are late features, but do not always indicate incurable disease
• Emergency presentation with obstruction (15%, usually at the splenic flexure), perforation (<5%) or other reason (anaemia, jaundice) occurs in 30%
• Iron deficiency anaemia in middle-aged men or post-menopausal women suggests a caecal neoplasm until proven otherwise (p. 313)
• Colorectal cancer is an unusual cause of a persistent pyrexia

Investigations

Patients with rectal bleeding, change in bowel habit, or iron deficiency anaemia (especially in post-menopausal women) must always be investigated for colonic cancer. Once the diagnosis is established, operability must be assessed.

Initial investigations

The whole colon should be examined by barium enema or colonoscopy, preferably preoperatively, but if necessary postoperatively, because tumours may be multiple in about 3%. The terms 'synchronous' (more than one tumour at one time) and 'metachronous' (a second tumour after resection of the first) for multiple tumours are sometimes used.
• Rigid sigmoidoscopy—any patient with rectal bleeding
• Blood tests:
 anaemia may be the only feature of caecal tumours. ESR is often normal

raised ALP may be due to hepatic or bony metastases. Elevated
γGT or AST indicates hepatic origin
• Air contrast barium enema:
  usual initial colonic investigation for patients with an altered
    bowel habit (single contrast examinations are obsolete)
  radiological features of cancer are strictures with shouldering
    ('apple core'), or irregular filling defect in the bowel wall
    (Fig. 9.1)
  colonoscopy is necessary if a barium enema is normal or views
    were poor in a patient with persistent rectal bleeding
• Colonoscopy:
  increasingly used as the initial colonic investigation for patients
    with rectal bleeding, polyp(s) seen on sigmoidoscopy, or those
    with a strong family history of colorectal cancer
  detects polyps or cancer that has been missed at barium enema
    in 20–30% with rectal bleeding
  provides a histological diagnosis which is desirable before
    surgery, but not essential if the radiological appearances are
    typical

Subsequent investigations
• Ultrasound:
  —to exclude hepatic metastases in all patients before surgery
  —intracavitary rectal ultrasound is valuable for assessing tumour
    stage in rectal cancer, but is not widely available
• Chest X-ray:
  —look for lung metastases
• Other preoperative tests include ECG and blood crossmatch,
  depending on the age of the patient

Management
Management depends on the site and extent of the tumour,
although surgery is almost always necessary to prevent obstruction
or relieve bleeding. Palliative laser therapy is occasionally used if
surgery is contraindicated, but may not be locally available. The
site and prospect of a possible colostomy should be discussed
with the patient. Good bowel preparation and prophylactic
antibiotics (intravenous metronidazole 500 mg and cefuroxime
750 mg three times daily) are needed before elective colorectal

9.3   Colorectal cancer

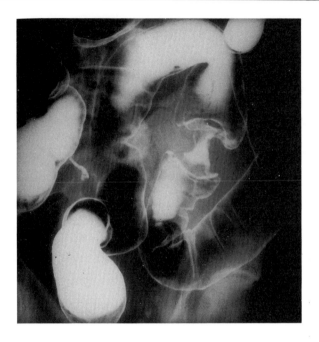

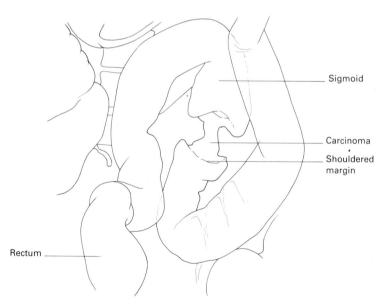

Fig. 9.1 Colorectal cancer. Barium enema showing a typical annular carcinoma in the mid-sigmoid colon.

surgery. Antibiotics should be started on induction and continued for 48 h.

Rectum
• Most need anterior resection (rectal excision and anastomosis, usually with a stapling gun) or abdominoperineal resection if anastomosis is impossible
• Small tumours <10 cm from the anus can often be removed by local excision in the elderly

Transverse/distal colon
• Transverse or left hemicolectomy is indicated
• Emergency operations for obstruction need two or three stages (decompression, resection and anastomosis). A colostomy decompresses the bowel, relieves symptoms and can be closed later

Caecum/ascending colon
• Right hemicolectomy is appropriate during elective or emergency surgery

Adjuvant therapy
• Chemotherapy does not appear to improve survival, but further trials are in progress
• Radiotherapy is only useful for fixed rectal tumours which cannot be cured by resection. The value of pre- versus postoperative radiotherapy is being compared

Recurrent or inoperable disease
• An aggressive approach to detection and treatment of recurrence is justified in young patients
• Surveillance colonoscopy after surgical removal of the primary tumour is advised for younger patients, since there is an increased risk of recurrent polyps and cancer. Suitable intervals are 6 months after surgery, then at 3-year intervals, although the benefit remains unproven
• Resection of isolated hepatic metastases in young patients should be considered, at a specialist centre, because survival may be improved. Ultrasound screening, probably every 6–12 months, is needed for detection of metastases

___

- Carcinoembryonic antigen measurements are unreliable, because they fail to rise in a third with recurrent tumour, but are helpful if positive
- Symptoms of obstruction or recurrent rectal bleeding must be relieved even when a cure is not possible. Local ethanol injection or laser photocoagulation may help, but palliative surgery may be needed

Screening
Screening aims to detect cancer at a treatable stage. The target groups and method of screening remain controversial.

Screening by colonoscopy every 3 years is widely accepted for high-risk groups (such as patients with polyps, familial adenomatous polyposis, cancer family syndrome (p. 292), a first-degree relative with colorectal cancer aged <45 years, extensive ulcerative colitis (p. 259), or after resection of colorectal cancer). These represent a minority of all patients with colorectal cancer. Faecal occult blood screening in these high-risk groups is not worthwhile, because it has a low negative predictive value.

General population screening selects motivated patients and may detect less aggressive tumours earlier, without altering the outcome, but does appear to identify more resectable cancers. Good trials are in progress.

A plan for average-risk patients who enquire about screening is shown in Fig. 9.2.

Prognosis
Histopathological criteria of spread and differentiation are the most useful guide. Adaptations of Duke's classification are most widely used.
- Dukes' A (tumour limited to the bowel wall)—82% 5-year survival
- Dukes' B (tumour penetrating the wall, but no lymph nodes)—62% 5-year survival
- Dukes' C (lymph node involvement)—30% 5-year survival
- Well differentiated tumours have a better prognosis than poorly differentiated tumours at any stage

Other factors
- Age—older patients have a higher operative mortality. Young

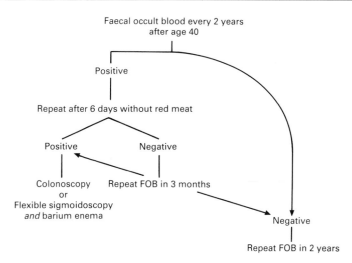

Fig. 9.2 Colorectal cancer screening for patients not in a high-risk group
FOB = faecal occult blood.

patients may have more aggressive tumours, but this is disputed
• Sex—women have a better prognosis than men
• Duration of symptoms—inversely related to prognosis, except in obstruction, when survival is halved, or perforation, when 5-year survival is <10%

9.4 Colonic diverticular disease
Colonic diverticula are present in 50% aged >70 years in Europe, but most are asymptomatic. The term 'diverticular disease' is in common usage, but is hardly appropriate for describing the presence of uncomplicated diverticula. 'Colonic diverticulosis' avoids the connotations of the word 'disease', which may worry patients unnecessarily. Symptomatic diverticulosis may become complicated by inflammation or abscess (diverticulitis).

Asymptomatic diverticulosis
• Diverticula can be considered an incidental finding on barium enema when there are no abdominal symptoms (a patient being investigated for iron deficiency anaemia, for instance), or when symptoms that are present are uncharacteristic

---

Symptomatic diverticulosis

Symptoms
Colonic symptoms in the elderly are more likely to be due to diverticulosis than irritable bowel syndrome, but colorectal cancer must always be considered. Common features are:
• Colicky left iliac fossa pain relieved by defaecation, in regular episodes continuing for weeks or months. Pain is sometimes central or in the right iliac fossa, and persistent
• Constipation (which is thought to cause diverticula), with pellety stools, often covered in mucus
• Bloating and flatulence
• Dyspepsia is common, but is more likely to be due to a coexisting hiatal hernia and gall stones ('Saint's triad')
• Rectal bleeding, recently altered bowel habit, right-sided or upper abdominal pain, diarrhoea, or tenesmus must not be attributed to diverticulosis without investigation

Diagnosis
• Characteristic symptoms, normal blood tests (full blood count, ESR) and diverticula on barium enema (Fig. 9.3) are sufficient for diagnosis
• Rigid sigmoidoscopy should always be performed before a barium enema, because the rectum can be more closely examined. A biopsy should always taken, because histology may show disease (Crohn's disease, microscopic colitis) even when the rectal mucosa looks normal
• Flexible sigmoidoscopy alone is sufficient for diagnosis when symptoms are typical, and avoids the need for both rigid sigmoidoscopy and a barium enema. It may not be readily available and is inadequate if there is anaemia, because the whole colon must be examined
• Colonoscopy is only indicated when a barium enema shows distortion of the bowel wall in association with diverticula (Fig. 9.3), but should be performed by an experienced colonoscopist because of the risk of perforation. Carcinoma, Crohn's disease, ischaemia or a pericolic abscess from diverticulitis may be impossible to distinguish radiologically from muscle hypertrophy or stricture

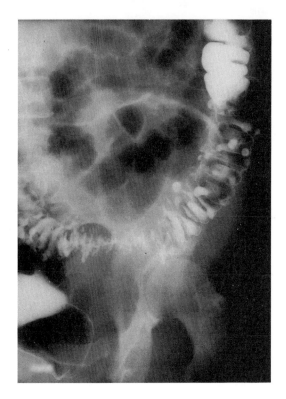

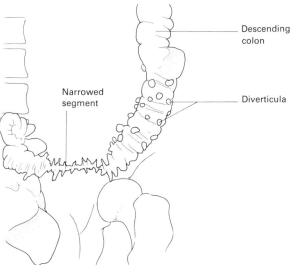

Fig. 9.3 Radiological appearance of colonic diverticular disease. Barium enema showing a narrowed segment in the sigmoid colon due to diverticular disease; thickened muscle is compressing the necks of the diverticula and the redundant mucosa is restricting the lumen.

Management

• Increasing dietary fibre (p. 385) relieves pain if constipation is present, but existing diverticula do not regress
• Antispasmodic agents (dicyclomine 10–20 mg, mebeverine 135 mg, or peppermint oil 2 capsules three times daily) may help pain
• Stimulant laxatives should be avoided for treating constipation because these may increase colonic pressure and provoke pain. Osmotic laxatives (lactulose 30–100 ml/day) are preferred

Complicated diverticulosis

Diverticulosis may be complicated by inflammation or abscess (diverticulitis), perforation, bleeding, or obstruction.

Inflammation

Diverticulitis is recognized by pain, fever, leucocytosis and an elevated ESR. Prior symptoms of diverticulosis are often absent. Colonoscopy is contraindicated in the acute stage, but may be done when symptoms settle if diverticulitis cannot be distinguished from a carcinoma or Crohn's disease on the barium enema.
• Pericolic abscess is suggested when a mass is palpable. It may present with obstruction
• Perforation may present with peritonitis, pelvic, paracolic, or subphrenic abscess. Chronic pyrexia, ill health and weight loss may be the only features in the elderly or debilitated
• Portal pyaemia with liver abscesses is often due to diverticulitis in the elderly
• Fistulae (vesicocolic, ileocolic) are more commonly due to diverticulitis than Crohn's disease in the elderly, but are rare
    Management of diverticulitis needs admission to hospital, blood cultures, intravenous fluids, antibiotics (metronidazole 500 mg and cefuroxime 750 mg three times daily) and analgesia (intramuscular pethidine 50–100 mg every 4 h). Osmotic laxatives (lactulose 30 ml/day) are often needed to avoid, or treat, constipation. Surgery is necessary for abscesses, perforation or fistulae.

Bleeding

Recurrent rectal bleeding is uncommon and usually occurs without other symptoms of diverticulosis. Iron deficiency anaemia is never due to uncomplicated diverticulosis. Carcinoma, ulcerative colitis, Crohn's disease and angiodysplasia must be excluded by colonoscopy, but angiography during active bleeding may be necessary to detect the site of bleeding (p. 18). Management is initially conservative (p. 18) unless the patient is on anticoagulants, when fresh frozen plasma is needed. Subsequent anticoagulation then needs a sound reason (such as a prosthetic valve).

Obstruction
Colonic obstruction may be due to inflammation or a fibrotic stricture, but carcinoma co-existing with diverticulosis is more common.

Indications for surgery
Surgery is only indicated for complications of diverticulosis (Table 9.2). Colectomy or myotomy for symptomatic diverticulosis is very rarely necessary, and only after medical treatment has been vigorously tried and other causes of symptoms have been excluded.

Table 9.2 Indications for surgery in colonic diverticulosis

Infection:
recurrent diverticulitis
paracolic or pelvic abscess
peritonitis
Perforation
Fistulae:
colovesical
colovaginal
ileocolic
Obstruction
Major haemorrhage

• Recurrent diverticulitis is unusual, but can be cured by resection and primary anastomosis between attacks
• Abscesses are best localized by ultrasound and drained percutaneously. Colonic resection is rarely necessary, because perforated diverticula causing an abscess usually seal spontaneously
• Patients with perforated diverticula and peritonitis need adequate rehydration and parenteral antibiotics (metronidazole 500 mg and cefuroxime 750 mg three times daily) before emergency

laparotomy. Resection of the affected colon and a double-barrelled colostomy is probably best, but when it is not possible to mobilize an inflamed mass of sigmoid colon, resection with closure of the rectal stump and a colostomy (Hartmann's procedure) is then necessary
• Fistulae are treated by sigmoid colectomy and closure of the bladder or vaginal connection
• Obstruction can be managed conservatively if incomplete (p. 33), but total colonic obstruction needs decompression by a transverse colostomy, with later resection of the stricture

Prognosis
• Treating symptomatic diverticulosis with increased dietary fibre appears to reduce the complication rate to around 5%

9.5   Intestinal ischaemia
Intestinal ischaemia includes small intestinal ischaemia, but this is rare compared to ischaemic colitis. Vascular disease may be acute or chronic, but does not always involve arterial occlusion. Focal ischaemia (due to vasculitis) or venous infarction are rare.

Vascular anatomy
The gut is supplied by the coeliac axis, superior mesenteric artery and inferior mesenteric artery (Fig. 9.4). The stomach and rectum (supplied by coeliac axis and inferior mesenteric vessels, respectively) are well protected by oesophageal and internal iliac anastomoses respectively. Branches of the superior and inferior mesenteric arteries anastomose through a variable marginal artery, which means that the splenic flexure is at particular risk from ischaemia. Ischaemic colitis is usually microvascular, with no apparent large-vessel disease.

Causes
Although there are many causes (Table 9.3, p. 306), intestinal ischaemia is rare and there are only four clinical syndromes: acute, chronic and focal intestinal ischaemia, which usually affect the small intestine, and ischaemic colitis.

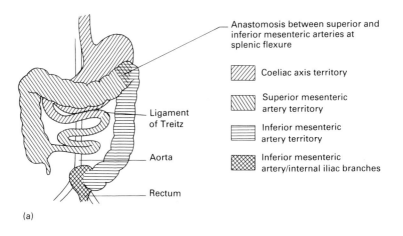

Anastomosis between superior and
inferior mesenteric arteries at
splenic flexure

▨ Coeliac axis territory

▧ Superior mesenteric
   artery territory

☰ Inferior mesenteric
   artery territory

▨ Inferior mesenteric
   artery/internal iliac branches

Ligament
of Treitz

Aorta

Rectum

(a)

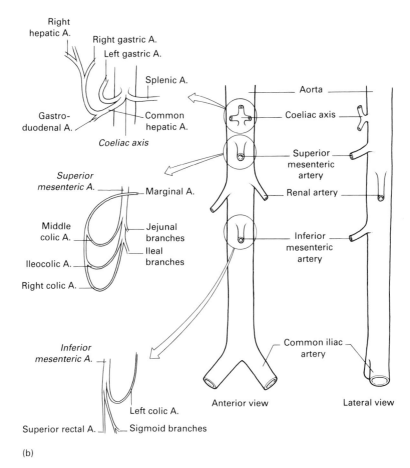

Right
hepatic A.

Right gastric A.

Left gastric A.

Splenic A.

Gastro-
duodenal A.

Common
hepatic A.

Coeliac axis

*Superior
mesenteric A.*

Marginal A.

Middle
colic A.

Jejunal
branches

Ileal
branches

Ileocolic A.

Right colic A.

*Inferior
mesenteric A.*

Left colic A.

Superior rectal A.

Sigmoid branches

Aorta

Coeliac axis

Superior
mesenteric
artery

Renal artery

Inferior
mesenteric
artery

Common iliac
artery

Anterior view

Lateral view

(b)

Fig. 9.4 Mesenteric vascular supply. (a) Vascular territories. (b) Vascular
anatomy.

9.5   Intestinal ischaemia

Table 9.3 Causes of intestinal ischaemia

Common	Uncommon	Rare
Atheroma:	Systemic emboli:	Thrombosis:
stenosis	atrial thrombus	polycythaemia
thrombosis	bacterial endocarditis	sickle cell
embolization	Non-occlusive infarction:	oral contraceptive
	cardiac failure	antithrombin III deficiency
	septicaemia	protein C deficiency
	trauma	microvascular
	anaphylaxis	Vasculitis:
		rheumatoid arthritis
		polyarteritis nodosa
		systemic lupus
		Takayasu's disease
		Behçet's disease
		Miscellaneous:
		aortic dissection
		infiltration by tumour
		iatrogenic (catheters)

Acute ischaemia (see p. 30)

Chronic ischaemia
Chronic small intestinal ischaemia is *very* rare.

Clinical features
- Abdominal pain 20–60 min after eating ('mesenteric angina')
- Weight loss, because the patient becomes afraid to eat
- Audible epigastric bruit, but this is often absent and may be normal in thin adults

Management
The diagnosis should be suspected in an elderly arteriopath when other causes of post-prandial pain and weight loss have been excluded. Mesenteric angiography may show a stenosis at the origin of the superior mesenteric artery, but reveals nothing about arterial flow. Doppler ultrasound may be helpful, if available.

Nifedipine 10 mg before meals can be tried, but often has little effect. Small, frequent meals are advisable. Arterial reconstructive surgery should be restricted to specialist units.

9.5 Intestinal ischaemia

Focal ischaemia

Trauma, radiation, vasculitis, or drugs (enteric-coated potassium) may cause focal ischaemic damage. These cause a small intestinal stricture that presents as subacute obstruction; bleeding or perforation rarely occur. Diagnosis is made by small bowel radiology. Management is surgical, to exclude other causes (Table 7.10, p. 240) and to relieve the obstruction.

Strangulated herniae also cause focal ischaemia, but present acutely. The exception is a Richter's hernia (ischaemia of part of the herniated bowel, which subsequently returns to the abdominal cavity), because initial symptoms may resolve temporarily.

Ischaemic colitis

Ischaemic colitis can be acute, chronic or focal, but is classified separately because it is more common and presents differently from small intestinal ischaemia. It is often left sided

Clinical features

Patients are usually elderly arteriopaths with a history of myocardial infarction, peripheral vascular disease or hypertension.
• Diarrhoea may precede rectal bleeding, or vice versa. The onset of either is usually sudden
• Abdominal pain is usual but not invariable, unlike small intestinal ischaemia. It is often left sided
• Toxic dilatation occurs rarely
• Symptoms may occur for days or weeks before presentation, although patients with colonic gangrene present within hours and cannot be distinguished clinically from those with acute small intestinal ischaemia

Diagnosis

• Sigmoidoscopy shows a normal rectal mucosa and blood, or profuse blood-stained mucus, coming from above. The appearances may look like Crohn's disease or ulcerative colitis, with pronounced mucosal oedema, but colonoscopy is not advised because of the risk of perforation
• Biopsies show ulceration and a polymorphonuclear infiltrate. Haemosiderin-laden macrophages are characteristic, but uncommon

9.5 Intestinal ischaemia

• A plain abdominal X-ray often shows an abnormal segment, usually at the splenic flexure, with mucosal oedema ('thumb-printing', Fig. 9.5)

• A frequent dilemma is to distinguish ischaemic colitis from acute Crohn's colitis (Table 9.4). It is normally possible to exclude ulcerative colitis, because the rectum is not inflamed, but occasionally the rectal mucosa can look congested

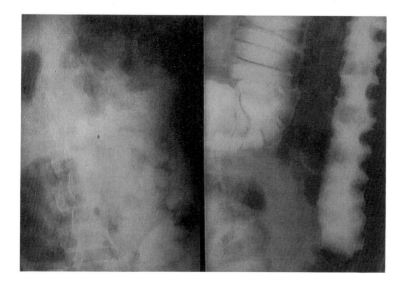

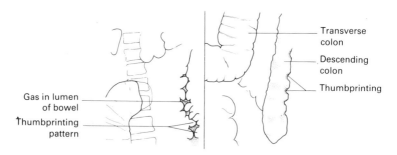

Fig. 9.5 Radiological appearance of ischaemic colitis. Radiographs in acute ischaemic colitis. In the plain film (left) gas outlines smooth indentations of the mucosa in the descending colon—thumbprinting. This is shown on barium enema (right).

9.5 Intestinal ischaemia

- An unprepared, single contrast barium enema may help resolve the dilemma, although the radiological features are often visible on a plain abdominal X-ray. Air contrast barium enema in the acute stage may increase the risk of perforation, and colonoscopy is contraindicated if there is peritonism

Table 9.4 Features favouring a diagnosis of ischaemic colitis

History:
   age >60 years
   vascular disease (angina, hypertension, previous myocardial infarction, claudication)
   diabetes
   onset with sudden pain, then bleeding

Signs:
   no abdominal mass
   no perianal or extraintestinal features of Crohn's disease

Radiology:
   single affected segment
   often localized around the splenic flexure
   thumb-printing (mucosal oedema, distinguished from mucosal islands by being larger)
   symmetrical stricture

Endoscopy:
   variable appearance, from mild reddening, local ulceration to gangrene

Histology:
   intramucosal haemorrhage
   fibrosis
   haemosiderin (uncommon)

Management

It is often not possible to distinguish colonic gangrene from acute small intestinal ischaemia as the cause of an abdominal catastrophe, but resuscitation with intravenous fluids and laparotomy are indicated for both conditions (p. 30).

Resolution is the rule for most patients with ischaemic colitis. Intravenous fluids and transfusion to maintain the haemoglobin at 10 g/dl are indicated, until bleeding, pain and diarrhoea improve. Deterioration is an indication for blood cultures, intravenous antibiotics and plain abdominal X-ray; if colonic dilatation has developed (diameter >6.0 cm), colectomy is indicated.

Most recover completely and recurrence is surprisingly rare. Follow-up barium enema is unnecessary if symptoms resolve. About 25% develop a colonic stricture, which needs resection. Colonoscopic dilatation of a localized stricture may be an alternative at a specialist centre, because these patients are often a poor operative risk.

9.6 Anorectal conditions

Haemorrhoids
Haemorrhoids are dilatations of the normal rectal submucosal venous plexus, which develop due to straining at stool. They are often associated with redundant mucosa or perianal skin. The traditional classifications into internal or external, first-, second- or third-degree haemorrhoids are better replaced by descriptive terms (such as bleeding, temporarily or permanently prolapsed, thrombosed).

Bleeding
• Bright red blood often spurts round the pan after defaecation, or smears the outside of the stool. This type of bleeding does *not* exclude a rectal carcinoma or proctitis
• Anaemia should never be attributed to haemorrhoidal bleeding without investigation

Haemorrhoidal prolapse
• Prolapse is recognized by the patient, but has to be distinguished from a polyp, rectal prolapse or skin tag by rectal examination
• Permanent prolapse often causes discomfort from venous engorgement, or mucous discharge and pruritis. Pain does not occur without a fissure, thrombosis or infection

Thrombosis
• Rapid onset; severe perianal pain may take several days to resolve
• A perianal haematoma is due to thrombosis of a venous saccule

Management
• A serious cause of rectal bleeding *must* be excluded by sigmoidoscopy, and colonoscopy, or flexible sigmoidoscopy with a barium enema if aged >40 years

• A high-fibre diet is suitable for most patients, to soften the stool (p. 385)
• Persistent hard stools suggest that dietary fibre intake remains insufficient (possibly due to poor tolerance) and can be temporarily relieved by lactulose 30–100 ml/day
• Surgical intervention is only indicated for persistent symptoms (Table 9.5)

Table 9.5 Management of haemorrhoids

Situation	Management
All patients	High-fibre diet (p. 385)
Severe bleeding	Local sclerosant injection, repeated after 6 weeks
Prolapse	Elastic band ligation
Thrombosis	Local ice pack to relieve oedema Lignocaine 1% gel (no more than 3 days) Lactulose 30–100 ml/day Injection or ligation after recovery
Recurrence	Haemorrhoidectomy, if injection or ligation is unsuccessful (<10%)

Fissures and fistulae

Anal fissure
• A linear breach in the anal mucosa, often associated with a skin tag (sentinel pile) or anal polyp
• Pain during defaecation is characteristic, often with bleeding
• Diagnosis is made by inspection of the anal margin when gently parting the buttocks. Rectal examination is painful, but possible after applying lignocaine 2% gel perianally and into the anal canal by means of a bacteriology swab
• Management is directed at relieving constipation (dietary fibre, with lactulose). Surgical division of the internal anal sphincter (lateral sphincterotomy), or anal stretch, is indicated when fissures recur

Perianal fistulae
• Perianal fistulae result from chronic infection. Acute infection causes an abscess

9.6   Anorectal conditions

• Most are non-specific, but an underlying cause should be suspected for extensive, bilateral or recurrent fistulae. Crohn's disease, diabetes, or tuberculosis should be considered
• Types of fistulae are shown in Fig. 9.6
• The fistula track should be identified with a probe and sinogram before surgery

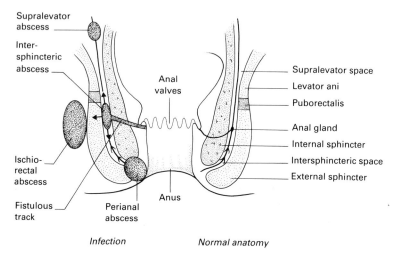

Fig. 9.6 Perianal fistulae and abscesses. Infection starts in the anal glands and may spread vertically, horizontally, or circumferentially. An abscess is an acute, localized collection of pus, whilst a fistula, which connects two epithelial surfaces, is the chronic phase of the same disease process.

Pruritus ani

Perianal itching has many causes (Table 9.6). Questions about cleansing, rectal or vaginal discharge, local ointments (for 'piles'), skin disorders, or family members with the condition are relevant.

Examination must include inspection for skin disease, digital assessment of sphincter tone and proctosigmoidoscopy.

Urine testing for glycosuria, Sellotape slide for threadworm (*Enterobius vermicularis*) and skin scrape for fungi are often helpful. Skin biopsy, high vaginal swab or anorectal manometry (for sphincter dysfunction) are rarely indicated.

Treatment is directed at the cause. Careful washing after defaecation is most important. Topical hydrocortisone 1% twice daily for 2 weeks provides symptomatic relief, but reassessment rather than re-prescription is indicated for persistent symptoms.

Table 9.6 Causes of pruritus ani

Common	Uncommon	Rare
Poor hygiene	Rectal discharge	Eczema
Haemorrhoids	(sphincter dysfunction)	Lichen sclerosus
Fissure	Fistula	Paget's disease
Threadworm	Fungal infection (diabetes)	Bowen's disease
	Contact dermatitis	Vaginal discharge
	Spurious diarrhoea	

Proctalgia fugax

Paroxysmal perineal pain lasting a few minutes, often felt deep in the rectum or after defaecation and perhaps waking the patient at night, has no organic cause. It is common in house officers and other people under stress. Rectal or puborectalis spasm have been suggested as causes. Avoidance of constipation and temazepam 10–20 mg at night may be helpful.

9.7 Investigation of iron deficiency anaemia

Patients with iron deficiency anaemia, often detected during a full blood count for non-specific symptoms, are a common gastroenterological problem. Iron deficiency should *not* be attributed to an uncomplicated peptic ulcer, hiatus hernia, NSAIDs, oesophagitis, or haemorrhoids without investigation of the colon. Iron deficiency in post-menopausal women, or men beyond middle age, suggests a caecal neoplasm until proved otherwise.

Investigation of the oesophagus, stomach, duodenum and whole colon is needed, and it is most convenient to perform upper gastrointestinal endoscopy and colonoscopy during one visit to the endoscopy unit. Otherwise initial investigation is guided by the symptoms; rectal bleeding is an indication for rectal examination, sigmoidoscopy and barium enema, whereas if dyspepsia is present, then upper gastrointestinal endoscopy is reasonable first.

For asymptomatic patients, or those with non-specific symptoms, the following plan is suggested.

9.7 Investigation of iron deficiency anaemia

Essential investigations

History
A careful history is mandatory. Ask about:
- Evidence of bleeding—menstrual loss in women
- Diet—frequency of meat intake, vegetarian (no meat), vegan (no dairy products either)
- Weight loss—suggests carcinoma, malabsorption
- Diarrhoea—coeliac disease, Crohn's disease
- Easy bruising—bleeding diathesis

Examination
- Signs of iron deficiency—cheilosis, koilonychia (see Table 13.4, p. 374)
- Mouth and lips—for telangiectases (hereditary haemorrhagic telangiectasia can present as iron deficiency in adults)
- Abdominal mass—neoplasm, Crohn's disease
- Rectal—faecal occult blood
- Sigmoidoscopy and rectal biopsy (p. 246)

Blood tests
A hypochromic (MCH <27 pg), microcytic (MCV <80 fl) anaemia (Hb <14 g/dl (men), <12 g/dl (women)) can be due to chronic disease, thalassaemia trait, or sideroblastic anaemia, as well as iron deficiency.
- Full blood count and film—hypochromic microcytosis and target cells when severe. Thrombocytosis indicates inflammation, or acute-on-chronic bleeding. Occasional macrocytes (dimorphic film) or Howell–Jolly bodies (hyposplenism) suggest coeliac disease
- Serum iron and total iron binding capacity (TIBC)—low serum iron (<10 μmol/l) and high TIBC (>70 μmol/l) confirms iron deficiency. Low iron and low TIBC (<45 μmol/l) suggests chronic disease. Normal values suggest a haemoglobinopathy and is an indication for measuring HbA$_2$ (normal <2%). Serum ferritin should be measured in complex cases (such as diagnosing iron deficiency in chronic disease)
- Folate, vitamin B$_{12}$, albumin—if malabsorption suspected
- Prothrombin time (13–15 sec) or ratio (INR 1.0 : 1.1)—should be within 30% of normal range before jejunal biopsy

9.7   Investigation of iron deficiency anaemia

Upper gastrointestinal endoscopy
• Preferable to a barium meal, because biopsies can be taken
• Low duodenal biopsies should always be taken to exclude coeliac disease at an early stage if the endoscopy does not reveal the cause of iron deficiency

Colonoscopy
• Convenient to perform immediately after upper gastrointestinal endoscopy, under the same sedation
• Allows biopsies to be taken of any colonic lesions and the cause to be treated if bleeding is due to polyps or angiodysplasia

Barium enema
• Only if colonoscopy is not readily available, because patients will be subjected to a further procedure (colonoscopy and polypectomy), should polyps be detected
• Good views of the caecum are important to exclude a neoplasm

Further investigations
The cause of iron deficiency anaemia which has not been diagnosed after the investigations above can present a very difficult problem. Before repeating any of the investigations, it is wise to retake the history and to review the results, to ensure that obvious causes (dietary insufficiency, menstrual loss) or pitfalls (haemoglobinopathy) have not been overlooked.

For patients who are asymptomatic, it is then reasonable to stop iron therapy and to repeat the full blood count after 3–6 months; if anaemia recurs, then further investigation is warranted.

For symptomatic patients, those needing repeat transfusions, or in whom there is clear evidence of gastrointestinal blood loss (recurrent rectal bleeding or positive faecal occult blood), then the following investigations are suggested.

Colonoscopy
• Good preparation is essential if angiodysplasia or telangiectasia are to be seen, usually in the ileocaecal region

9.7 Investigation of iron deficiency anaemia

Small bowel radiology
• Crohn's disease is usually associated with a high platelet count and raised ESR, but occasionally presents with iron deficiency and weight loss, especially in adolescents

Bone marrow
• Sideroblastic anaemia should be excluded, after discussion with the haematologists

^{51}Cr-labelled red cell scan
• Chronic blood loss is occasionally located to one region of the intestine (proximal or distal colon, or small intestine). Careful colonoscopy, or surgery and operative endoscopy may then be indicated to identify the vascular malformation that usually causes the bleeding

Meckel's diverticulum scan
• Bleeding from ulcerated, heterotopic gastric tissue rarely causes anaemia in adolescents or adults. A diverticulum may also be visible on small bowel radiology

Laparotomy
• Laparotomy is rarely helpful unless there are clues to the source of blood loss beforehand. Referral to a specialist centre is advisable before 'blind' laparotomy

10 Irritable Bowel Syndrome

10.1 Clinical features

The term 'irritable bowel syndrome' is used to described a heterogeneous group of abdominal symptoms for which no organic cause can be found. This does not mean that the symptoms are all psychological; most are probably due to disorders of bowel motility which are poorly defined because diagnostic tests are lacking. Although the group is distinguished by the lack of pathology or mortality, the morbidity from persistent symptoms is often substantial.

Typical features
The diagnosis can be made with confidence if five or more features are present:
- Age 20–40 years
- Abdominal pain
- Bloating
- Altered bowel habit (constipation alternating with looseness)
- Pellety or ribbon-like stools
- Duration >6 months
- Obsessional personality
- Unremarkable examination, although general abdominal tenderness is common
- Insufflation of air on sigmoidoscopy reproduces pain
  Less common manifestations:
- Nausea
- Dyspareunia
- Pain in the back, thigh or chest
- Urinary frequency
- Depression

Symptom patterns
Symptoms occasionally follow an episode of acute gastroenteritis ('post-dysenteric irritable bowel syndrome'). More commonly there is no precipitating factor, although stress frequently exacerbates the condition.

Predominant pain
- Central, right or left iliac fossa pain, less commonly in several sites. It is often poorly localized
- Daily pain alone for >3 months is rarely organic

10   Irritable Bowel Syndrome

10.1 Clinical features

- Persistent ache, often with sharp exacerbations
- Relieved by defaecation, but sometimes follows defaecation
- Worse at times of stress, or during menstruation in women

Predominant diarrhoea
- Morning frequency, often with urgency
- Usually with pain

Predominant constipation
- Especially women
- Sense of incomplete evacuation (tenesmus)
- Associated with the passage of mucus, but never blood

Non-ulcer dyspepsia (p. 75)

Markers of organic disease (Table 10.1)

Table 10.1 Markers distinguishing organic disease from irritable bowel syndrome

Age >40 years
History <6 months
Periodic pain, with episodes of complete relief
Anorexia
Weight loss
Mouth ulcers
Rectal bleeding
Abnormal investigations

Investigations
The aim is to exclude organic disease by the minimum number of appropriate tests.

All patients
- Urine test for protein or blood caused by renal tract disease
- Full blood count, ESR and liver enzymes will identify many organic causes of similar symptoms
- Stool culture if diarrhoea is present
- Sigmoidoscopy and rectal biopsy are always indicated.
Proctoscopy, to identify anterior mucosal prolapse, is always indicated if there is a sensation of incomplete evacuation after defaecation (p. 289)

Indications for a barium enema
• Typical features with any marker of organic disease (Table 10.1) (especially if age >40 years)
• Typical features with rectal bleeding at any age
• Barium enema may be deferred until diet or drugs are found to be ineffective if the history is <6 months and age <40 years

Further investigations
Additional tests should be avoided unless there are unusual features or markers of organic disease; there is no need to arrange an ultrasound just because the pain is in the right upper quadrant, nor an endoscopy just because the pain is epigastric. Gall stones, hiatus hernia or colonic diverticulosis may be incidental to the patient's symptoms.
• Endoscopy is justified when the pain is clearly related to meals (dyspepsia), retrosternal (heartburn) or periodic
• Ultrasound of the pancreas and biliary tree is appropriate when upper abdominal pain is episodic and the endoscopy is normal. Pelvic ultrasound is indicated for lower abdominal pain related to periods
• Small bowel radiology is necessary when there is weight loss or abdominal pain and diarrhoea, to exclude Crohn's disease
• Diarrhoea without pain is investigated as in Fig. 7.1 (p. 211). Mild symptoms from hypolactasia, coeliac disease, or small intestinal bacterial overgrowth may be misattributed to an irritable bowel, especially after an episode of gastroenteritis
• Motility tests (such as transit studies or intestinal manometry) are not diagnostic of irritable bowel syndrome, probably because the condition represents more than one motility disorder. Many show increased sensitivity to rectal balloon distension, but this also occurs in proctitis and other diseases

10.2 Management

Approach
Taking the history and examining the patient in a careful, sympathetic and thorough manner makes subsequent explanation and reassurance very much easier. The 'there's nothing wrong, it's all in the mind' approach helps nobody.

10.2 Management

Explanation

A provisional diagnosis and initial explanation can usually be given on the first visit. Helpful descriptions (unfortunately without much objective pathophysiological evidence) include:

• Explaining that small volume, hard faeces cause the bowel muscle to contract harder

• Describing the pain as bowel spasm, similar to muscle cramp

• Suggesting that the bowel is more sensitive than normal, and that some foods may trigger spasm in many patients

• Describing the typical features of an irritable bowel (often recognized by the patient, with relief) and relation to stress in some people (like pre-exam diarrhoea)

• A diagram illustrating colonic segmentation (haustra) may assist explanation

On a subsequent visit, with the results of normal investigations, it is important to make a definitive diagnosis of irritable bowel syndrome and explain the likely pattern of symptoms.

• Symptoms often continue for months or years, but ultimately resolve

• Symptoms can be relieved, but not always cured

• There is no risk of cancer or serious disease

• Explain that there *is* something wrong, but that it is not a disease and the bowel is 'out of tune' or 'more sensitive' than normal

Diet

Food intolerance

• Many patients have a specific food intolerance (terminology explained on p. 230) that can be reproducibly identified by an exclusion diet (p. 390). An exclusion diet improves symptoms in about two-thirds of patients

• Once the food has been identified (often lettuce, onions, chocolate or additives), avoidance brings relief. The food can often be reintroduced without relapse after 12 months, for unexplained reasons

• Coffee, tea or alcohol may exacerbate diarrhoea

High-fibre diet

• Indicated when constipation is a prominent feature

- Fibre intake should be increased gradually. Mixed unrefined sources of fibre (fruit, vegetables, wholemeal bread) are more palatable than adding bran to food (p. 287), but may not be sufficient
- A high-fibre diet (p. 385) may make flatulence, diarrhoea or bloating worse

Drugs

Drugs are only used to treat symptoms and none are universally successful. About one-third of patients will get better on any particular drug. Many patients prefer to manage without drugs. The efficacy of one drug in an individual often varies with time.

Pain

Antispasmodics have an anticholinergic action and are less likely to work when constipation predominates.

- Mebeverine 135 mg three times daily is dramatically effective in a few, gives some relief to many, but may have no effect. Alternative drugs (alverine citrate 60 mg, or dicyclomine 20 mg, three times daily) may help different patients
- Peppermint oil (1–2 capsules three times daily) is useful for patients who have constipation and bloating, since it has no anticholinergic action, or those who dislike 'drugs'
- It is worth trying different drugs, because benefit is often temporary, or unpredictable

Constipation

- A high-fibre diet is preferable to 1–2 tablespoons of coarse bran daily, but this can be tried if the diet does not produce a soft stool
- An osmotic laxative (magnesium sulphate 10–30 ml/day, or lactulose 30–100 ml/day) can be added if bran alone is ineffective. Stimulant laxatives (p. 287) may make pain worse

Diarrhoea

- Loperamide, up to 12 mg/day, relieves frequency and urgency
- Codeine phosphate is best avoided, because long-term use may cause dependency
- Amitriptyline 10–25 mg three times daily may help persistent diarrhoea, partly through its anticholinergic effect

---

• Diarrhoea that is not readily controlled is an indication for investigation (Fig. 7.1, p. 211)

Other drugs
• Dyspeptic symptoms may respond to metoclopramide or antacids (p. 76)
• Anxiolytics or antidepressants may benefit some patients

Prognosis
• Symptoms disappear or improve in about half after 12 months; <5% become worse and the remainder remain unchanged
• Intermittent symptoms are likely, but these are usually due to identifiable stress or a change in diet and can be controlled
• There is no mortality

10.3 Clinical dilemmas

Persistent symptoms
• Usually due to a failure to treat constipation adequately, or to alter the diet
• Personality is important. Psychologically distressed patients select themselves by presenting for treatment. Explanations to provide insight and assistance in coping with symptoms are more likely to reduce visits than a dismissive approach. Clinical depression may be present and should be treated
• Further investigation is not justified unless the symptom pattern has changed or clinical signs (such as weight loss) have developed

Symptoms with identifiable disease
• Features of the irritable bowel syndrome are not uncommon in patients with identifiable gastrointestinal disorders (such as gall stones, colonic diverticula, hiatus hernia and even ulcerative colitis)
• Whilst judgement is necessary to decide which symptoms are related to the known disease, continuous abdominal discomfort, bloating or symptoms that do not fit with the common pattern of the disease are more likely to be due to an irritable bowel and are best treated with sympathetic explanation and reassurance

11 Gastrointestinal Infections

11.1 Acute gastroenteritis

Gastroenteritis is caused by infection within the lumen of the gastrointestinal tract which usually results in diarrhoea and abdominal pain of acute onset and short duration, frequently with vomiting. It is often not possible or necessary to identify the organism, but it is important to recognize when investigation is indicated (p. 329).

Causes

Viruses are the commonest cause of gastroenteritis worldwide, whilst many bacteria exert their effect through toxins (Table 11.1); others are invasive. In adults in the UK, the causes and approximate frequencies are:

- Non-specific (culture-negative)—50%
- *Campylobacter* sp.—20%
- *Salmonella* sp.—15% (zoonotic organisms, spread from infected animals to man; *not* those causing enteric fever)
- *Shigella* sp.—5%
- *Cl. difficile*—5%
- Miscellaneous—5%

Table 11.1 Common causes of acute gastroenteritis

Bacterial	Viral	Toxins	Other
Salmonella sp.	Rotavirus	*E. coli*	*Giardia lamblia*
Shigella sp.*	Echovirus	*Staphylococcus aureus*	*Cryptosporidium* sp.
Campylobacter sp.	Norwalk	*Vibrio cholerae*	*Isospora belli*
Yersinia	agent	*Cl. difficile*	Alcohol[†]
*enterocolitica**		*Bacillus cereus*	Heavy metals[†]
*Cl. perfringens**		*Vibrio parahaemolyticus*	
E. coli		*Cl. botulinum*	
Aeromonas sp.			

* Action partly through toxin production.
[†]Symptoms may be similar to infective causes.

Clinical features

General

- History of travel, or eating unusual or suspect food (reheated chicken, seafood, take-away food, mass catering, conference dinners)
- The incubation period depends on the cause (see Table 11.2, p. 333)
- Other people are often affected

327

11.1 Acute gastroenteritis

- Diarrhoea—may be bloody (*Shigella* sp., *Campylobacter* sp., entero-invasive *E. coli,* Table 7.3, p. 214)
- Crampy abdominal pain—often severe in the young or elderly, especially with *Campylobacter* sp.
- Vomiting—particularly with *B. cereus*
- Systemic features (fever, headache, myalgia) are common in *Shigella* sp., *Campylobacter* sp., or *Y. enterocolitica* infections
- Resolution usually within 24–96 h

Susceptible patients
- Elderly or very young
- Hypogammaglobulinaemia
- Gastric hypoacidity—but does not appear to be a major problem with H_2 receptor antagonists, or proton pump inhibitors
- Total gastrectomy
- Immunocompromised—chemotherapy, AIDS (p. 343)
- Hyposplenic—invasive salmonellosis is more common

Sequelae
Sequelae are uncommon.
- Persistent diarrhoea may be due to:
  —secondary hypolactasia (especially post-viral, in children)
  —persistent infection (*Salmonella* sp., *Giardia lamblia,* immunocompromised)
  —unmasked latent disease (ulcerative colitis, coeliac disease)
  —post-dysenteric irritable bowel syndrome
- Asymptomatic carrier—following *Salmonella* sp. enteritis
- Reactive arthritis:
  —or a full Reiter's syndrome (asymmetrical polyarthritis, orogenital ulceration, conjunctivitis) can occur after *Y. enterocolitica* or *Campylobacter* sp. infection and may be confused with Crohn's disease or ulcerative colitis.
  —may also occur after *Salmonella* sp. and rarely after *Shigella* sp. infection in the susceptible
- Erythema nodosum:
  —after *Y. enterocolitica* or *Campylobacter* sp. infection
- Septicaemia:
  —in the immunocompromised, elderly or functionally hyposplenic (sickle cell disease, coeliac disease, splenectomy)
  —usually the cause of *Salmonella*-associated deaths
  —focal infections (cholecystitis, meningitis) are very rare

- Infective colitis:
  - —diffuse mucosal changes may mimic ulcerative colitis (p. 269), but glandular architecture is preserved
  - —*Campylobacter* sp., *Y. enterocolitica*, *Salmonella* sp., *Shigella* sp. or *E. coli* 0157 are often the cause
- Toxic dilatation:
  - —more commonly due to undiagnosed ulcerative colitis than *Campylobacter* sp., *Y. enterocolitica* or *E. coli* 0157 enteritis
- Neuropathy:
  - —may complicate *Cl. botulinum* (12–72 h), tetrahydropurine toxin (*G. breve*) from shellfish, or heavy-metal poisoning

Investigations

Uncomplicated acute gastroenteritis does not need investigation. When investigation is indicated (see below), stool culture and microscopy for cysts and trophozoites of *Giardia lamblia* and *Entamoeba histolytica* must be performed, with subsequent tests depending on the circumstances. Formed stool is unlikely to harbour pathogens. Investigation may be necessary for public health reasons (such as contact with a *Salmonella* sp. carrier in the food industry).

Indications for investigation

- Elderly
- More than one person affected
- Symptoms persisting for more than 4 days
- Associated bleeding, or other sequelae (above)
- Acute gastroenteritis in a residential establishment

Subsequent investigation

- Repeat stool culture if the first specimen is negative and symptoms persist, including faecal assay for *Cl. difficile* toxin
- Stool examination for virus by electron microscopy is not necessary, except in outbreaks of culture-negative diarrhoea, or in children
- Persistent diarrhoea (>3 weeks) is an indication for sigmoidoscopy, biopsy and referral to a gastroenterologist (Fig. 7.1, p. 211)
- Arthritis is an indication for joint aspiration if there is a fever or leucocytosis, rheumatoid factor to confirm a seronegative

arthropathy, antibodies to *Y. enterocolitica* and X-ray if a large
joint is involved
• Severely ill patients need admission to hospital, full blood count,
electrolytes to assess dehydration, blood cultures and plain
abdominal X-ray to exclude colonic dilatation (p. 36)

Management of specific infections

General
• Ensure adequate fluid intake
• Oral rehydration solutions (Dioralyte 500–3000 ml/day) for
the elderly, very young, dehydrated, or if diarrhoea is severe
• Meticulous hand hygiene and a personal towel
• Personal eating and drinking utensils probably do little to
prevent spread of infection, except in *Shigella* sp. infections, but
remains customary advice
• Antidiarrhoeal agents should be avoided if possible, although
clearance of pathogens is probably not delayed. Loperamide 4 mg,
then 2 mg after each loose motion, usually relieves diarrhoea if
symptom control is needed, but should never be given to children
because fatal paralytic ileus has been reported
• Metoclopramide 10 mg intramuscular injection up to three times
daily controls vomiting. Dystonic reactions (more common in the
elderly and adolescents) do not occur with rectal domperidone
30–60 mg three times daily
• Intravenous 0.9% saline, alternating with 5% dextrose, each with
20 mmol/l KCl, is indicated for rehydrating severely ill patients.
Judge adequate rehydration by good urine output, but watch for
possible overload in the elderly

Salmonella sp.
• Do *not* give antibiotics, unless there is extra-intestinal infection
• Septicaemia or invasive salmonellosis is treated with intravenous
ciprofloxacin 200 mg 12 hourly until the patient is eating, then oral
ciprofloxacin 750 mg twice daily for 4 weeks. Trimethoprim is the
alterative drug of choice
• Notify the disease (p. 346)
• Faecal excretion continues for 4–8 weeks and very rarely up to
6 months
• Repeat stool samples are advisable when infection could affect
the patient's job (food handlers, nurses). Three negative samples

are advised before restarting work in these occupations, but the risk from a patient with formed stools is extremely low. Good education in personal hygiene is equally important.
- There is no specific treatment for asymptomatic carriers. Gall stones may be a nidus of infection and cholecystectomy is then advisable, with antibiotic cover (intravenous amoxycillin 500 mg three times daily, or ciprofloxacin 200 mg over 30 min twice daily, for 48 h) to kill spilled organisms

Shigella sp.
- It is often possible to manage patients without antibiotics
- Amoxycillin 500 mg three times daily for 5 days (or ciprofloxacin 500 mg orally, or 200 mg over 30 min intravenously twice daily) for patients with virulent species (*Sh. shiga* or *Sh. dysenteriae*), the severely ill, or those at the extremes of life, in whom the dose of antibiotics should be adjusted
- Repeat stool samples are needed for the same reasons as *Salmonella* sp. enteritis
- Bacteria can survive for several hours on hands or towels. Outbreaks in residential establishments are an indication for disposable towels, and disinfection of hands, lavatory seats and taps

Campylobacter sp.
- Antibiotics are usually unnecessary. Erythromycin 500 mg four times daily for 1 week is probably only effective if started very early in the infection or in the severely ill. Ciprofloxacin (200 mg intravenously or 750 mg orally, twice daily) is an alternative
- Excretion often continues for weeks after recovery, but no treatment is needed.

Y. enterocolitica
- Stool culture is positive in the acute stage, but antibody titres are necessary to confirm the diagnosis if presentation is delayed for more than 2 weeks
- Tetracycline 250 mg four times daily for 2 weeks is indicated (but not in pregnancy, lactation or childhood), but this does not affect established post-infective arthritis

E. coli 0157
- Haemorrhagic colitis caused by this organism is treated with oral co-trimoxazole 960 mg twice daily, ciprofloxacin (as above), or

intravenous gentamicin 80 mg three times daily for severely ill patients

Cryptosporidium sp.
- No treatment is needed, since infection is usually self-limiting except in the immunocompromised (p. 346)

Giardia lamblia
- Tinidazole 2 g as a single dose (p. 228) or metronidazole 800 mg three times daily for 3 days. Metronidazole 2.4 g as a single dose also appears to be effective

Viruses
- Cause 60% of children's infectious diarrhoea; probably account for many episodes of culture-negative infectious diarrhoea in adults
- General measures alone are sufficient

Cl. difficile
- Causes acute or persistent diarrhoea after antibiotic treatment, sometimes with no bleeding or systemic upset. Pseudomembranous colitis represents the severe end of the spectrum (p. 280)
- Metronidazole 400 mg three times daily for 1 week is indicated. Vancomycin 125–250 mg four times daily for 1 week can be used for resistant or recurrent infections
- Other antibiotics must be stopped immediately, if possible

Other toxins
- Food poisoning (Table 11.2) and travellers' diarrhoea (p. 213) need general measures alone, except at the extremes of life

Food poisoning
Bacteria either produce a toxin in food and rapidly cause symptoms, or cause enteric infection after ingestion (Table 11.2). Other organisms may also be transmitted through food (hepatitis A, *Listeria monocytogenes*, parasites).

11.2 Other gastrointestinal infections

Post-infective and tropical enteropathy
A variety of infections, including *Giardia lamblia, E. coli, Klebsiella pneumoniae* and some viruses, may be followed by enterocyte

11.2 Other gastrointestinal infections

Table 11.2 Bacteria involved in food poisoning

Organism	Incubation (h)*	Food at risk	Duration
B. cereus†	1–5	Fried or reheated rice	12–24 h
Staph. aureus	2–6	Unrefrigerated meat, milk	6–24 h
V. parahaemolyticus	12–18 (<48)	Crabs, shellfish	2–5 days
Cl. perfringens	8–22	Cooled stewed meat	12–48 h
Salmonella sp.	12–24 (<48)	Undercooked poultry, eggs	1–7 days
Cl. botulinum‡	18–36 (<96)	Fermented canned food	months

* All times are very approximate.
† A non-vomiting type, causing diarrhoea, has a longer (8–20-h) incubation and may be acquired from ice cream, meat or vegetables.
‡ Paralysis progresses rapidly after initial gastrointestinal upset. Antitoxin (20 ml intramuscular injection and 20 ml intravenously after an intradermal test dose of 0.1 ml) is given when the diagnosis is suspected, with intravenous penicillin 2 MU four times daily to kill remaining bacteria. Ventilation is indicated if vital capacity <1000 ml.

damage that can be asymptomatic. It may progress to partial villous atrophy and cause malabsorption. Post-infective tropical malabsorption, or tropical sprue is not necessarily the direct sequel of infection by one of these specific organisms. Clinical features, investigations and treatment are covered on pp. 226–227.

Tuberculosis
Intestinal tuberculosis is caused by *Mycobacterium tuberculosis* or *M. bovis* after ingestion (swallowed sputum or infected milk), or after blood-borne spread from another focus.

Clinical features
The diagnosis should always be considered in Indian, African, South-East Asian, or South/Central American patients with chronic gastrointestinal symptoms, even in second-generation immigrants. Presentation several years after the patient arrives from abroad is common.
Ileocaecal tuberculosis
• Clinically similar to Crohn's disease, with recurrent abdominal pain, pyrexia, weight loss or diarrhoea
• A mass is palpable in 40%, and lymphocytosis is common but by no means always present

Tuberculous peritonitis
- Ascites, weight loss and ill health. A 'doughy' feeling on abdominal palpation is rare
- Clinical suspicion and a diagnostic tap are essential, although laparotomy is often needed to establish the diagnosis (p. 25)

Tuberculous adenitis
- Mesenteric adenitis may cause acute abdominal pain, similar to appendicitis

Perianal tuberculosis
- Similar to Crohn's disease
- Colonic tuberculosis is very rare

Diagnosis
- About 30% have an abnormal chest X-ray; sputum samples may then be diagnostic. Most have no pulmonary disease. Gastric washings for *Mycobacterium* sp. are overrated and unpleasant
- A positive Mantoux test simply indicates previous exposure or past vaccination. A strongly positive test (>10 mm induration following 0.1 ml 1:1000 tuberculin) favours active infection, but is often negative in peritonitis
- Small bowel radiology will demonstrate ileocaecal tuberculosis, but cannot distinguish this from Crohn's disease, lymphoma, or severe *Strongyloides stercoralis* infection
- Laparotomy is indicated to establish the diagnosis when doubt exists. In an African or Indian patient with radiological ileocaecal distortion, tuberculosis can be assumed to be the cause unless there is no response to treatment after 2 months
- Culture of biopsy specimens is necessary to determine drug sensitivities. *M. bovis* is insensitive to pyrazinamide
- Ascitic fluid adenosine deaminase levels (p. 25), or peritoneal biopsy with an Abrams needle, may be diagnostic for tuberculous peritonitis, but laparotomy is often necessary to establish the diagnosis

Management
- The same regimen as for pulmonary tuberculosis is used, although evidence for efficacy is often difficult to monitor
- Quadruple therapy for 2 months (isoniazid 300 mg/day, rifampicin 450 mg/day, pyrazinamide 1250 mg/day, ethambutol 750 mg/day, for a 50-kg patient); followed by isoniazid and rifampicin alone for 4 months

- *M. bovis* should be treated with rifampicin and isoniazid for 9 months, as well as ethambutol for the initial 2 months
- Pyridoxine 10 mg/day is unnecessary, unless higher doses of isoniazid are used or paraesthesiae occur
- Response is judged by clinical improvement, weight gain, reversal of anaemia and fall in ESR. Intestinal parasites often coexist and may contribute to anaemia
- Routine liver function tests are unnecessary during antituberculous chemotherapy, unless there is pre-existing liver disease, or results are borderline at the start of treatment
- Abnormal liver function tests may be due to drugs (isoniazid, rifampicin), tuberculosis or other disease (cirrhosis). Drugs should be continued unless deterioration occurs. Biopsy is then indicated to establish the cause
- Follow-up for 2 years after recovery and stopping treatment is recommended
- Notification and contact tracing are essential (p. 346)

Typhoid and paratyphoid (enteric fever)
About 200 cases a year of *S. typhi*, *S. paratyphi A* , or *S. paratyphi* B infection occur in Britain. Paratyphoid produces similar, but usually less severe features than typhoid.

Clinical features
- Fever—stepwise progression is characteristic, but rarely seen
- Headache is typical
- Constipation—initially, but diarrhoea develops later
- Relative bradycardia—rarely in brucellosis as well
- Rash ('rose-spots')—after a few days, often overlooked
- Complications, in the third week or before, include intestinal haemorrhage, perforation and death. Asymptomatic carriers are rare

Diagnosis
- Leucopenia is common, but may also occur with dengue fever, malaria, or rarely in brucellosis
- Blood cultures in the first week; bone marrow culture is the most reliable test and may be positive even after prior antibiotic treatment
- Urine or faecal culture in the second week
- Serology (Widal test) is of no value in acute illness

Management
- Chloramphenicol 1 g (oral or intravenous) six hourly for 2 weeks. Multiple antibiotic resistance is increasing, especially from the Indian sub-continent, and ciprofloxacin 200 mg intravenously or 750 mg orally, twice daily, is then indicated. Care in children, for whom alternatives are trimethoprim or amoxycillin
- Isolation of excreta (urine, faeces), to prevent cross-infection
- Notification is necessary (see Table 11.7, p. 346) and contacts must be traced
- Three negative stool cultures off treatment are necessary before the patient returns to work. The district Consultant for Communicable Diseases will advise (p. 346)

Amoebiasis (*Entamoeba histolytica* infection)
Amoebiasis is prevalent throughout the tropics and sub-tropics, and asymptomatic cyst excretion is common (>10% worldwide, 1% in Europe).

Clinical features
- >90% of infections are asymptomatic
- Amoebic dysentery—similar to ulcerative colitis (p. 269), with proctocolitis or, rarely, a fulminant course which has a bad prognosis. It may also simply cause watery diarrhoea
- Non-dysenteric colonic disease—strictures, an inflammatory mass (amoeboma), appendicitis, abscess, perianal or skip lesions are less common, but can simulate Crohn's disease (p. 251)
- Invasive amoebiasis—hepatic abscess (acutely or focally tender hepatomegaly in an ill patient, p. 179) may rupture into the pleural, peritoneal, or pericardial cavity, with serious consequences. Other organs are rarely affected

Diagnosis
- Microscopy of fresh, warm stools to identify red-cell consuming (haematophagous) amoebae is diagnostic. Cyst excretion alone may be incidental. Three negative stool specimens virtually exclude the diagnosis
- Biopsies or mucosal scrapings should also be examined for trophozoites (amoebae with pseudopodia adjacent to the mucosa)
- Negative serology (several methods) is common in early disease and should not negate a clinical diagnosis of amoebiasis. Serology

is never positive in asymptomatic cyst carriage except after past
active disease.

A positive test confirms previous exposure, or active
disease; antibodies may be markedly elevated in invasive
amoebiasis

• Ultrasound and markedly elevated antibodies to *Entamoeba
histolytica,* or trophozoites in a fresh faecal sample, establish
the diagnosis of amoebic liver abscess. Percutaneous aspiration of
viscous, reddish ('anchovy-sauce') fluid is characteristic but is
rarely needed and may be complicated by a
pyogenic abscess

Management
• Metronidazole 800 mg three times daily for 10 days is effective
for all types of amoebiasis, but should usually be followed by
diloxanide 500 mg three times daily for 10 days to eliminate cyst
passage, because recurrent invasive disease sometimes occurs
• Three repeat stool specimens, to confirm clearance, are advisable
• Asymptomatic cyst excretors should receive a full course of
metronidazole, followed by diloxanide

Schistosomiasis
Schistosomiasis is endemic in Asia, much of the Middle East,
Africa, St Lucia and South America. Chronic schistosomiasis
usually affects the indigenous population, who may then travel and
present to doctors in non-endemic areas.

Visitors to endemic areas rarely develop severe chronic
schistosomiasis as a heavy worm burden takes many years to
accumulate, but may suffer schistosome dermatitis, or rarely
acute schistosomiasis (Katayama fever). Swimming in sea water
or chlorinated swimming pools is safe, even in endemic areas,
because the parasite needs the fresh water snail to develop. It is
not infectious, for the same reason.

Diagnosis is made by detecting excretion of ova in faeces. As a
rule schistosomiasis does not cause symptoms unless there is heavy
excretion of ova, even if serological tests are positive.

Schistosome dermatitis
An itchy papular rash affects exposed skin (swimmers' itch) within
24 h and resolves with 72 h, but is most unusual after primary
exposure.

Acute schistosomiasis (Katayama fever)
Fever, rigors, anorexia, diarrhoea, hepatosplenomegaly, urticaria and cough develop 20–60 days after heavy initial exposure. Diagnosis is suspected by an eosinophilia and confirmed by finding schistosome ova in faeces; serology becomes positive later. Steroids have been used in conjuction with praziquantel.

Chronic schistosomiasis
Schistosoma japonicum in Asia, and *S. mansoni* in other areas, may cause bloody diarrhoea or hepatosplenomegaly and portal hypertension. *S. haematobium* in the Middle East predominantly affects the urinary tract. Schistosomal colitis causes granulomatous inflammatory nodules, visible on sigmoidoscopy and confirmed by rectal biopsy, which also shows ova. Portal hypertension may cause recurrent haematemesis, but not encephalopathy except in the terminal stages, because hepatic fibrosis is pre-sinusoidal and hepatocellular function is preserved until very late in the disease (p. 153). Chronic liver disease in an Asian patient with light excretion of ova may still be due to hepatitis B, but granulomas on liver biopsy suggest schistosomiasis.

Treatment is indicated for chronic schistosomiasis with praziquantel, but is best undertaken by specialists, preferably following quantitative egg counts. Praziquantel 40 mg/kg as a single dose is effective in *S. mansoni,* and 25 mg/kg for 3 days in *S. japonicum.* Portal hypertension is likely to improve and surgical portal–systemic shunting should be a last resort, although surgery gives a better prognosis than in patients with cirrhosis.

11.3 Other parasitic infections
Infection by parasites, often several, is the norm in many parts of the world.

Classification
A simple classification is shown in Table 11.3.

Clinical features

General
• Infections are usually asymptomatic, but can cause low-grade debility or specific features (see p. 340)

11.3 Other parasitic infections

Table 11.3 Classification of common gastrointestinal parasites

Protozoa	Nematodes	Cestodes	Trematodes
Giardia lamblia	Roundworm:	Tapeworm:	Liver flukes:
Cryptosporidium sp.	*Ascaris lumbricoides*	*Taenia solium* (cysticercosis)	*Clonorchis sinensis*
Entamoeba histolytica	Hookworm:	*Taenia saginata*	*Opisthorchis viverrini*
Leishmania sp.	*Necator americanus*	*Hymenolepis nana*	*Fasciola hepatica*
	Ancylostoma duodenale	*Diphyllobothrium latum*	*Schistosoma* sp.:
	Threadworm:	Hydatid:	*Schistosoma mansoni*
	Enterobius vermicularis	*Echinococcus granulosus*	*Schistosoma japonicum*
	Whipworm:		
	Trichuris trichiura		
	Strongyloides stercoralis		
	Trichinella spiralis		

11.3 Other parasitic infections

- Gastrointestinal upset—nausea, bloating, or diarrhoea are common but non-specific when symptoms occur, but this affects a minority only
- Weight loss—indicates heavy infection or a complication, but this is unusual

Specific

- Anaemia—iron deficiency (*Necator americanus, Ancylostoma duodenale, Trichuris trichiuria*), vitamin B_{12} deficiency (*Diphyllobothrium latum*, from raw fish)
- Asthma—during larval migration (*Ascaris lumbricoides, Strongyloides stercoralis*)
- Colitis—often with granulomas (*Entamoeba histolytica, Trichuris trichiuria, Schistosoma mansoni* or *S. japonicum*)
- Cutaneous—urticaria (*Strongyloides stercoralis* 'cutaneous larva migrans'), or dermatitis (*Schistosoma* sp. 'swimmer's itch')
- Encystment—muscle, brain (*Taenia solium, Trichinella spiralis*)
- Fever—transient (*Trichinella spiralis, Schistosoma* sp.), or fulminant septicaemia (*Strongyloides stercoralis* hyperinfection in immunocompromised patients)
- Obstruction—intestinal, biliary (*Ascaris lumbricoides*, hydatid)
- Portal hypertension (*Schistosoma* sp., *Clonorchis sinensis*)
- Pruritus ani—(*Enterobius vermicularis*)
- Steatorrhoea—(*Strongyloides stercoralis*)

Visible faecal worms

This may be the only manifestation of infection and usually prompts a rapid visit to the doctor in the UK. The worm may have been retained for inspection.
- 0.5 cm long and 0.1 cm diameter, thicker at one end than the other: *Trichuris trichiuria* (whipworm), or *Enterobius vermicularis* (threadworm)
- 10–30 cm long, like a white earthworm: *Ascaris lumbricoides*
- 2->20 cm long, segmented: *Taenia saginata* or *Taenia solium*. *Diphyllobothrium latum* is a single, long (up to 25 m) worm that is very rare in Britain. Usually only a few segments of tapeworm are noticed
- All other worms excreted in faeces are microscopic

Diagnosis

Eosinophilia

- >0.44 × 10⁹/l. The number of eosinophils should be expressed in absolute terms, not as a percentage
- Common marker of infection with helminths, but not protozoa, usually >0.8 × 10⁹/l in active infection
- Other causes include:
  drug hypersensitivity
  atopy
  bronchopulmonary aspergillosis
  pulmonary infiltrates and eosinophilia
  vasculitis (polyarteritis)
  lymphoma (rarely)
  chronic active hepatitis (rarely)
  Crohn's disease (very rarely)
  eosinophilic leukaemia (very rare)

Examination of faecal sample

- Faecal examination of ova or cysts is the only way of differentiating infections. Repeated stool samples and concentration techniques may be necessary, and should be discussed with the laboratory
- Perianal skin is heavily infected during *Enterobius vermicularis* infection, which can be detected by a Sellotape slide (Sellotape applied to the anal margin and examined under a microscope for 0.5–1 cm long worms)

Serological tests

- Not available for most parasitic infections
- ELISA or other tests for *Entamoeba histolytica*, *Schistosoma* sp., *Echinococcus granulosus* (hydatid disease), *Leishmania* sp. and *Trichinella spiralis* virtually exclude the disease if negative, except in the early stages. Serological tests are not a reliable index of active infection. Treatment is, however, indicated in the UK for patients with positive serology and a compatible clinical history

Management of specific parasites

The recommendations in Table 11.4 are for sporadic infection in non-endemic areas. General measures, including hand hygiene for

11.3 Other parasitic infections

Table 11.4 Drugs for gastrointestinal parasites

Parasite	First choice	Second choice
Protozoa:		
Giardia lamblia	Tinidazole 2 g stat	Mepacrine 100 mg t.d.s. 7 days
Entamoeba histolytica	Metronidazole 800 mg t.d.s. 10 days	Diloxanide furoate 500 mg t.d.s. 10 days
Cryptosporidium sp.	None	
Leishmania sp.	Sodium stibogluconate 10 mg/kg for 30 days[†]	Pentamidine[†]
Nematodes:		
Ascaris lumbricoides	Mebendazole 100 mg b.d. 3 days	[†]
Necator americanus	Mebendazole 100 mg b.d. 3 days	[†]
Ancylostoma duodenale	Same	[†]
Enterobius vermicularis	Mebendazole 100 mg stat['] (repeated after 2 weeks)	[†]
Trichuris trichiuria	Mebendazole 100 mg b.d. 3 days	Albendazole 4 mg/kg stat*
Strongyloides stercoralis	Thiabendazole 1.5 g b.d. 3 days	[†]
Trichinella spiralis	Mebendazole 100 mg t.d.s. 7 days	Thiabendazole 1.5 g b.d. 7 days
Cestodes:		
Taenia sp.		
cysticercosis	Praziquantel 10 mg/kg stat	[†]
adult tapeworm	Niclosamide 2 g stat	[†]
Diphyllobothrium latum	Same	[†]
Hymenolepis nana	Same	[†]
Echinococcus sp.	Albendazole*[†]	Praziquantel[†]
Trematodes:		
Clonorchis sinensis	Praziquantel 25 mg/kg t.d.s. 2 days	
Opisthorchis viverrini	Same	
Fasciola hepatica	Same	
Schistosoma japonicum	Same	
Schistosoma mansoni	Praziquantel 40 mg/kg stat[†]	

* Named patients only, from SmithKline Beecham.
[†] Specialist advice required.
' General measures (hygiene) are as important.
(stat: single dose; b.d.: twice daily; t.d.s.: three times daily)

nematode infections (especially *Enterobius vermicularis*), or treatment of anaemia, are also important. Other members of the family should have stools examined for parasites.

Treatment of complications (such as *Strongyloides stercoralis* hyperinfection) should be in consultation with specialists.

11.4 Immunocompromise

Human immunodeficiency viruses (HIV-1 and HIV-2) are the predominant cause of acquired immune deficiency in all parts of the world, but other immunocompromised patients (following chemotherapy) are also susceptible to opportunistic gastrointestinal infections.

Acquired immune deficiency syndrome (AIDS)

Acute HIV infection has unusual, specific gastrointestinal features, but most opportunistic infections that become pathogenic such as *Cryptosporidium* sp., cytomegalovirus (CMV) (Tables 11.5 and 11.6) suggest AIDS.

The term 'gay bowel syndrome' is now rarely used, but refers to infections causing proctocolitis or diarrhoea in homosexual men who are not necessarily immunocompromised. Any infection in Tables 11.5 or 11.6 is an indication for measuring immunoglobulins and HIV status, only *after* counselling.

HIV enteropathy

Diarrhoea for which no causative organism can be found is common in AIDS and AIDS-related complex (ARC). This is attributed to HIV enteropathy causing partial villous atrophy, with histological crypt hypoplasia and polymorph infiltration. It contributes to malabsorption, weight loss or susceptibility to infection.

Table 11.5 Differential diagnosis of diarrhoea in AIDS

Moderate	Severe	Bloody
Giardia lamblia	*Cryptosporidium* sp.	Herpes simplex virus
Salmonella sp.	*Isospora belli*	*Chlamydia trachomatis*
Campylobacter sp.	Cytomegalovirus	Cytomegalovirus
Mycobacterium sp.		*Campylobacter* sp.
Gonorrhoea		*Entamoeba histolytica*
HIV enteropathy		*Shigella* sp.

11.4 Immunocompromise

Table 11.6 Gastrointestinal complications of AIDS

Clinical problem	Site	Cause
Sore mouth	Oropharyngeal	*Candida* sp. Gonorrhoea Herpes simplex
Mouth ulcer(s)	Oropharyngeal	Herpes simplex Syphilis Kaposi's sarcoma* Acute HIV infection
Painful dysphagia	Oesophageal	*Candida* sp. Cytomegalovirus* Acute HIV infection
Diarrhoea (see Table 11.5)		
Constipation	Rectal stricture	*Chlamydia* sp. Lymphogranuloma venereum
Abdominal pain	Subacute obstruction	*Mycobacterium* sp.* Intestinal lymphoma* Kaposi's sarcoma*
	Gall bladder	Cytomegalovirus*
Rectal bleeding	Ulcer/tumour	Syphilis Lymphogranuloma venereum Kaposi's sarcoma* Anorectal carcinoma
	Other	Thrombocytopenia (drug-induced)
Jaundice	Liver	Hepatitis B, B + D, or C Drugs

* Highly suggestive of AIDS in the presence of immunodeficiency for which no other cause can be found.

A lactose-free diet will diminish symptoms associated with hypolactasia, but there is no other specific treatment apart from antidiarrhoeal agents (p. 213). Severe diarrhoea is usually caused by a superimposed infection.

Candida sp.
• Oropharyngeal candidiasis causes a sore mouth, or painful dysphagia if there is oesophageal involvement (p. 55)
• Diagnosis is by sight (white oral plaques, not to be confused with oral hairy leukoplakia) and confirmed by swab (hyphae demonstrated by Gram stain)

• Oral candidiasis is treated initially with nystatin suspension 1 ml four times daily, which should be given prophylactically in AIDS after an episode of oral candidiasis
• Oesophageal candidiasis is treated with oral fluconazole 50 mg daily for 7–14 days or ketoconazole 200 mg daily for 14 days. Specialist advice is recommended

Herpes simplex virus type 1 HSV-1
• Proctitis occasionally occurs. Extensive oropharyngeal ulceration or disseminated herpetic infection is more common in the immunocompromised. There is often a past history of genital herpes (HSV-2)
• Cellular inclusion bodies in a rectal biopsy specimen distinguish herpetic proctitis from Crohn's disease
• Antibodies to HSV (and other viruses, including hepatitis B) may be absent in immunodeficiency. This is a poor prognostic sign
• Oral acyclovir 200 mg five times daily is effective, but intravenous treatment (5–10 mg/kg over 1 h, three times daily) is needed for sick patients. Maintenance therapy (same oral dose) is indicated for frequent relapse

Cytomegalovirus (CMV)
• Proctocolitis is recognized by bloody, watery diarrhoea and superficial mucosal ulceration at sigmoidoscopy, in association with choroidoretinitis or pneumonitis. Oesophagitis causes odynophagia
• Diagnosis is confirmed by intranuclear eosinophilic inclusion bodies in a rectal biopsy specimen
• Treatment with dihydroxypropoxymethylguanine (DHPG) is available at specialist centres, but disseminated infection is usually fatal. Other drugs are being developed

Chlamydia sp.
• Chlamydial proctitis closely resembles Crohn's disease
• Biopsy occasionally demonstrates chlamydial inclusion bodies, which can be distinguished from CMV or HSV inclusion bodies by electron microscopy. Microimmunofluorescent antibody tests establish the diagnosis

• Tetracycline 500 mg four times daily is effective, but may have to be continued for several weeks

Cryptosporidium sp. and Isospora belli
• Intractable watery diarrhoea causes weight loss and dehydration in the immunocompromised patient. *Cryptosporidium* sp. in normal individuals is a cause of traveller's diarrhoea, which is severe but transient (Table 7.3, p. 214)
• Oocysts are readily identified in stool
• Spiramycin 1 g three times daily for 3 weeks is sometimes effective for cryptosporidiosis; there is no alternative, although azidothymidine may help. Co-trimoxazole 960 mg twice daily for 3 weeks is indicated for *Isospora belli*

11.5 Notification
Diseases affecting the gastrointestinal tract that are notifiable by law are shown in Table 11.7. The Medical Officer for Environmental Health (telephone number and address on the notification form, or from the local Health Authority offices), should be telephoned first and then sent the notification form, for which a small fee is payable. Some districts in Britain now have a Consultant in Communicable Diseases; the local Microbiology

Table 11.7 Notifiable and prescribed gastrointestinal disorders

Common	Rare
Hepatitis—any type*	Tuberculosis*
Food poisoning—any type	Leptospirosis*
Dysentery—bacillary *(Shigella* sp.)	Amoebiasis
	Typhoid
	Paratyphoid
	Cholera
	Lead poisoning*
	Toxic jaundice (hydrocarbons)*
	Ancylostomiasis[†]
	Brucellosis[†]
	Vinyl chloride portal fibrosis[†]
	Hepatic angiosarcoma[†]
	Beryllium (hepatic granuloma)[†]
	Arsenic and other heavy metals[†]

[†] Not statutorily notifiable, but a prescribed disease in certain occupations.
* A prescribed disease in certain occupations.

Department will know. The environmental health departments of local councils in Britain deal with commercial establishments, rather than patients.

Prescribed diseases have an industrial origin for which compensation may be payable if the claimant has worked in a specified occupation. The Employment Medical Adviser at the Health and Safety Executive (Appendix 1) will advise.

12 Procedures and Investigations

12.1 Houseman's checklist

The explanation given in each section is designed to help those unfamiliar with the procedures to describe them to patients. The history and examination must be documented in the notes before any invasive procedure. A pre-printed history sheet saves time when there is direct access to endoscopy from general practitioners. Resuscitation equipment must be immediately available for any procedure that involves sedation.

Upper gastrointestinal endoscopy

Indications
- Diagnostic:
  dyspepsia, especially when age >40 years (p. 72)
  haematemesis (p. 10)
  weight loss (to do low duodenal biopsies, p. 217)
  iron deficiency anaemia (p. 315)
  persistent vomiting (p. 79)
  biopsy of gastric lesions detected by barium meal (p. 86)
  biopsy of duodenal mucosa for coeliac disease (p. 352)
- Therapeutic:
  dilatation of oesophageal (and sometimes pyloric) strictures (p. 56)
  palliation of oesophageal cancer (p. 59)
  sclerotherapy of bleeding oesophageal varices (p. 13)
  injection, thermocoagulation or laser photocoagulation of other
    bleeding lesions (p. 11)

Preparation
- Nil by mouth for at least 4 h (longer after a large meal)
- Water only for 8 h and nil by mouth for 4 h, if pyloric obstruction is suspected
- Delay for 24 h after any upper gastrointestinal barium study (such as a barium swallow for dysphagia); barium can block the suction channel of the endoscope
- Written consent, after explanation

Explanation
- Intravenous sedation (often midazolam 2.5–10 mg) is given
- The pharynx is sprayed with lignocaine 1% if the patient is particularly anxious, or has a pronounced gag reflex

12.1 Houseman's checklist

- The flexible endoscope, the size of a small finger, is gently passed
into the oesophagus and steered through the stomach into the
duodenum (a diagram helps patients to understand)
- Breathing is not impaired, but a probe (from a pulse oximeter)
may be strapped to a finger for measuring blood oxygen saturation
- The procedure takes about 5 min
- Eating or drinking is allowed after the procedure as soon as the
patient wishes, unless local anaesthetic spray has been used, in
which case sensation must have recovered (about 30 min)
- Findings and instructions should be given in the presence of a
relative or friend after the procedure, or written down, because
amnesia often follows sedation

Complications
- Sore throat occurs, but is transient
- Amnesia following sedation sometimes persists for hours, even
after the patient appears to have recovered. Patients must not be
allowed to drive or perform a responsible job without assistance for
24 h (looking after children, operating machinery)
- Perforation (<0.1%)
- Cardiorespiratory arrest or death (<0.1%) is rare, but patients
with cardiorespiratory disease should have nasal oxygen (2 l/min)

Jejunal biopsy
Low duodenal biopsies (from the second part of the duodenum) at
upper gastrointestinal endoscopy are satisfactory for most purposes
(p. 217). Whilst a normal biopsy excludes coeliac disease, duodenal
villi can appear stunted when overlying Brunner's glands; jejunal
biopsy is then indicated if there is any doubt about the diagnosis.
Unusual causes of malabsorption, including giardiasis, lymphoma,
Whipple's disease, or amyloidosis can also be diagnosed by jejunal
biopsy (p. 233). Multiple jejunal biopsies can be obtained with a
Quinton hydraulic biopsy instrument at specialist centres; this is helpful
if there is doubt about the diagnosis after using simpler techniques.
Jejunal aspirates can be taken for microscopy and culture.

Indications
- Diagnostic:
    diagnosis of coeliac disease and repeated, after 3–6 months on a
    gluten-free diet, to confirm response (p. 223)

persistent diarrhoea (Fig. 7.1, p. 211)
folate deficiency
iron deficiency for which other causes cannot be found (p. 315)
weight loss
diagnosis of giardiasis, if stool examination normal (p. 228)
diagnosis of small bowel bacterial overgrowth (p. 229)

Preparation
- Platelet count >100 × 10^9/l
- Clotting studies (INR <1.3, or prothrombin time <22 sec)
- Nil by mouth for 4 h
- Consent, after explanation

Explanation
- Performed in X-ray department, or where fluoroscopy is available
- The pharynx is sprayed with lignocaine 1%. Sedation is rarely necessary
- A fine-bore tube (3-mm diameter) attached to the biopsy capsule is swallowed, whilst the patient is standing. When 60 cm has been swallowed, the patient lies down and the position is checked fluoroscopically. The tube is steered into the jejunum (Meditech catheter), or passes spontaneously (Crosby–Watson capsule) and the biopsy is triggered by suction, after which it is removed
- The procedure takes between 15 min (Meditech) and 60 min (Crosby–Watson)
- The biopsy is painless
- Eating or drinking is allowed 30 min after the anaesthetic spray

Complications
- Sore throat is occasionally reported, but is transient
- Bleeding occurs <0.1%. Perforation has been reported in malnourished patients, but is extremely rare
- Retained capsule is extremely uncommon. The tube is cut as short as possible and the remainder should pass spontaneously

Colonoscopy

Indications
- Diagnostic:
  rectal bleeding, especially when recurrent, or after a normal or

---

inadequate barium enema (p. 295)
iron deficiency anaemia (p. 315)
persistent diarrhoea (Fig. 7.1, p. 211)
biopsy of a lesion detected by barium enema
assessment of patients with Crohn's disease (p. 246) or ulcerative
colitis (p. 267)
surveillance for colorectal cancer in selected patients (p. 297)
• Therapeutic:
polypectomy
diathermy or laser photocoagulation of angiodysplasia
dilatation of colonic strictures in selected patients (p. 310)
decompression of pseudo-obstruction (p. 36)

Preparation
• Low-residue diet (no fruit, vegetables, or bread) for 36 h and
nothing solid for 12 h before the procedure
• Sodium picosulphate and magnesium citrate (Picolax), 2 sachets
24 h before the procedure. Many alternative preparations are
available and the local endoscopy unit will have a preferred
preparation
• Flexible sigmoidoscopy is performed after 2 phosphate enemas
alone and often allows examination up to the splenic flexure
• Consent, after explanation

Explanation
• Sedation is given (such as intravenous midazolam 2.5–10 mg),
sometimes with intravenous pethidine 50–100 mg as well
• The flexible colonoscope (diameter of a large finger) is passed per
rectum, around the colon. Fluoroscopy is sometimes helpful
• The procedure takes 15–30 min
• The patient goes home accompanied, an hour or two after the
procedure

Complications
• Abdominal discomfort after the procedure is common, but rarely
remembered. It can be reduced if gas, which is insufflated during
the procedure, is aspirated during withdrawal of the colonoscope
• Incomplete examination occurs in 5–20%, depending on operator
experience. A barium enema or repeat examination is then
indicated

12.1 Houseman's checklist

- Perforation is rare (0.2%), but more common in acute colitis, extensive diverticulosis or ischaemic colitis, which are relative contraindications to colonoscopy. Haemorrhage after biopsy or polypectomy is even less common

ERCP (endoscopic retrograde cholangiopancreatography)

Indications (p. 195, and Figs 4.2, 6.5, pp. 119, 196)

Preparation
- Platelet count >100 × 10^9/l
- Clotting studies (INR <1.3, prothrombin time <22 sec)
- Nil by mouth for 4 h
- Pethidine 75–100 mg and metoclopramide 10 mg are given by intramuscular injection 30 min before the procedure, with intramuscular gentamicin 80 mg if there is obstructive jaundice
- Consent, after explanation

Explanation
- The procedure is performed in the X-ray department
- Sedation (such as intravenous midazolam 5–10 mg) is given
- A side-viewing endoscope is passed into the duodenum. A fine catheter is inserted through the ampulla, into the pancreatic duct and then into the bile duct. Contrast is injected and X-rays taken
- Therapeutic procedures include sphincterotomy (5-mm incision in the ampulla), pre-cut sphincterotomy (when the bile duct cannot be cannulated), stent insertion (through a stricture), or stone retrieval (basket, balloon, lithotripsy, direct dissolution)
- The procedure takes 20–60 min
- The patient goes home the same day, unless a therapeutic procedure has been performed

Complications
- Complete examination is possible in >90%, but more than one attempt may be needed, especially for therapeutic procedures
- Acute pancreatitis—2%
- Haemorrhage after sphincterotomy—1%, requiring prompt surgery
- Cholangitis—2%
- Death—<0.5%

12   Procedures and Investigations

12.1 Houseman's checklist

Liver biopsy

Indications
* Diagnostic:
  persistently elevated (>2-fold) liver enzymes 6 months after viral
    hepatitis (p. 162)
  asymptomatic elevation of liver enzymes (Fig. 5.7, p. 181),
    especially in alcohol abuse (p. 174)
  clinical suspicion of cirrhosis (p. 172), chronic active hepatitis
    (p. 164) or carcinoma (p. 177)
  biopsy of hepatic lesions detected by ultrasound
  investigation of unexplained pyrexia (to detect granulomas, p. 169,
    miliary tuberculosis, lymphoma, or systemic vasculitis)
  abnormal liver function in relatives of patients with familial
    hepatic disease (haemochromatosis, Wilson's disease)
* Ascites or emphysema are relative contraindications

Preparation
* Platelet count $>100 \times 10^9/l$
* Coagulation studies (INR <1.3, prothrombin time <22 sec).
Give a single dose of vitamin K 10 mg and re-check clotting 48 h
later if coagulation is disordered; otherwise infuse 2–4 units of
fresh frozen plasma immediately prior to biopsy
* Consent, after explanation
* Liver biopsy should not be performed after midday, so that
observations can be done, or complications recognized, when staff
are readily available
* Ultrasound or CT scan-guided liver biopsy is helpful for focal
lesions, but needs to be discussed and co-ordinated with a
radiologist

Explanation
* The procedure is performed on the ward. Sedation is not usually
necessary
* Lignocaine 2% is carefully infiltrated down to the capsule
between the 8–10 ribs, where there is dullness to percussion in the
mid-axillary line. A 2 mm nick in the skin is made with a scalpel
* Breathing is rehearsed (breath must be held in full expiration
during biopsy)
* Biopsy with a fine needle (Trucut, or Menghini) takes a few
seconds

- After the biopsy the patient lies on the right side for 2 h and then in bed for 6 h. Pulse and blood pressure are measured every 15 min for 1 h, every 30 min for 2 h and then hourly up to 8 h. Observation overnight in hospital is usual
- Transjugular or laparoscopic biopsy are specialist techniques when percutaneous biopsy is contraindicated (due to disordered coagulation or ascites) or impossible

Complications
- Local pain (often pleuritic or in the shoulder) is common, but usually relieved by oral paracetamol 2 tablets every 4 h
- Pneumothorax is rarely clinically apparent and does not need drainage unless breathing is compromised
- Bleeding, requiring transfusion or operation—<0.5%
- Death—<0.1%, may follow inappropriate biopsy (colon, pancreas, gall bladder, inferior vena cava) or tear in the liver capsule

Percutaneous transhepatic cholangiogram (PTC)

Indications
- Diagnostic:
  cholestatic jaundice with a dilated biliary tree (p. 195)
- Therapeutic:
  relief of jaundice, in conjunction with ERCP (p. 195)
  decompression of an obstructed biliary tree (percutaneous catheter drainage for up to 72 h), prior to a definitive procedure

Preparation
- As for liver biopsy
- Pethidine 50–100 mg, metoclopramide 10 mg and gentamicin 80 mg by intramuscular injection are given 30 min before the procedure

Explanation
- The procedure is performed by a radiologist. Sedation is often helpful
- A fine needle is inserted into the liver, in the 8th or 9th intercostal space. Contrast is gently injected as the needle is

withdrawn under fluoroscopy, until an intrahepatic duct is delineated. Contrast is then injected to outline the biliary tree and X-rays taken
• The procedure takes 15–30 min
• Observation after the procedure is the same as for liver biopsy

Complications
• Local pain is relieved by paracetamol
• Biliary leak is rare, even in obstructive jaundice, and resolves spontaneously. Analgesia (intramuscular pethidine 50–100 mg) may be necessary
• Cholangitis is very rare, unless percutaneous stent insertion or joint PTC/ERCP have been attempted

12.2 Radiology

Requests
Salient clinical features, rather than a statement of the suspected diagnosis, help the radiologist interpret X-rays. Stating the specific question to be answered by the radiological investigation is also helpful. Potential complicating factors (diabetes, epilepsy, pacemakers) should be mentioned, especially for contrast or invasive procedures.

Discussion with the radiologist about the most appropriate imaging technique saves the patient unnecessary investigation and allows the radiologist to proceed at his discretion, depending on the findings (from ultrasound to CT scan, for example). A visit to the X-ray department and 'please' or 'thank you' on the request form are simple courtesies that pay dividends.

Plain film checklist
Plain, supine abdominal and erect chest X-rays are indicated for any patient with acute abdominal pain (p. 21). Erect abdominal X-ray is only needed to detect fluid levels when there is doubt about the diagnosis of intestinal obstruction.

On a plain abdominal X-ray, look for:
• Sub-diaphragmatic gas, or clear delineation of liver, kidneys or spleen (perforated viscus, p. 24)

- Intestinal diameter:
  small intestine >2.5 cm (obstruction)
  colon >6.0 cm (obstruction, toxic dilatation, Fig. 1.3 p. 37)
- Mucosal pattern:
  thickened wall (acute ulcerative colitis or Crohn's disease)
  mucosal islands (small radio-opaque projections into the lumen
    in acute colitis, p. 38)
  thumb-printing (large radio-opaque projections, ischaemic colitis,
    Fig. 9.5, p. 308)
  gas in the wall (impending perforation, pneumatosis coli)
- Gas pattern:
  displaced or separated loops of small bowel (mass effect,
    inflammation)
  segment of jejunum ('sentinel loop' in acute pancreatitis)
  fluid levels (obstruction, on an erect abdominal film)
  central distribution of normal small bowel (ascites)
  gas in the biliary tree (cholangitis, recent passage of stone)
- Faecal distribution:
  throughout the colon (constipation)
  distal extent (ulcerative colitis, stricture)
- Calculi:
  along the line of the transverse processes (renal/ureteric)
  right upper quadrant (gall stones)
  phleboliths, calcified lymph nodes, foreign bodies, or artefacts
    may be included in the differential diagnosis

Contrast studies
Double contrast studies of upper and lower gastrointestinal tracts
are routine, and single contrast studies have few indications
(p. 265). In a double contrast study, barium coats the mucosa and
gas provides the contrast. Effervescent tablets are swallowed, or air
is insufflated, to put the mucosa under slight tension. Barium is
used unless perforation is suspected, when Gastrografin or non-
ionic agents (such as Omnipaque) are indicated.

Oesophagus (Figs 2.3, 2.4 and 2.5; pp. 56, 61 and 64)

Stomach and duodenum (Figs 3.1 and 3.3; pp. 73 and 92)

Small bowel
- Barium follow-through is more widely used than small bowel

enema, but may give less information, especially distally, due to dilution
• Both require bowel preparation, with a low-residue diet and laxative, to enhance intestinal transit during the procedure
• Large films of the abdomen are taken at 30-min intervals until the barium reaches the caecum. Enhanced films of areas of interest (terminal ileum) are then taken (Figs 7.3 and 8.1; pp. 218 and 247)
• Small bowel enema is more troublesome and needs duodenal intubation, but produces better mucosal definition. It is indicated when mucosal changes may be subtle (Crohn's disease, polyps, diverticula), or if a follow-through examination is unsatisfactory
• Reflux of barium through the ileocaecal valve on a barium enema sometimes defines the terminal ileum very well and should not be overlooked

Large bowel
• Barium enema should only be done after digital rectal examination, sigmoidoscopy and biopsy. It is sensible to wait 72 h after rectal biopsy before a barium enema, but the risk of perforation is small
• Preparation is the same as for colonoscopy. Elderly patients (>75 years) may need admission for the preparation and procedure
• A smooth-muscle relaxant (intravenous hyoscine butylbromide 20 mg) may be needed to decrease colonic spasm
• Large films are taken every 10–15 min until the barium reaches the caecum, followed by films of areas of interest (lateral views to show the rectum and posterior rectal space, enhanced views of the flexures or caecum). The procedure takes 20–30 min
• A single contrast enema, without preparation, is indicated when there is doubt about the diagnosis of acute colitis or obstruction. The extent of colitis shown by a single contrast barium enema can be misleading, although it should help distinguish ulcerative, Crohn's and ischaemic colitis (p. 308)
• If the caecum is not clearly shown, a peroral pneumocologram (oral barium and rectal air insufflation) avoids a repeat barium enema

Mesenteric angiography
• Intra-arterial digital subtraction angiography needs less contrast than conventional techniques, for equivalent definition

• Low ionic contrast media (such as Omnipaque) cause fewer side effects and do not contain iodine, but are much more expensive. They are indicated for patients at increased risk of reactions (asthma, diabetes, cardiac failure, other allergies) or, with care, if there is a history of sensitivity to traditional contrast agents
• Mesenteric anatomy is shown in Fig. 9.4 (p. 305)

Other imaging techniques

Ultrasound
• Indicated for the investigation of abdominal pain (gall stones, pancreatitis), jaundice, abnormal liver function tests (Fig. 5.7, p. 181), hepatomegaly or abdominal masses. Pelvic ultrasound and Doppler examination of blood flow in large vessels are also useful (p. 154). Diagnostic biopsy or therapeutic aspiration can be performed under ultrasound control
• An ideal, non-invasive investigation for thin patients
• Whilst reliable in experienced hands, the interpretation is subjective and intestinal gas can prevent adequate views
• Preparation involves nothing to eat for 4 h if the gall bladder is to be imaged. Failure of the gall bladder to contract after a fatty meal suggests chronic cholecystitis (p. 22) and influences non-surgical management of gall stones (p. 191)
• Ultrasound of other areas of the abdomen needs no preparation, apart from the pelvis, when the bladder should be full
• Intraoperative ultrasound and endosonography of the rectum, oesophagus or duodenum give better resolution and more accurate information about the margins of tumour infiltration than transcutaneous ultrasound, but the techniques are not widely available

Computerized tomography (CT scan)
• Indicated if ultrasound is not technically possible (fat patients, excessive bowel gas), or if doubt about the diagnosis persists
• CT scan is better than ultrasound for demonstrating retroperitoneal structures (except the pancreas), common bile duct stones, or for fat patients, but still needs skilled interpretation
• Contrast (oral and intravenous) is given to facilitate definition
• Preparation is the same as for ultrasound

Magnetic resonance imaging (MRI)
• Potentially excellent for discriminating benign from malignant hepatic or pancreatic lesions, but indications are still being assessed
• Implants of magnetic materials (clips, prosthetic valves, pacemakers) are contraindications, depending on the type

Isotope studies
• Investigation of choice in acute cholecystitis, protein-losing enteropathy, or Meckel's diverticulum, but reserved for cases of doubt in other conditions (Table 12.1)
• Discussion with the Nuclear Medicine Department is advised, because not all tests may be locally available
• No preparation is necessary, but isotope studies should be avoided in children, or women of child-bearing age, especially if they may be pregnant

Table 12.1 Indications for gastrointestinal isotope studies

Condition	Scan	Page
Acute cholecystitis, biliary colic	^{99}Tc HIDA	22, 23
Active bleeding	^{99}Tc sulphur colloid	18
Obscure bleeding	^{99}Tc red cell	
	^{51}Cr red cell	316
Meckel's diverticulum	^{99}Tc pertechnate	18
Protein-losing enteropathy	^{51}Cr albumin	217
Steatorrhoea	^{14}C triolein	368
Crohn's disease activity	^{111}In white cell	249
Terminal ileal absorption	^{75}SeHCAT	213
	$^{57/58}$Co vitamin B$_{12}$	220
Budd–Chiari syndrome	^{99}Tc pertechnate	156
Gastric emptying	^{99}Tc scrambled egg	363

12.3 Function tests
The reliability of results depends on familiarity with the procedure and if such tests are necessary, the patient is best referred to a centre where they are regularly performed. Details of the tests are available in larger textbooks (Appendix 2) and only an outline is given here.

12.3 Function tests

Gastric function

Gastric acid secretion
The purpose is to measure basal, maximal and sometimes cephalic-stimulated secretion.
• Instructions to the patient:
—no antacids, H_2 receptor antagonists or anticholinergics for 5 days
—nothing to eat and only water to drink for 8 h before the test
—a nasogastric tube is used to aspirate gastric juice
• Basal acid secretion is measured for 1 h
• Maximal acid secretion is measured after 6 µg/kg pentagastrin intramuscular injection (= 0.42 mg for 70 kg)
• Cephalic-stimulated secretion is measured when the integrity of the vagal nerves needs to be assessed (p. 107), after sham feeding, which is safer than insulin infusion
• Measurements of volume (ml), pH (units), titratable acidity (mmol/l), acid output (mmol/h, calculated as volume (l) × titratable acidity) are made for each collection period, by prior arrangement with the Biochemistry Department
• Interpretation:
basal acid output is the sum of the four collections (in mmol/h). Normal is 0–5 mmol/h
peak acid output is the sum of the two consecutive highest collection periods (in mmol/h) after pentagastrin. Normal is 1–45 (mean 22) mmol/h for men and 1–30 (mean 12) mmol/h for women
maximal acid output is the single highest observed acid output

Gastric motility
Gastroparesis due to autonomic neuropathy (diabetes, amyloidosis) occasionally causes recurrent vomiting (p. 79). A barium meal provides subjective information about gastric emptying, but isotope studies provide a quantitative measurement.
• Drugs that affect motility (metoclopramide, domperidone, cisapride, anticholinergics, opiates) are avoided for 72 h. Fluids only for 12 h and nil by mouth for 4 h is usual before the test
• A radiolabelled meal (such as 100 g scrambled egg) is eaten, followed by gamma camera counting for about 90 min. Normal emptying is 20–30% solids and 40–50% liquids within 60 min, but ranges vary between laboratories

Pancreatic function
The principal indication is for symptoms of exocrine insufficiency (p. 121), with minimal or no changes on ERCP. Pancreatic supplements should be stopped 5 days before the test.

Direct (intubation) tests
• A double lumen tube (with gastric and duodenal ports) is positioned under fluoroscopic control after an overnight fast
• Basal and secretin-stimulated (1 unit/kg infused over 1 h) secretion of bicarbonate are measured by duodenal aspiration at 15-min intervals. Enzyme assay of lipase, amylase or trypsin may be performed, but normal values vary widely between laboratories
• Mean duodenal pH should be >6.0. Lower values indicate reduced bicarbonate secretion, rapid gastric emptying or acid hypersecretion
• Maximum HCO_3 <50mmol/l, or output <15 mmol/h is abnormal, although about 20% with a 'normal' result have pancreatic disease
• The Lundh test meal is a test of digestion (trypsin activity is measured in duodenal aspirate after a standard meal), but false positives are more common than with the secretin test (above)

Indirect tests (without duodenal intubation)
• The benzoyl-tyrosyl-*p*-aminobenzoic acid (btPABA) test involves two 6-h urine collections on consecutive days after test capsules containing control PABA and btPABA
• A PABA excretion index >82% is normal (indicating splitting of the bt peptide from PABA), but drugs (thiazides, paracetamol) or food (prunes) can produce false negatives
• A ^{14}C-labelled btPABA test can be performed in a single day
• The fluorescein dilaurate test involves two 10-h urine collections after a capsule of fluorescein dilaurate on the test day and one of fluorescein alone, as a control
• Urinary fluorescein is measured by spectrophotometer, which may be easier than PABA measurements in some laboratories
• An excretion index of <20% is abnormal. False negatives are very rare, but false positives not uncommon. Repeat testing is indicated for equivocal (20–30%) values

12.3 Function tests

Intestinal function

Intestinal absorption
- 5 g D-xylose, followed by a 5-h urine collection, or a 60-min blood xylose corrected for body surface area (blood xylose × measured surface area/1.73), is a non-specific test of carbohydrate malabsorption
- <22% urinary excretion, or 60-min corrected blood xylose <0.56 mmol/l are abnormal, but 20% untreated coeliac disease have a normal value and it should not be relied upon to detect abnormal absorption, or to avoid jejunal biopsy
- Rapid gastric emptying or intestinal transit, renal dysfunction or incomplete urine collection all give false positive results
- Sensitivity is improved by adding 3-O-methyl-D-glucose 1.0 g and measuring the plasma 60-min xylose: 3-mGlc ratio, but jejunal biopsy is still necessary to define the cause of malabsorption

Intestinal permeability
- Isotonic lactulose 5 g and L-rhamnose 0.1 g in 250 ml water, followed by a 5-h urine collection and calculation of the lactulose: rhamnose ratio, detects abnormal intestinal permeability, but may not be locally available. The test is sensitive but not specific
- The normal ratio is <0.04, and higher values indicate small intestinal disease (coeliac disease, Crohn's disease, tropical sprue, malnutrition)
- Other double sugar tests (lactulose/mannitol) depend on available assay techniques, but single marker tests (polyethyleneglycol or ^{51}Cr-EDTA) may give false results for the same reasons as the xylose absorption test

Terminal ileum
- Isotopic (^{75}SeHCAT or $^{57/58}$Co vitamin B_{12}) absorption tests have a high negative predictive value (a normal test reliably excludes disease), but specificity is poor
- The tests are sometimes useful when serum vitamin B_{12} is low or diarrhoea is unexplained, and the terminal ileum looks normal on contrast radiology
- Function tests are unnecessary when there are visible changes in the terminal ileum on small bowel radiology with a low serum vitamin B_{12} or persistent diarrhoea, because treatment with vitamin B_{12} replacement or cholestyramine is indicated

12.4 Other tests

Manometry

Manometry is a specialist procedure that is best performed at a referral centre. The principal indications for oesophageal manometry are dysphagia or chest pain of uncertain cause (p. 66), and for anorectal manometry are defaecation disorders (p. 289). Only patients with persistent or disabling symptoms should be referred. Manometry is not difficult to do, but considerable expertise is needed for useful interpretation of the results.

Oesophageal

• A catheter is swallowed and pressure recorded either by continuous perfusion or by intraluminal transducers. A sleeve sensor is best for measuring lower oesophageal sphincter (LOS) pressure, because focal sensors become displaced during swallowing. Intraluminal transducers are expensive, but are the only method for ambulatory recordings
• A normal recording shows sequential progression of the peristaltic wave (pressure is measured at 5-cm intervals) and relaxation of the LOS
• Either the pressure generated (amplitude can be >80 mmHg in oesophageal spasm) or the wave progression (failure of relaxation of the LOS in achalasia) may be abnormal. Provocative stimuli (edrophonium, acid perfusion) are sometimes used to trigger oesophageal contraction

Anorectal

• A multilumen tube, with a distal balloon and three side ports connected to pressure transducers, is inserted 10 cm into the rectum. Myoelectric recordings from the external anal sphincter or puborectalis can be measured simultaneously through needle electrodes. Perineal sensation is best assessed by measuring the current threshold at which a tingling sensation is felt between two cutaneous electrodes
• The rectum is distended by inflating the distal balloon (50–200 ml air)
• Normal recordings show relaxation of the internal sphincter during rectal distension and a rebound increase in pressure during deflation

• Absent sphincter relaxation during rectal distension (aganglionosis, p. 286), abnormal sphincteric tone (in faecal incontinence) or abnormal rectal sensation (desire to defaecate at high or low rectal volumes) may be detected
• Colonic and small intestinal manometry are research techniques at present

pH monitoring
24-h pH monitoring is best done at a referral centre, because whilst the technique is not difficult, interpretation can be complex. It is indicated for persistent symptoms of gastro-oesophageal reflux or undiagnosed chest pain, in the absence of visible oesophagitis (p. 66). Drugs for the treatment of gastro-oesophageal reflux should be stopped >5 days before testing.
• 24-h monitoring is performed with a pH-sensitive transducer placed 5 cm above the oesophagogastric junction, attached to an electronic recorder carried at the waist
• Frequency, time and duration that pH <4.0 are measured. Alkaline reflux is defined as pH >7.0
• Symptoms and position (lying or standing) are recorded by the patient
• Results are expressed as a percentage of the total recording time that oesophageal pH is below a certain level (usually <4)
• Normal individuals have about 20 episodes when pH <4 during 24 h, totalling <2% of the recording time, and rarely at night
• Symptoms due to reflux must correlate with abnormal oesophageal pH, but biliary reflux can confound results since pH may be high during symptoms

Breath tests
The choice of test depends on availability. Isotopes should be avoided in women of child-bearing age. The main advantage is that breath tests are non-invasive, but interpretation can be impossible after small intestinal resection. Other techniques (such as jejunal aspiration for small intestinal overgrowth) are more sensitive.

Hydrogen breath test
• Indicated for the diagnosis of bacterial overgrowth (lactulose or

glucose, p. 228) or hypolactasia (lactose) (p. 229), and to measure mouth–caecum transit (lactulose)
- Unabsorbed sugar is fermented by bacteria to hydrogen (and methane), which is absorbed into the circulation and exhaled via the lungs
- 50 g lactulose, glucose or lactose is given. 30 ml end-expiratory air is then collected (in a modified Haldane–Priestley tube) at 20-min intervals for 3 h, and analysed in a hydrogen analyser
- >20 ppm hydrogen after <2 h is abnormal for lactulose or lactose, and diagnoses bacterial overgrowth or hypolactasia respectively. The time of a step rise indicates arrival at the caecum, but interpretation can be difficult with rapid transit

^{14}C tests
- Exhaled $^{14}CO_2$ is low (<0.0005%) after ^{14}C-lactose in hypolactasia
- $^{14}CO_2$ is high (>0.0007%) after ^{14}C-glycocholate in bacterial overgrowth
- $^{14}CO_2$ is low (<0.0005%) after ^{14}C-triolein in fat malabsorption (p. 217)

Gut hormones
- All tests are performed after an overnight fast, most easily when the patient attends for endoscopy (p. 100), or during the assessment of secretory diarrhoea (Fig. 7.2, p. 212)
- Any H_2 receptor antagonists, or omeprazole, must be stopped for 2 weeks before gastrin levels are measured. High gastrin levels are otherwise impossible to interpret, although patients most likely to have Zollinger–Ellison syndrome (p. 104) are also those most likely to be taking these drugs. Symptomatic treatment with antacids for these 2 weeks is trying for the patient and doctors
- 10 ml blood is taken into a heparinized tube with 200 μl aprotinin (4000 IU/ml) (Trasylol)
- The sample is immediately taken to Biochemistry for separation and freezing
- A supraregional assay service (Appendix 1) measures gastrin, glucagon, vasoactive intestinal polypeptide, somatostatin or pancreatic polypeptide. Calcitonin should be measured in patients with unexplained diarrhoea, to exclude extremely rare cases of medullary thyroid carcinoma

13 Nutrition

13.1 Nutritional assessment

Nutritional assessment of any patient, particularly one with gastrointestinal disease, is essential. Dietary inadequacy, appetite disorders and general or specific malabsorption all contribute to nutritional deficiency. Neglecting the nutritional status of ill patients compromises survival. Starvation in hospital may follow surgery, prolonged investigation or gastrointestinal symptoms, combined with apprehension and unappetizing food.

The aim of assessment is to recognize general (protein–calorie) malnutrition (Table 13.1), as well as specific deficiencies (Tables 13.2–13.4, pp. 373 and 374).

Table 13.1 Assessment of protein–calorie malnutrition

Readily assessed	Objective measurements

History:
  anorexia
  dietary history (dietitian)
  calorie intake (dietitian)
  food and fluid chart (in-patient)
	Weight loss >10% in <3 months
	
	Blood tests:
	  albumin <35 g/l
	  lymphocytes <1.5 × 10^9/l
	  transferrin <2 g/l

Examination:
  muscle wasting
  oedema
  angular stomatitis
	Skin tests:
	  mid-triceps skin fold < 8 mm (M)
	                    <17 mm (F)
	  mid-arm circumference <30 cm (M)
	                        <26 cm (F)

Weight and height (Appendix 3):
  below minimum weight for height
  body mass index <19 kg/m^2
	negative tuberculin test

General malnutrition
• No single measurement is sufficient
• Height, weight and serum albumin (or total protein) may be the simplest measures available, but do not accurately reflect nutritional status. Hepatic, renal or intestinal disease will contribute to a low albumin or total serum protein
• Malabsorption, which may occur in the absence of diarrhoea, must not be overlooked (p. 215)
• The body mass index (Quetelet index) is most often used to assess obesity—the malnutrition of affluence. It is calculated according to the formula:

$$\text{Body mass index} = \frac{\text{Weight (kg)}}{\text{Height}^2 \text{ (m)}}$$

13.1 Nutritional assessment

- The relation to mortality is shown in Fig 13.1

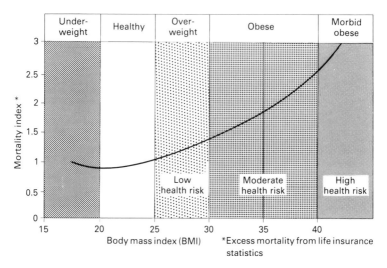

Fig.13.1 Relationship between obesity and mortality. Body mass index is explained in the text. (Adapted from Bray G.A. *International Journal of Obesity* 1978; **2**: 99–114, with permission.)

Specific deficiencies

- Deficiencies of vitamins and minerals are usually mixed, so clinical presentation is rarely classic (Tables 13.2–13.4 and p. 216)
- Diagnosis depends on the clinical context. Clues to the type of nutritional deficiency may be provided by chronic hepatic disease, malabsorption or malnutrition due to inadequate diet in housebound elderly, alcoholics, vegans (vitamin B_{12}), or Asians (vitamin D)
- Normal values of many of the less common tests vary between laboratories and the technique used. It is often unnecessary to do specific vitamin or trace element tests, but simply to treat suspected deficiency generously (see Tables 13.14–13.16, pp. 392 and 393)

Indications for nutritional support

The decision to provide nutritional support depends on the nutritional status (Table 13.1, p. 371) and nature of the illness (Table 13.5). A decision concerning nutritional support is mandatory if eating has not been possible for 3 days or dietary intake has been inadequate for 5 days.

13 Nutrition

13.1 Nutritional assessment

Table 13.2 Recognition of fat-soluble vitamin deficiencies in adults

Substance	Clinical	Diagnostic tests
Vitamin A	Night blindness Xerophthalmia, keratomalacia	Dark adaptation time
Vitamin D	Bone pain, proximal myopathy	Alkaline phosphatase Low Ca, low P Pelvic X-ray (Looser's zones, bone biopsy
Vitamin K	Bruising	Prothrombin time, or INR >1.3
Vitamin E	Spinocerebellar degeneration	White cell vitamin E

Table 13.3 Recognition of water-soluble vitamin deficiencies in adults

Substance	Clinical	Diagnostic tests
Thiamine (B_1)	Neuropathy, ophthalmoplegia psychosis, cardiac failure All alcoholics admitted to hospital	Red cell transketolase
Riboflavin (B_2)	Angular stomatitis, mucosal fissures (lips, genitalia) Normochromic anaemia, apathy, ataxia	Red cell glutathione reductase activity
Pyridoxine (B_6)	Sideroblastic anaemia, neuropathy, hyperoxaluria	Aminotransferase activity
Nicotinamide (niacin)	Dermatitis, diarrhoea, dementia, weight loss	Urinary metabolites
Folate	Macrocytic anaemia Alcoholic patients	Red cell folate <640 ng/l
Vitamin B_{12}	Macrocytic anaemia, painful neuropathy, ataxia, poor proprioception, paresis	Serum vitamin B_{12} <150 ng/l
Vitamin C	Poor wound healing, gum hyperplasia, bleeding, perifollicular, or subperiosteal haemorrhages	White cell ascorbic acid, or urinary excretion <10% after 1 g ascorbate

13.1 Nutritional assessment

Table 13.4 Recognition of mineral deficiencies in adults

Substance	Clinical	Diagnostic tests
Iron	Microcytic anaemia, glossitis, cheilosis, koilonychia	Serum iron < 11 μmol/l (F) <14 μmol/l (M), iron binding capacity >75 μmol/l, serum ferritin <15 μg/l
Calcium	Weakness, proximal myopathy, perioral paraesthesiae, tetany, Chvostek (jaw) and Trousseau (arm) signs	Serum calcium <2.20 mmol/l (add 0.02 × (40-serum albumin) to correct for albumin level)
Phosphate	Proximal myopathy	Serum phosphate <0.80 mmol/l
Magnesium	Myopathy not responding to calcium replacement	Serum magnesium <0.70 mmol/l
Zinc	Anorexia, crusting red rash, diarrhoea, depression, anaemia, candidiasis	Serum zinc <6 μmol/l (may be low in any acute illness)
Copper	Hypochromic anaemia not responsive to iron, low white cell count, osteoporosis	Red cell superoxide dismutase activity
Selenium	Cardiac failure	Glutathione peroxidase activity, serum Se

Table 13.5 Indications for nutritional support

General	Specific
Weight loss >10% in <3 months	Multiple injuries
Albumin <35 g/l	Burns
No food intake >3 days	Chronic sepsis (abscess)
Inadequate dietary intake >5 days	Acute pancreatitis
	Intestinal fistulae
	Short bowel syndrome
	Crohn's disease (adolescents)
	Complications of major surgery
	Dysphagia
	Persistent vomiting
	Malignancy
	Children or adolescents with chronic disease

13 Nutrition

13.1 Nutritional assessment

Nutritional requirements
- Four factors must be considered:
  energy
  nitrogen
  electrolytes
  trace elements/vitamins
- The nutritional status of the patient, severity of disease and catabolic rate determine the engery/nitrogen balance required (Table 13.6). High energy and nitrogen intakes are not needed in

Table 13.6 Daily nutritional requirements

Catabolic state	Low	Intermediate	High
Energy:			
(kJ/kg/24 h)*	125	125–150	150–250
(kcal/kg/24 h)	30	30–35	35–60
Nitrogen (g/kg/24 h)†	0.16	0.2–0.3	0.3–0.5
K (mmol/l/g N)	5	5	7
Phosphate (mmol/24 h)	20	20–30	30–50

Requirements for all catabolic states:

	Enteral	Parenteral
Electrolytes:		
Na	1 mmol/kg/24 h	1 mmol/kg/24 h
K	5 mmol/g N	5 mmol/g N
Ca	20 mmol/24 h	7–14 mmol/24 h
Mg	14 mmol/24 h	3–28 mmol/24 h
Trace elements (μmol/24 h):		
Fe	180–320	20–70
Zn	230	40–200
Mn	45–90	5–35
Cu	30–45	10–70
Cr	1–4	0.5–1
F	80–200	50
I	1–2	1–7
Se	0.6–2.6	0.4
Mo	0.2	0.2

* Energy is also measured in kilocalories (1 kcal = 4.2 kJ), but kcal is frequently shortened to cal, which is confusing.
† The non-protein energy: nitrogen ratio is not widely used any more, but is approximately 1000 kJ/g N (250 kcal/g N) in low catabolic and 550 kJ/g N (135 kcal/g N) in high catabolic states.

most situations, unless the patient is profoundly catabolic or has major nutrient losses, as in burns
• In low catabolic states such as starvation, paralysis or disease preventing an adequate oral intake, replacement with a normal energy/nitrogen balance is needed, with electrolyte, trace element or vitamin supplements if specific deficiencies are present
• In high catabolic states, including fever, sepsis, major surgery, trauma and burns, energy expenditure and hence requirements are increased by 10–100%

Feeding route
• Enteral feeding (see below) is the preferred method and should always be used if the gut is functioning, by whatever access is possible (sip feed supplements, fine-bore nasogastric tube, percutaneous endoscopic or surgical gastrostomy, or jejunostomy)
• Parenteral feeding should only be used when enteral feeding is impossible due to gut failure (see Table 13.9, p. 379)

13.2 Enteral feeding
Enteral feeding includes feeding with specially formulated feeds by sips, fine-bore nasogastric tube, or by enterostomy (gastro- or jejunostomy).

Indications (see Table 13.7.)

Table 13.7 Indications for enteral nutrition

Gastrointestinal disease:
malabsorption
short bowel
enteral fistulae
Catabolic states:
burns
sepsis
Anorexia:
any prolonged (>5 days) illness
especially elderly
before/after surgery
cancer and its therapy
stroke patients with loss of gag reflex

Choice of feed

There are either general purpose or elemental feeds, with many proprietary preparations. Elemental feeds are only indicated for severe malabsorption (short bowel, pancreatic insufficiency). Energy and nitrogen balance (Table 13.6, p. 375), volume, osmolality, palatability and cost must be considered. Most preparations contain appropriate amounts of vitamins (except folate) and trace elements, unless there are specific deficiencies, when supplements will be needed. Most are also gluten and lactose free.

General purpose

• Fresubin (3.8 g protein, 420 kJ energy/100 ml) is a suitable preparation. It is palatable when chilled as a sip feed and appropriate for fine-bore tube feeding
• 1500–2000 ml/day is needed for moderately catabolic patients
• Many hospitals have a local prescribing policy to limit the choice of enteral feeds and other preparations on account of cost. Ensure, or Clinifeed Favour have a similar balance of protein, energy, vitamins and trace elements to Fresubin

Elemental feeds

• Elemental feeds are pre-digested, containing nutrients in a directly absorbable form
• Elemental feeds are unpalatable and hyperosmolar. They are expensive and the indications for their use are extremely limited (such as active Crohn's disease refractory to steroids, p. 256)
• A fine-bore tube is needed and the feed must be introduced slowly to avoid side effects (diarrhoea, abdominal cramps, nausea)
• Elemental-028 powder (1550 kJ/100 g) for reconstitution is a suitable choice of elemental feed (about 500 g/day). Vitamins and trace elements are included, but folate may be insufficient

Techniques

Sip feeds, in addition to meals

• Suitable for most patients needing nutritional supplements. Any nutritious drinks, cooled or warmed for palatability, are suitable, or more expensive proprietary preparations (Fortisip) may be used
• Patients who cannot eat are unlikely to drink sufficient liquid supplements (1500–2000 ml/day) for all their nutritional

requirements. Fine-bore nasogastric feeding is then needed, with a balanced proprietary preparation (such as Fresubin)

Fine-bore tube feeding
• Polyurethane tubes with a stylet are easily inserted (start extracting the stylet when the tube is halfway down)
• Weighted tubes offer little advantage, except for nasojejunal feeding when patients have impaired gastric motility
• The position must be checked, either by sharply injecting 5 ml air whilst listening at the epigastrium ('bubble test'), or by aspirating and testing with litmus paper. An X-ray is necessary if there is *any* doubt about the position, especially in unconscious patients, but this is rare

Gastrostomy and jejunostomy feeding
• Surgically sited gastrostomy or jejunostomy tubes are an alternative to parenteral nutrition when proximal obstruction prevents nasogastric feeding. Percutaneous endoscopic gastrostomy is possible at specialist centres

Regimen
• Continuous drip feeding enhances absorption and reduces complications. A pump is invaluable for regulating the feed
• Starter regimens are rarely necessary if gastrointestinal function is normal. Starting at a slower rate, with additional water to maintain fluid balance, is better than diluting the feed. Bolus feeding is a cause of diarrhoea or bloating

Complications (Table 13.8)

Table 13.8 Complications of enteral nutrition

Problem	Management
Abdominal distension	Reduce rate of infusion
Tube obstruction	Inject water (1 ml syringe), or replace tube
Tube misplacement	X-ray position in unconscious patients
Oesophageal erosions	Use a soft, fine-bore tube
Hyperglycaemia	Insulin (common in septicaemia)
Electrolyte imbalance	Check serum K weekly, phosphate and zinc after 3 weeks
Low folate	Folate supplements after 3 weeks

• Diarrhoea with enteral feeding is usually due to bolus feeding or antibiotics. It can be alleviated by continuous feeding (if necessary at a slow rate to start with) and loperamide 8–16 mg/day, or codeine phosphate 60–180 mg/day. Do not stop the feeding

13.3 Parenteral feeding
Parenteral feeding is much more demanding than enteral feeding, and is hazardous unless it is done well. Meticulous asepsis and care of the catheter are essential, if life-threatening complications are to be avoided.

Indications
The gastrointestinal tract is inaccessible or not functioning normally in unusual circumstances (Table 13.9). The indications for nutritional support are the same as for enteral feeding (Tables 13.5 and 13.7, p. 374 and 376), when associated with gut failure.

Table 13.9 Circumstances requiring parenteral nutrition

Problem	Comment
Complete dysphagia	Fine-bore tubes pass most strictures. Tube placement with a paediatric endoscope is sometimes necessary
Intestinal osbtruction:	
mechanical	Perioperative
ileus	Postoperative
Short bowel:	When enteral feeding is insufficient
intestinal fistulae	
extensive disease	Elemental feeds may be an alternative for Crohn's disease (p. 256)
resection	Home parenteral feeding is for specialists
Acute pancreatitis	Fig. 1.2 (p. 29)

Choice of feed

3-litre bags
• 3-litre bags are much safer and easier to use than separate bottles of lipid emulsion and glucose/amino acid solutions, because the risk of infection is lower. This is especially true for occasional users
• Some hospitals make up their own 3-litre bags under aseptic conditions

13 Nutrition

13.3 Parenteral feeding

• Ready made bags are available commercially and can be adapted to a patient's daily nutritional requirements (Appendix 1)

Individual constituents

Nitrogen is provided by an amino acid solution, with equal proportions of energy from glucose and a fat emulsion. There are four steps in calculating the constituents for an individual patient.

• Daily nitrogen requirements must be decided first (Table 13.6, p. 375). Nitrogen loss calculated from 24 h urinary urea (1 mole urea contains 28 g nitrogen) is not very reliable

• The amount of energy required must then be calculated, depending on the weight of the patient and the underlying disease (pp. 375 and 376)

• Additional electrolytes are added to the 3-litre bag if needed, according to the results of electrolyte and Actrapid insulin given intravenously (1–2 U/h) according to blood glucose monitoring (Table 13.11, p. 382)

• Vitamins and trace elements are added as Solvito N 1 vial daily (water-soluble vitamins), Vitlipid N 10 ml/24 h (fat-soluble vitamins) and Addamel 10 ml/24 h (trace elements), or equivalent preparations. Many amino acid solutions are low in phosphate and this needs to be corrected (Addiphos contains 40 mmol phosphate, but also contains 30 mmol K and 30 mmol Na/20 ml)

A suitable temporary regimen for moderately catabolic patients (weight about 70 kg) if no 3-litre bag is available is shown in Table 13.10. Extra KCl may need to be added (total 45 mmol/24 h in the regimen shown) to the dextrose infusion, especially if serum K <4.0 mmol/l.

Table 13.10 Suitable parenteral feeding regimen for moderately catabolic patients

	Solution	Amount (ml)	N (g)	Energy (kJ)	Additive	Duration (h)
Line 1:	Vamin 14	1000	14.1	1500	Addamel 10 ml	24
Line 2:	Intralipid 10%	1000	—	4200	Vitlipid 10 ml	12
					Solvito N Ivial*	
	Dextrose 20%	1000	—	3360	Addiphos 10 ml	12

* Add Solvito N to Vitlipid, then both to Intralipid.

Techniques

Tunnelled central venous lines
• The cannula is inserted under local anaesthetic, in the operating theatre or anaesthetic room. The catheter runs subcutaneously for about 5 cm before entering the subclavian or internal jugular vein
• The cannula is connected to a 10 cm extension tube, which is both sutured and taped onto the skin, to avoid tugging directly on the cannula
• The position is checked by X-ray (catheters are faintly radio-opaque). The tip should lie about 1 cm proximal to the atrium

Catheter care
• The skin entry site and any connections must be checked and sprayed with Povidone–iodine twice daily
• 1 cm wide Elastoplast strips should be used to secure the extension tube, but should not cover the connections or entry site
• The value of a dressing is debatable. Dressings hide the entry site, create a warm, moist environment for bacterial growth and, when changed, increase the risk of infection. Some transparent dressings (such as Opsite) adhere tenaciously to plastic tubing. No dressing at all is preferable if the site can be checked and sprayed twice daily
• The catheter must only be used for parenteral feeding and not for giving drugs or taking blood. A triple lumen catheter is advisable for sick patients, the other channels being used to monitor CVP and give drugs if needed.
• The giving set must be changed daily. A 3-way tap is sometimes inserted between the extension tube and giving set, to lock off the catheter, but this increases the temptation to inject drugs through this route
• Should a pyrexia develop and other causes have been excluded, the catheter must be removed and the tip sent for culture

Peripheral nutrition
Peripheral intravenous nutrition is useful when it is desirable to maintain nutrition, but when enteral feeding is temporarily inappropriate and can be expected to start within 1 week. It is not an alternative to central venous feeding when parenteral feeding is needed for longer periods, because thrombophlebitis is common.

A nitrate patch applied over the vein distal to the cannula may decrease thrombophlebitis. Modern commercial solutions (such as Vitrimix) are less hypertonic than solutions for central venous delivery, but additives cannot be given, although they are still far better than no nutrition at all.

Monitoring

Guidelines are shown in Table 13.11. More frequent estimations (especially of electrolytes and glucose) are often necessary in the first week, but when feeding is stable the frequency can be reduced. Baseline measurements must be taken before treatment; measurement of magnesium, folate and zinc are often forgotten. Microbiology specimens (sputum, urine, drains, blood, faeces, catheter tips) are done as clinically indicated. Accurate fluid balance is vital.

Table 13.11 Monitoring during parenteral nutrition

Measurement	Daily	Twice weekly	Weekly	Fortnightly
Electrolytes	+			
Urea	+			
Full blood count	+			
Glucose*	+			
Check entry site	+			
Fluid balance	+			
Weight		+		
Albumin		+		
Liver function tests		+		
Calcium		+		
24-h urinary urea		+		
Magnesium			+	
Phosphate			+	
Zinc			+	
Iron				+
Folate				+

* Frequent bedside monitoring to adjust insulin infusion.

Complications

The complication rate depends on the experience of the person inserting the line, and subsequent catheter care (Table 13.12). Designated people should be responsible for inserting feeding lines and checking catheter care. Few British hospitals have an ideal

Table 13.12 Complications of parenteral nutrition

Mechanical:
  pneumothorax
  air embolus
  catheter displacement
  major venous thrombosis
  pulmonary embolus

Septic:
  septicaemia
  endocarditis

Metabolic:
  fluid overload
  hyperglycaemia
  electrolyte imbalance

Hepatic:
  abnormal liver function tests*
  jaundice

Deficiencies:
  phosphate
  trace elements
  essential fatty acids (linoleic, arachidonic)
  vitamins, especially folate

* Usually mild, transient and predominantly cholestatic.

nutritional team consisting of a doctor, nurse, dietitian and pharmacist. The advantages are that a nutritional team can agree on standard procedures and policy, as well as offering expertise, advice, or training.

13.4 Therapeutic diets

Badly planned, badly presented or poorly understood diets result in poor compliance and are not worth prescribing. An imaginative dietitian is invaluable for helping patients maintain special diets.

Weight-reducing diet

Obesity (the malnutrition of affluence) contributes to the cause of osteoarthritis, diabetes, cardiovascular disease and many other diseases, directly increasing the risk of death (Fig. 13.1, p. 372). Mortality in patients more than 25% overweight is increased by 500% in diabetics, and 160% in patients with ischaemic heart disease.

Principles
- Indicated for overweight (>110% recommended weight for height) and obese (>120%) patients (body mass index >25 kg/m^2). See Appendix 3
- A realistic target weight should be set (Appendix 3) and steady, moderate weight loss planned (about 0.5 kg/week)
- Low fat and sugar, but high complex carbohydrate (fibre) intake is recommended. Fat has twice the energy density of protein or carbohydrate
- Early weight loss is largely due to loss of body water due to breakdown of glycogen. Inappropriately low carbohydrate intake can lead to a breakdown of lean body mass (protein). Prolonged, steady dieting is necessary for any substantial loss of body fat
- Energy expenditure must exceed intake until the target weight is reached
- Eating patterns must be permanently changed, or weight will be regained
- Regular supervision, a weight chart posted in a prominent place, support from a skilled dietitian or slimming organizations (especially those that charge) improves success
- The minimum daily energy intake that includes essential nutrients without supplements is about 3000 kJ (700 kcal)
- Patients >120 kg usually have a *high* metabolic rate (>8000 kJ) and even higher food intake, despite frequent denials about excessive eating

Constituents of 4700 kJ (1100 kcal) diet
- Daily allowance:
  skimmed milk 1 pint
  butter or margarine 15 g, or low-fat butter substitute 25 g
  as much vegetables/salad as wanted
  three pieces of fruit
  unlimited water, tea, coffee, low-calorie fizzy drinks/squashes
- Protein—any two of the following, each day:
  lean meat 100 g (liver, pork, veal, steak, beef, lamb, no fat)
  fish or shellfish 100 g (not in batter)
  beans or pulses 175 g
  cottage cheese 100 g
  hard cheese 50 g
  two eggs (no more than four eggs/week)

- Carbohydrate (unrefined, high fibre)—a total of 6–10 portions of any of the following:
  wholemeal bread one slice
  one potato medium-sized
  breakfast cereal (not sugar coated) 25 g
  one Weetabix or Shredded Wheat
  pasta or rice 25 g (before cooking)

Other approaches to obesity
- Dietary compliance is invariably required with any anti-obesity drug treatment
- Appetite suppressants—only when excessive appetite limits the effect of diet, for a maximum 6 months. All have serious side effects (blood disorders, pulmonary hypertension). D-fenfluramine 60 mg/day is currently the only non-amphetamine
- Thermogenic drugs—thyroxine, ephedrine, or caffeine are not recommended, because protein, rather than fat, is mobilized and side effects are unacceptable. Lipolysis-specific β-agonists are under trial
- Mechanical devices—for patients who cannot achieve dietary compliance and only if concomitant disease requires urgent weight loss, or if obesity poses a danger to life:
  —jaw wiring—efficacious, but weight regained when jaws unwired
  —nylon waist cord—after weight loss, to prevent regain in weight
  —gastric balloon—inserted endoscopically. Effective, but often poorly tolerated and deflation after several weeks is common
- Surgery—same indications as for mechanical devices:
  jejuno-ileal bypass has 5% mortality and 60% morbidity
  gastroplasty is effective, but mortality is 4% and morbidity 33%

High-fibre diet
Indicated for diverticular disease, most patients with constipation and some with irritable bowel syndrome. The potential for reducing the risk of colorectal cancer, cardiovascular disease, or gall stones has yet to be confirmed. A higher fibre intake (aiming for 30 g/day) is suitable for most Western people as a pattern of healthy eating.

Principles
- Fibre provides bulk, absorbs water and satisfies hunger. Intake should be increased gradually
- Excessive flatulence from bacterial fermentation is the main

disadvantage, but only intestinal strictures or neurogenic constipation (p. 287) are contraindications
• Additional bran is rarely needed if fibre-rich foods are eaten regularly and in sufficient quantity
• Fluid intake must be increased (to 1500 ml/day or more) to compensate for water retained by increased fibre

Guidelines
• Good sources of fibre are:
  wholemeal (not ordinary brown) bread
  wholegrain cereals (muesli, All Bran, Bran Flakes, Weetabix)
  porridge oats
  wholemeal flour
  wholemeal pasta
  fresh vegetables (beans, peas, green leafy vegetables)
  pulses (dried beans, lentils)
  fresh fruit (oranges, apples, peaches)
• Vegetables should be lightly cooked
• Unprocessed coarse bran can be added if dietary changes are insufficient: 1 tbsp/day, added to soups, cereals, stewed fruit, home baking
• Bran tablets are available, but not prescribable. Ispaghula husk granules (Regulan, Fybogel) are more convenient and expensive than dietary changes or unprocessed bran, but much less preferable

Gluten-free diet
Indicated for coeliac disease (p. 220).

Principles
• An *absolute* gluten-free diet is the only way to treat coeliac disease. Non-compliance is the commonest cause of persistent symptoms (p. 225)
• Gluten ingestion increases the risk of lymphoma and ulcerative jejunitis in coeliac disease, so the diet must be continued for life
• The Coeliac Society (Appendix 1) provides an excellent recipe book, with the gluten content of most foods

Guidelines
• Avoid:
  wheat, barley, oats, rye
  any products (bread, cakes, biscuits, pastry, crispbread)

wheat cereals (Weetabix, Puffed Wheat)
pasta
packet soups
gravy, Oxo cubes, curry powder, mustard, sauces
chocolate, ice cream, sweets
• Allowed:
any fish, meat, poultry, game (no breadcrumbs/batter)
any cheese, eggs, milk, dairy products
any vegetables, potatoes, rice, or fruit
Cornflakes, Rice Krispies
bread, cakes, or biscuits from gluten-free flour
• Essential gluten-free products are prescribable, including bread
(Juvela, Rite Diet), pasta (Aglutella, Aproten), biscuits (Nutricia)
and flour

Lactose-free diet
Indicated for hypolactasia, especially when diarrhoea persists after
acute gastroenteritis (p. 215), treatment of Crohn's disease (p. 260),
ulcerative colitis (p. 276), or after gluten exclusion in coeliac
disease (p. 225).

Principles
• Milk and liquid milk products are the only appreciable source of
lactose. Many dairy products contain insufficient lactose to cause
symptoms
• Hypolactasia may be temporary, so milk can be reintroduced later
• Variable tolerance to milk is often due to changes in colonic
absorptive capacity (p. 230)

Guidelines
• Avoid:
milk of any sort (cows', goats', sheeps', cream), except soya milk
yoghurt
cottage cheese
ice cream
• Allowed—anything else, including butter, cheese

Elemental diet (p. 377)

Low-residue diet
Indicated when intestinal strictures cause symptoms, or prior to

investigations (colonoscopy, barium enema, small bowel radiology) or colorectal surgery.

Principles
• Indigestible fibrous foods are kept to a minimum
• Nutritional supplements (p. 377) are often necessary for strictures in association with Crohn's disease

Guidelines
• Avoid:
high-fibre foods (p. 386)
• Allowed:
any meat, fish, poultry, or game (no stuffing)
milk, dairy products

Low-fat diet
Indicated for steatorrhoea due to chronic pancreatitis, cholestasis, or severe malabsorption, as well as hyperlipidaemia. No benefit has been shown for other types of hepatobiliary disease, although avoiding fatty foods (rather than a specific low-fat diet) decreases post-prandial discomfort in some patients with gall stones or hepatitis.

Principles
• Reduce total fat intake to 30–50 g/day, or until steatorrhoea is controlled
• Substitute polyunsaturated for saturated fats in hyperlipidaemia
• Fat is important for palatability and the diet must be prescribed carefully. Medium-chain triglyceride supplements are indicated if calorie intake is insufficient following fat restriction (shown by continued weight loss)

Guidelines
• Avoid:
all fried food
butter, margarine (in moderation)
any cheese (except cottage cheese)
whole, evaporated or condensed milk, cream
fatty meat (goose, duck, sausages, paté)
fatty fish (salmon, herrings)

salad cream, mayonnaise, salad dressing
any pastry or cakes
chocolate, marzipan, Ovaltine, nuts, olives
• Allowed:
skimmed milk
low-fat spreads
cottage cheese
chicken, turkey, liver, game
white fish, haddock, smoked fish
any vegetables or fruit
any bread or pasta and most cereals
Marmite, Oxo, herbs, spices

Low-protein diet
Indicated in acute hepatic encephalopathy (p. 147) or renal failure, but only continued if encephalopathy relapses after treatment of the provoking cause. Not indicated for cirrhosis without encephalopathy.

Principles
• The aim is an intake that avoids encephalopathy but maintains adequate nutrition (usually 40–50 g/day distributed evenly)
• The purpose is to decrease toxic products of bacterial action on nitrogenous compounds (ammonia, mercaptans, aromatic amino acids)

Guidelines
• Limit:
meat, fish, cheese, peas, lentils, nuts
eggs
• Allowed:
other vegetables (potatoes, greens, tomatoes, marrow)
200 ml/day milk (half a pint)
butter
bread

Low-salt diet
Indicated for refractory ascites or fluid retention in hepatic, cardiac or renal failure, although it is usually sufficient to avoid adding salt to food.

13.4 Therapeutic diets

Principles
- Normal intake often exceeds the recommended daily allowance (1 mmol/kg/day), because most salt is added to food to improve palatability
- The aim is to restrict intake to 40–60 mmol/day
- KCl (such as 'Lo Salt') is best avoided, especially if potassium-sparing diuretics are prescribed, and re-education about salt intake given instead

Guidelines
- Avoid:
  any salt added before, during or after cooking
  convenience foods (ready-made meals)
  bacon, gammon, ham, sausages, paté
  cheese
  Oxo, Marmite, bottled sauces
  crisps, savoury biscuits, peanuts, savoury snacks
- Allowed:
  bread (in moderation)
  butter or margarine (in moderation)
  any meat, fish, eggs, vegetables, fruit
  pasta, cereals
- Palatability is improved by lightly cooking vegetables, using herbs (dill, garlic, rosemary, chives) or sauces (onion, apple)

Exclusion diet (Table 13.13)
Indicated for food allergy, intolerance and the irritable bowel syndrome, especially if symptoms appear related to food. About half respond well and more are improved (p. 322). An experienced dietitian is needed to motivate the patient and to provide a systematic approach.

Principles
- The basic diet is continued for 2 weeks, with a diary kept of food eaten and symptoms experienced
- Foods are reintroduced one at a time after 2 weeks, if improvement has occurred. Further items are tried at intervals of 2 days
- Foods should be fresh or frozen, since many tinned or packet foods contain preservatives
- Intelligent co-operation by the patient is clearly essential

13.4 Therapeutic diets

Table 13.13 Constituents of an exclusion diet

Food	Not allowed	Allowed
Meat	Preserved tinned meats Corned beef, paté, salami Bacon, sausages	All other meats Chicken, lamb
Fish	Smoked fish (haddock, kippers) Shellfish (mussels, prawns)	White fish (cod, sole)
Vegetables	Potatoes (any kind) Onions (fresh or dried) Sweetcorn	All other vegetables Cabbage, sprouts, beans, carrots, peas
Fruit	Citrus (lemons, grapefruit, oranges, limes) Including fruit juice	All other fruits
Cereals	Wheat (bread, cakes, biscuits) Rye (crispbreads) Oats (porridge) Pulses Corn (cornflakes, cornflour)	Rice Tapioca Millet, buckwheat
Oils	Corn oil, vegetable oil	Sunflower, olive, soya oil
Dairy	Cows' milk Butter Cheese Eggs Yoghurt	Goats', soya milk Goats', sheeps' milk cheese
Drinks	Tea Coffee (fresh, decaffeinated) Alcohol Squashes	Apple, pineapple, tomato juices
Others	Chocolate Yeast Marmite Nuts Preservatives	Sugar Spices Honey Herbs Sea salt

Mineral and vitamin supplements

Indicated when there are specific deficiencies (Tables 13.2–13.4, pp. 373 and 374), or unexplained symptoms in association with severe malabsorption. Prophylaxis is indicated in profound cholestasis (primary biliary cirrhosis, PBC), short bowel syndrome or parenteral nutrition. Optimum amounts are often uncertain, but Tables 13.14–13.16 give guidance.

Parenteral administration is usually necessary, since deficiencies in gastrointestinal disease are due to failure of absorption.

13 Nutrition

13.4 Therapeutic diets

Table 13.14 Treatment of fat-soluble vitamin deficiencies in gastrointestinal disorders

Substance	Acute deficiency	Prophylaxis
Vitamin A	Retinol 100 000 U i.m. weekly	100 000 U i.m. monthly
Vitamin D	Calciferol 100 000 U i.m. weekly Oral alfacalcidol 1 μg daily is indicated in severe PBC	Calciferol 100 000 U i.m. monthly*
Vitamin K	Phytomenadione 10 mg i.v. for 3 days	10 mg i.m. monthly
Vitamin E	–	Vitamin E suspension 5 mg daily No parenteral preparation

i.m.: intramuscular injection; i.v.: intravenous injection; o.d.: once daily; b.d.: twice daily; t.d.s.: three times daily

Table 13.15 Treatment of water-soluble vitamin deficiencies in gastrointestinal disorders

Substance	Acute deficiency	Prophylaxis
Thiamine (B$_1$)	Parentrovite HP 10 ml slowly i.v. for 3 days	Parentrovite Weak 4 ml i.m. monthly
Riboflavin (B$_2$)	Same	Same (deficiency still possible despite Parentrovite)
Pyridoxine (B$_6$)	Same	Parentrovite Weak 4 ml i.m. monthly, or pyridoxine 10 mg daily (oral)
Nicotinamide (niacin)	Same	Parentrovite Weak 4 ml i.m. monthly
Folate	Folic acid 15 mg daily for 1 month, then 5 mg for 3 months to replenish stores	5 mg daily 15 mg daily in malabsorption No parenteral preparation
Vitamin B$_{12}$	Hydroxycobalamin 1000 μg i.m. daily for 5 days	1000 μg i.m. every 3 months
Vitamin C	Ascorbic acid 300 mg i.m. daily	Parentrovite Weak 4 ml i.m. monthly

13.4 Therapeutic diets

Table 13.16 Treatment of mineral deficiencies in gastrointestinal disorders

Substance	Acute deficiency	Prophylaxis
Iron	Ferrous sulphate 200 mg t.d.s. for 3 months Total dose iron infusion if oral iron not absorbed or tolerated	200 mg o.d.
Calcium	Calcium gluconate 10 ml i.v. (tetany), then 40 ml i.v./day	Calcium gluconate 2 tabs t.d.s.*
Phosphate	50 mmol/l i.v. over 12 h	Phosphate-Sandoz 2 tabs o.d.†
Magnesium	50 mmol $MgCl_2$ i.v. over 12 h	$MgCl_2$ solution 15 mmol/day
Zinc sulphate	200 mg tab t.d.s. for 2 weeks	200 mg o.d.
Trace elements (see below)		

* Effervescent calcium tablets also contain 4.5 mmol Na. Calcium should be monitored every 2 weeks, especially if vitamin D is given as well.
† Rarely required.

Principles
• Diagnostic tests are complicated or unreliable for many substances (Tables 13.2–13.4, pp. 373–374). Iron, vitamin B_{12} and folate are exceptions
• Mixed deficiencies are common
• Fat-soluble vitamins are deficient in cholestasis, but all vitamins and some trace elements become deficient in severe malabsorption
• Vitamins A or D, iron, calcium, zinc and copper are toxic in overdose, so response should be checked every 1–2 weeks

Guidelines
• Vitamins: see Tables 13.14 and 13.15
• Minerals: see Table 13.16
• Trace elements:
  copper, manganese, iodine, fluoride, chromium, selenium,
    molybdenum, nickel, cobalt, vanadium are ubiquitous
  Addamel 10 ml contains the daily requirements (including Ca,
    Mg but not P, and relatively deficient in Fe) for parenteral
    nutrition

supplementation is rarely necessary even in severe chronic
  malabsorption, but copper, iodine or selenium deficiency may
  occur
if zinc or magnesium supplements are required, monthly
  infusions (40 ml Addamel/l over 12 h) are justifiable
if trace elements are deficient then essential fatty acids may be
  too, so 500 ml Intralipid 20% should then also be given

Appendices

1   Useful addresses

Local organizations, which are listed in the telephone directory (Yellow Pages) under Social Service and Welfare Organizations, or Charitable and Benevolent Organizations, are especially helpful for:
* Alcohol abuse
* Services for the elderly
* Services for the disabled
* Drug abuse
* Hospices and cancer relief
* Bereaved

Adverse drug reactions
CSM, Freepost, London SW8 5BR
CSM Mersey, Freepost, Liverpool L3 3AB
CSM West Midlands, Freepost, Birmingham B15 1BR
CSM Northern, Freepost 1085, Newcastle NE1 1BR
CSM Wales, Freepost, Cardiff CF4 1ZZ
Dial 100 and ask for CSM Freephone

Al-Anon
61 Great Dover Street, London SE1 47F (Tel. 071 403 0888)
24 hour telephone service
Offers group support for close friends and relatives of problem drinkers. Local groups throughout the country

Alcoholics Anonymous
PO Box 1, Stonebrow House, Stonebrow, York YO1 2NJ (Tel. 0904 644026)

61 Great Dover Street, London SE1 47F (Helpline Tel. 071 352 3001)
Provides anonymous groups for the assistance of alcoholics and problem drinkers. Local numbers in the telephone directory.

Alcohol Concern (National Agency On Alcohol Misuse)
305 Grays Inn Road, London WC1X 8QF (Tel. 071 833 3471)
Concerned with prevention and treatment of alcoholism.

British Digestive Foundation
3 St Andrews Place, Regent's Park, London NW1 4LB (Tel. 071 486 0341)
Produces patient-orientated leaflets and supports research.

British Society of Gastroenterology
3 St Andrews Place, Regent's Park, London NW1 4LB (Tel. 071 387 3534)
Encourages education, training and audit in gastroenterology and gastrointestinal endoscopy.

Appendices

1   Useful addresses

British Association of Cancer United Patients (BACUP)
121–123 Charterhouse Street, London EC1 6AA (Tel. 071 608 1785; cancer
information service: 071 608 6661; cancer counselling service: 071 608 1038)
   Provides information and support for patients and relatives using a telephone
and written answer service by experienced cancer nurses.

Cancer Relief MacMillan Fund
Anchor House, 15–19 Britten Street, London SW3 3TZ (Tel. 071 351 7811)
   Provides nursing services. Local numbers in the telephone directory.

Cancer-Link
17 Britannia Street, London WC1X 9JN (Tel. 071 833 2451)
9 Castle Terrace, Edinburgh EH1 2DP (Tel. 031 228 5557)
   Patient-based, offering support on all aspects of cancer.

Coeliac Society
P.O. Box 220, High Wycombe, Bucks NG11 2HY (Tel. 0494 37278)
   Provides advice and counselling concerning the disease and diet, together
with holidays and social activities.

Colostomy Welfare Group
38–39 Eccleston Square, London SW1 1PB (Tel. 071 828 5175)
   Comprised of volunteers who are all colostomists who will visit in hospital or
at home, pre- and postoperatively.

Committee on Safety of Medicines
Market Towers, 1 Nine Elms Lane, London SW8 5NQ (Tel. 071 720 2188)
   Notification of adverse drug reactions and regulatory matters.

Department of Health
Alexander Fleming House, Elephant and Castle, London SE1 6BY
(Tel. 071 407 5522)
   Head office of the Chief Medical Officer and his staff

Dial UK
Victoria Buildings, 117 High Street, Claycross, Derbyshire CH5 9DZ,
(Tel. 0246 250055)
   Patient-based advice for the disabled, to live independently in the
community. Provides home helps, meals on wheels.

Drug Information (on any aspect of drug therapy)
Check details in latest BNF or Data Sheet Compendium first.

Aberdeen	Tel. 0224 681818	Extn 52316
Belfast	Tel. 0232 248095	Direct line
Birmingham	Tel. 021 378 2211	Extn 2296/2297
Bristol	Tel. 0272 282867	Direct line
Cardiff	Tel. 0222 759541	Direct line
Dundee	Tel. 0382 60111	Extn 2351
Edinburgh	Tel. 031 229 2477	Extn 2094/2416/2443
or	Tel. 031 229 3901	Direct line

Appendices

1 Useful addresses

Glasgow		Tel. 041 552 4726	Direct line
Guildford		Tel. 0483 504312	Direct line
Inverness		Tel. 0463 234151	Extn 288
	or	Tel. 0463 220157	Direct line
Ipswich		Tel. 0473 712233	Extn 4322/4323
	or	Tel. 0473 718687	Direct line
Leeds		Tel. 0532 430715	Direct line
Leicester		Tel. 0533 555779	Direct line
Liverpool		Tel. 051 236 4620	Extn 2126/2127/2128
London:			
Guy's Hospital		Tel. 071 955 5000	Extn 3594/5892
	or	Tel. 071 378 0023	Direct line
London Hospital		Tel. 071 377 7487	Direct line
	or	Tel. 071 377 7488	Direct line
Northwick Park		Tel. 081 869 2761	Direct line
Londonderry		Tel. 0504 45171	Extn 3262
Manchester		Tel. 061 225 2063	Direct line
	or	Tel. 061 276 6270	Direct line
Newcastle		Tel. 091 232 1525	Direct line
Oxford		Tel. 0865 742424	Direct line
Southampton		Tel. 0703 796908	Direct line
	or	Tel. 0703 796909	Direct line

Drug Abuse (Release)
169 Commercial Street, London E1 6BW (mailing address only)
(Helpline Tel. 071 603 8651)
24-h emergency Tel. 071 603 8654
Offers advice and information for patients charged with drug offences. It deals with the social, medical and legal problems arising from drug abuse.

Drug Abuse (Families Anonymous)
310 Finchley Road, London NW3 7AG (Tel. 071 731 8060)
Helps families and friends of drug abusers to relieve stress and aid recovery. Local support groups.

Employment Medical Advisory Services
1 Chepstow Place, Westbourne Grove, London W2 4TF (Tel. 071 229 3456)
Part of the Health and Safety Executive with local offices. Has a Prestel service (lead frame number 575) which has talkback facilities to enable users to send messages as well as giving general information.

Eating Disorders Association
Sackville Place, 44–48 Magdalen Street, Norwich NR3 1JE (Tel. 0603 621 414)
Offers mutual support and sharing of information. Concerned to promote research and statistical information.

Environmental Health—Medical Officer
Local names and addresses available from District Health Authority, local Microbiology Department, or Public Health Laboratory (PHLS).

Appendices

1 Useful addresses

Familial Adenomatous Polyposis
The Polyposis Registry, St Mark's Hospital, City Road, London EC1V 2PS
(Tel. 071 601 7958—direct line)
 Primarily research based, data collection and follow up.

Family Cancer Clinic
Department of Clinical Genetics, Royal Free Hospital Trust, Pond Street,
London NW3 2QG (Tel. 071 794 0500 extn 3702)
 Referral centre/advice on patients/families with multiple tumours.

Gastrointestinal Hormone Supraregional Assay Service
Hammersmith Hospital, DuCane Road, London W12 0HS (Tel. 081 740 3044)
 Specialist gut hormone assays available. Discuss the problem before sending
 samples.

Genetic Counselling
Telephone the Department of Medical/Clinical Genetics, at many teaching
hospitals.

Hospice Information Service
St Christopher's Hospice, Lawrie Park Road, Sydenham, London SE26 6DZ
(Tel. 071 779 9252)
 A resource link producing directories of hospices in the UK and overseas.

Hollister Stoma Care Advice Service
43 Castle Street, Reading, Berks RG1 7SN (Tel. 0800 521377)
 Offers confidential advice on any aspect of stoma care for patients and their
 carers.

Health Education Authority
Hamilton House, Mabledon Place, London WC1H 9TX (Tel. 071 631 0930)
 Official agency for health education for the general public.

Ileostomy Association of Great Britain and Ireland
Amblehurst House, Black Scotch Lane, Mansfield, Notts N18 4PF
(Tel. 0623 28099)
 Advisory service for people with ileostomies by way of hospital and home
 visits. Many of the volunteers are ileostomists themselves.

Kingston Trust
The Drove, Kempshott, Basingstoke, Hants RG22 5LU (Tel. 0256 52320)
 Provides homes for all types of stoma patients or those with other abdominal
 diseases in need of short stay or permanent accommodation.

Liver transplant units
Discuss possible transplantation as early as possible to allow full assessment.

Birmingham
Liver Unit, Queen Elizabeth Hospital, Birmingham B15 2TH
(Tel. 021 472 1311 extn 3428)

Appendices

1 Useful addresses

Cambridge
Transplant Co-ordinator, Addenbrookes Hospital, Hills Road, Cambridge
CB2 2QQ (Tel. 0223 217251—direct line)

Leeds
Transplant Co-ordinator, St James' University Hospital Trust, Becket Street,
Leeds LS9 7TF (Tel. 0532 433144 extn 4553)

London
Transplant Co-ordinator, Liver Unit, King's College Hospital, Denmark Hill,
London SE5 9RS (Tel. 071 274 6222—bleep 149 or Tel. 071 326 3254—direct
line)
Transplant Co-ordinator, Liver Unit, Royal Free Hospital, Pond Street, London
NW3 2QG (Tel. 071 794 0500—bleep)

Marie Curie Memorial Foundation
28 Belgrave Square, London SW1 1QG (Tel. 071 235 3325)
21 Rutland Street, Edinburgh EH1 2AE (Tel. 031 235 3325)
Runs 11 UK nursing homes and a nationwide domicilliary nursing service
especially night nursing. Provides urgent welfare needs in kind, advice and
general information.

Medical Advisory Service
10 Barley Mow Passage, Chiswick, London W4 4PH (Tel. 071 994 9874)
Telephone service run by nurses offering information and advice on medical
and health care by nurses, putting people in touch with the right organization.

National Association for Colitis and Crohn's Disease
98A London Road, St Albans, Hertfordshire AL1 1NX (Recorded message
Tel. 0727 44296)
Offers support and information for patients with inflammatory bowel disease
and their families.

National Society For Cancer Relief
30 Dorset Square, London NW1 (Tel. 071 402 8125)
See Cancer Relief MacMillan Fund.

Nursing services
Health Visitors
Community Nurses
District Nurses
Private Nursing Organizations
Local services listed under 'Nurses' in the telephone directory

Nutrition
(For commercial parenteral 3-litre bag service, 48 h notice is generally needed
before initiating feeding, but delivery is throughout the UK)

Appendices

1   Useful addresses

Supervisor, Compound Unit, Baxter Health Care Ltd, Caxton Way, Thetford, Norfolk IP24 3SE (Tel. 0842 763954)

Nutrition Product Manager, Kabi-Pharmacia, Daly Avenue, Knowlhill, Milton Keynes MK5 8PH (Tel. 0908 661101)

Poisons Information
Check in BNF or Data Sheet Compendium for latest details.

Belfast	Tel. 0232 240503
Birmingham	Tel. 021 554 3801
Cardiff	Tel. 0222 709901
Edinburgh	Tel. 031 229 2377
Leeds	Tel. 0532 430715 or Tel. 0532 432799
London	Tel. 071 635 9191 or Tel. 071 955 5095
Newcastle	Tel. 091 232 5131

Public Health Laboratory Service
1 Colindale Avenue, London NW9 5DF (Tel. 081 200 4400)
Central reference laboratory with local laboratories covering all districts, giving investigation services and advice.

Share-a-Care (National Register for Rare Diseases)
8 Cornmarket, Farringdon, Oxon
Puts people with rare diseases in contact with others who have the same disorder. A national register is compiled.

Tropical diseases
Offers clinical advice and information on immunization for foreign travel.

London
Hospital for Tropical Diseases, 4 St Pancras Way, London NW1
(Tel. 071 387 4411)

Liverpool
Liverpool School of Tropical Medicine, Pembroke Place, Liverpool L3 5QA
(Tel. 051 708 9393)

Portsmouth
Battenburg Avenue Clinic, North End, Portsmouth (Tel. 0705 664235)

Paediatric gastroenterology

Children's Liver Disease Foundation
40 Stoke Road, Guildford, Surrey GU1 4RS (Tel. 0483 300565)
Provides advice and emotional support for families with a child suffering from liver disease.

Cystic Fibrosis Research Trust
5 Blyth Road, Bromley, Kent BR1 3RS (Tel. 081 464 7211)
Provides support for parents, their children and adults suffering from cystic fibrosis.

Appendices

1 Useful addresses

Galactosaemia Support Group
31 Cotysmore Road, Sutton Coldfield, West Midlands B75 6BJ (no phone)

Helen House Hospice
37 Leopold Street, Oxford OX4 1QT (Tel. 0865 728251)
A hospice for children, providing terminal and short-term relief care.

National Advisory Service for Parents of Children with a Stoma
51 Anderson Drive, Valley View Park, Darvel KA17 0DE (Tel. 0560 22024)
Provides a support group for parents of children who have a stoma,
ileostomy, colostomy or urostomy. Includes Hirschsprung's disease.

National Reye's Syndrome Foundation
15 Nicholas Gardens, Pyrford, Woking, Surrey GU22 8SD (Tel. 09323 46843)
A support group for parents of children suffering from Reye's syndrome

National Society for Phenylketonuria
Worth Cottage, Lower Scholes, Pickles Hill, Keighley, North Yorkshire
BD22 0RR (Tel. 0535 44865)
Offers support for parents of children suffering from phenylketonuria
concerning their medical, social and educational welfare.

2   Further reading

A bibliography in a rapid reference book cannot be comprehensive. This section suggests general reference texts and refers to papers covering areas of controversy or particular complexity.

General texts

Bouchier IAD, Allan RN, Hodgson HJF, Keighley MRB. (1984) *Textbook of Gastroenterology.* Baillière Tindall, London.
Misiewicz JJ, Pounder RE, Venables CW, eds. (1992) *Diseases of the Gut and Pancreas,* 2nd edn. Blackwell Scientific Publications, Oxford. In press.
Sherlock S. (1989) *Diseases of the Liver and Biliary Systems,* 8th edn. Blackwell Scientific Publications, Oxford.

Alimentary emergencies

Webb WA. Management of foreign bodies of the upper gastrointestinal tract. *Gastroenterology* 1988; **94**: 204–16.
Hunt RH. Diagnosis and treatment of gastrointestinal bleeding: when, with what and by whom? *European Journal of Gastroenterology and Hepatology* 1990; **2**: 69–110.
Bouchier IAD. Management of oesophageal varices. *European Journal of Gastroenterology and Hepatology* 1990; **2**: 325–46.
Berry AR, Campbell WB, Kettlewell MGW. Management of major colonic haemorrhage. *British Journal of Surgery* 1988; **75**: 637–40.
Wilson C, Heads A, Shenkin A, Imrie CW. C-reactive protein, antiproteases and complement factors as objective markers of severity in acute pancreatitis. *British Journal of Surgery* 1989; **76**: 177–81.

Oesophagus

Gillebert G, Janssens J, Vantrappen G. Ambulatory 24 h intra-oesophageal pH and pressure recordings *vs* provocation tests in the diagnosis of chest pain of oesophageal origin. *Gut* 1990; **31**: 738–44.
Atkinson M. Barrett's oesophagus—to screen or not to screen? *Gut* 1989; **30**: 2–5.

Stomach and duodenum

McKinlay AW, Upadhay K, Gemmell CG, Russell RI. *Helicobacter pylori*: bridging the credibility gap. *Gut* 1990; **31**: 940–5.
Eckhardt VF, Giessler W, Kanzler G, Remmele W, Bernhard G. Clinical and morphological characteristics of early gastric cancer. *Gastroenterology* 1990; **98**: 708–14.
Allum WH, Hallisey MT, Kelly KA. Adjuvant chemotherapy in operable gastric cancer. *Lancet* 1989; **ii**: 571–4.

Pancreatic disease

Poston GJ, Williamson RCN. Surgical management of acute pancreatitis. *British Journal of Surgery* 1990; **77**: 5–12.
Ihse I. Pancreatic pain. *British Journal of Surgery* 1990; **77**: 121–2.

Appendices

2 Further reading

Kocjan G, Rode J, Lees WR. Percutaneous fine needle aspiration cytology of the pancreas: advantages and pitfalls. *Journal of Clinical Pathology* 1989; **42**: 341–7.

Carter DC. Cancer of the pancreas. *Gut* 1990; **31**: 494–6.

Liver disease

Sharon N, Alexander GJM. Hepatitis C, D and E virus infection. *Baillière's Clinical Gastroenterology* 1990; **4**: 749–74.

Editorial. Diuretics or paracentesis for ascites? *Lancet* 1988; **ii**: 775.

Maddrey WC, Van Thiel DH. Liver transplantation: an overview. *Hepatology* 1988; **8**: 948–9.

Biliary disease

Bouchier IAD. New drugs: gall stones. *British Medical Journal* 1990; **300**: 592–6.

Paumgartner G. Shock wave lithotripsy of gallstones. *American Journal of Roentgenology* 1989; **15**: 153:335–424

Cuschieri A, Dubois F, Mouiel, J *et al.* The European experience with laparoscopic cholecystectomy. *American Journal of Surgery* 1991; **161**: 385–7.

Small intestine

Corazza GP, Menozzi MG, Strocchi A, *et al.* The diagnosis of small bowel bacterial overgrowth. *Gastroenterology* 1990; **98**: 302–9.

Holmes GKT, Prior P, Lane MR, Pope D, Allan RN. Malignancy in coeliac disease—effect of a gluten-free diet. *Gut* 1989; **30**: 333–9.

Ulcerative colitis and Crohn's disease

Kirsner RG, Shorter JB, eds. (1988) *Inflammatory Bowel Disease*, 3rd edn. Lea & Febiger, Philadelphia.

Jewell DP. Pathogenesis of inflammatory bowel disease. *European Journal of Gastroenterology and Hepatology* 1990; **2**: 235–65.

Jewell DP. Timing and indications for colectomy in severe ulcerative colitis. *Gastroenterology International* 1991; (in press).

Ireland A, Jewell DP. Sulphasalazine and the new salicylates. *European Journal of Gastroenterology and Hepatology* 1989; **1**: 43–50.

Giafter MH, North G, Holdsworth CD. Controlled trial of polymeric versus elemental diet in the treatment of active Crohn's disease. *Lancet* 1990; **335**: 816–19.

Large intestine

Houlston RS, Murday V, Harcopos C, Williams CB, Slack J. Screening and genetic counselling for relatives of patients with colorectal cancer in a family cancer clinic. *British Medical Journal* 1990; **301**: 366–8.

Buyse M, Zeleniuch-Jacquotte A, Chalmers TC. Adjuvant therapy of colorectal cancer. *Journal of the American Medical Association* 1988; **259**: 3571–8.

Hughes K, Scheele J, Sugarbaker PH. Surgery for colorectal cancer metastatic to the liver. *Surgical Clinics of North America* 1989; **69**: 339–59.

Appendices

2   Further reading

Irritable bowel syndrome
Nanda R, James R, Smith H, Dudley CRK, Jewell DP. Food intolerance and
the irritable bowel syndrome. *Gut* 1989; **30**: 1099–104.

Gastrointestinal infections
Farthing MJG, Keusch GT. (1990) *Enteric Infection*. Chapman & Hall, London.
Qadri SM. Infectious diarrhoea. *Postgraduate Medical Journal* 1990; **88**:
169–84.
Christensen ML. Human viral gastroenteritis. *Clinical Microbiology Reviews*
1989; **2**: 51–89.
Gazzard BG. HIV disease and the gastroenterologist. *Gut* 1988; **29**: 1497–505.
Griffin PM, Olmstead LC, Petras RE. *Escherichia coli* 0157:H7-associated
colitis. *Gastroenterology* 1990; **99**: 142–9.

Investigations
Cotton PB, Williams CB. (1990) *Practical Gastrointestinal Endoscopy*, 3rd edn.
Blackwell Scientific Publications, Oxford.
Read NW, ed. *Gastrointestinal Motility: Which Test?* (1989) Wrightson
Biomedical Publishing, Petersfield.

Nutrition
Editorial. Dietary recommendations: how do we move forward? *British Journal
of Nutrition* 1990; **64**: 301–5.
Grant A, Todd E. (1987) *Enteral and Parenteral Nutrition*, 2nd edn. Blackwell
Scientific Publications, Oxford.

3   Height and weight charts

- 'Overweight' is defined as 10–19% above the upper limit for either men or women
- 'Obesity' is ≥20% above the upper limit
- The desirable weight for height shown in Table A3.1 is based on actuarial data for longevity and good health and should form the basis of advice on body weight
- The body mass index (BMI) (weight(kg)/height^2 (metres), normal range 20–25 kg/m^2) is explained on p. 371. See Fig. 13.1, p. 372

  BMI is a more sensitive index of the relationship between body weight and disease and is becoming the accepted standard of reference. Table A3.2 shows values of BMI according to height and weight data.

Table A3.1(a) Height and weight chart for men

Height		Weight					
		Small frame		Medium frame		Large frame	
cm	ft. ins	kg	st. lb	kg	st. lb	kg	st. lb
158	5.2	57.6–60.3	9.2–9.8	59.0–63.5	9.5–10.1	62.1–67.5	9.12–10.10
160	5.3	58.5–61.2	9.4–9.10	59.9–64.4	9.7–10.3	63.0–68.9	10.0–10.13
163	5.4	59.4–62.1	9.6–9.12	60.8–65.3	9.9–10.5	63.9–70.2	10.2–11.2
165	5.5	60.3–63.0	9.8–10.0	61.7–66.6	9.11–10.8	64.8–72.0	10.4–11.6
168	5.6	61.2–63.9	9.10–10.2	62.6–68.0	9.13–10.11	65.7–73.8	10.6–11.10
170	5.7	62.1–65.3	9.12–10.5	63.9–69.3	10.2–11.0	67.1–75.6	10.9–12.0
173	5.8	63.0–66.6	10.0–10.8	65.3–70.7	10.5–11.3	68.4–77.4	10.12–12.4
175	5.9	63.9–68.0	10.2–10.11	66.6–72.0	10.8–11.6	69.8–79.2	11.1–12.8
178	5.10	64.8–69.3	10.4–11.0	68.0–73.4	10.11–11.9	71.1–81.0	11.4–12.12
180	5.11	65.7–70.7	10.6–11.3	69.3–74.7	11.0–11.12	72.5–82.8	11.7–13.2
183	6.0	67.1–72.0	10.9–11.6	70.7–76.5	11.3–12.2	73.8–84.6	11.10–13.6
185	6.1	68.4–73.8	10.12–11.10	72.0–78.3	11.6–12.6	75.6–86.4	12.0–13.10
188	6.2	69.8–75.6	11.1–12.0	73.8–80.1	11.10–12.10	77.4–88.7	12.4–14.1
191	6.3	71.1–77.4	11.4–12.4	75.2–81.9	11.13–13.0	79.2–90.9	12.8–14.6
193	6.4	72.9–79.2	11.8–12.8	77.0–84.2	12.3–13.3	81.5–93.2	12.13–14.11

From 1983 Metropolitan Life Insurance Company height and weight tables, for men aged 25–59 in shoes and wearing indoor clothing.

Table A3.1(b) Height and weight chart for women

| Height | | Weight | | | | | |
| cm | ft. ins | Small frame | | Medium frame | | Large frame | |
		kg	st. lb	kg	st. lb	kg	st. lb
147	4.10	45.9–50.5	7.4–7.13	49.1–54.5	7.11–8.9	53.1–59.0	8.6–9.5
150	4.11	46.4–50.9	7.5–8.1	50.0–55.4	7.13–8.12	54.0–60.3	8.8–9.8
152	5.0	46.8–51.8	7.6–8.3	50.9–56.7	8.1–9.0	54.9–61.7	8.10–9.11
155	5.1	47.7–53.1	7.8–8.6	51.8–58.1	8.3–9.3	56.3–63.0	8.13–10.0
158	5.2	48.6–54.5	7.10–8.9	53.1–59.4	8.6–9.6	57.6–64.4	9.2–10.3
160	5.3	50.0–55.8	7.13–8.12	54.5–60.8	8.9–9.9	59.0–66.2	9.5–10.7
163	5.4	51.3–57.2	8.2–9.1	55.8–62.1	8.12–9.12	60.3–68.0	9.8–10.11
165	5.5	52.7–58.5	8.5–9.4	57.2–63.5	9.1–10.1	61.7–69.8	9.11–11.1
168	5.6	54.0–59.9	8.8–9.7	58.5–64.8	9.4–10.4	63.0–71.6	10.0–11.5
170	5.7	55.4–61.2	8.11–9.10	59.9–66.2	9.7–10.7	64.4–73.4	10.3–11.9
173	5.8	56.7–62.6	9.0–9.13	61.2–67.5	9.10–10.10	65.7–75.2	10.6–11.13
175	5.9	58.1–63.9	9.3–10.2	62.6–68.9	9.13–10.13	67.1–76.5	10.9–12.2
178	5.10	59.4–65.3	9.5–10.5	63.9–70.2	10.2–11.2	68.4–77.9	10.12–12.5
180	5.11	60.8–66.6	9.8–10.8	65.3–71.6	10.5–11.5	69.8–79.2	11.1–12.8
183	6.0	62.1–68.0	9.11–10.11	66.6–72.9	10.8–11.8	71.1–80.6	11.4–12.11

From 1983 Metropolitan Life Insurance Company height and weight tables, for women aged 25–59 in shoes and wearing indoor clothing.

3 Height and weight charts

Table A3.2 Body mass index ready reckoner

	Body mass index	Weight (kg) (to the nearest 1 kg)									
Dangerously	**45**	101	104	107	110	112	115	118	121	124	127
overweight	**44**	99	102	104	107	110	113	115	118	121	124
	43	97	99	102	105	107	110	113	116	118	121
	42	95	97	100	102	105	108	110	113	116	119
	41	92	95	97	100	102	105	108	110	113	116
Seriously	**40**	90	92	95	97	100	102	105	108	110	113
overweight	**39**	88	90	93	95	97	100	102	105	108	110
	38	86	88	90	93	95	97	100	102	105	107
	37	83	86	88	90	92	95	97	100	102	104
	36	81	83	85	88	90	92	95	97	99	102
	35	79	81	83	85	87	90	92	94	96	99
	34	77	79	81	83	85	87	89	91	94	96
	33	74	76	78	80	82	85	87	89	91	93
	32	72	74	76	78	80	82	84	86	88	90
	31	70	72	74	75	77	79	81	83	85	88
Overweight	**30**	68	69	71	73	75	77	79	81	83	85
	29	65	67	69	71	72	74	76	78	80	82
	28	63	65	66	68	70	72	74	75	77	79
	27	61	62	64	66	67	69	71	73	74	76
	26	59	60	62	63	65	67	68	70	72	73
Acceptable	**25**	56	58	59	61	62	64	66	67	69	71
	24	54	55	57	58	60	61	63	65	66	68
	23	52	53	55	56	57	59	60	62	63	65
	22	50	51	52	54	55	56	58	59	61	62
	21	47	49	50	51	52	54	55	57	58	59
	20	45	46	47	49	50	51	53	54	55	56
Underweight	**19**	43	44	45	46	47	49	50	51	52	54
	18	41	42	43	44	45	46	47	48	50	51
	17	38	39	40	41	42	44	45	46	47	48
Height	m	1.50	1.52	1.54	1.56	1.58	1.60	1.62	1.64	1.66	1.68
	ft ins	4.11	5.0	$5.0\frac{3}{4}$	$5.1\frac{1}{2}$	$5.2\frac{1}{4}$	5.3	$5.3\frac{3}{4}$	$5.4\frac{1}{2}$	$5.5\frac{1}{2}$	5.6

Appendices

3 Height and weight charts

Table A3.2 (*continued*)

	Body mass index	Weight (kg) (to the nearest 1 kg)													
Dangerously overweight	45	130	133	136	139	143	146	149	152	156	159	162	166	169	173
	44	127	130	133	136	139	143	146	149	152	156	159	162	166	169
	43	124	127	130	133	136	139	142	146	149	152	155	159	162	165
	42	121	124	127	130	133	136	139	142	145	148	152	155	158	161
	41	119	121	124	127	130	133	136	139	142	145	148	151	154	158
Seriously overweight	40	116	118	121	124	127	130	133	135	138	141	144	148	151	154
	39	113	115	118	121	124	126	129	132	135	138	141	144	147	150
	38	110	112	115	118	120	123	126	129	132	134	137	140	143	146
	37	107	110	112	115	117	120	123	125	128	131	134	136	139	142
	36	104	107	109	112	114	117	119	122	125	127	130	133	136	138
	35	101	104	106	108	111	113	116	119	121	124	126	129	132	134
	34	98	101	103	105	108	110	113	115	118	120	123	125	128	131
	33	95	98	100	102	105	107	109	112	114	117	119	122	124	127
	32	93	95	97	99	101	104	106	108	111	113	116	118	120	123
	31	90	92	94	96	98	100	103	105	107	110	112	114	117	119
Overweight	30	87	89	91	93	95	97	99	102	104	106	108	111	113	115
	29	84	86	88	90	92	94	96	98	100	103	105	107	109	111
	28	81	83	85	87	89	91	93	95	97	99	101	103	105	108
	27	78	80	82	84	86	88	89	91	93	95	98	100	102	104
	26	75	77	79	81	82	84	86	88	90	92	94	96	98	100
Acceptable	25	72	74	76	77	79	81	83	85	87	88	90	92	94	96
	24	69	71	73	74	76	78	80	81	83	85	87	89	90	92
	23	67	68	70	71	73	75	76	78	80	81	83	85	87	88
	22	64	65	67	68	70	71	73	75	76	78	79	81	83	85
	21	61	62	64	65	67	68	70	71	73	74	76	77	79	81
	20	58	59	61	62	63	65	66	68	69	71	72	74	75	77
Underweight	19	55	56	58	59	60	62	63	64	66	67	69	70	72	73
	18	52	53	55	56	57	58	60	61	62	64	65	66	68	69
	17	49	50	52	53	54	55	56	58	59	60	61	63	64	65
Height	m	1.70	1.72	1.74	1.76	1.78	1.80	1.82	1.84	1.86	1.88	1.90	1.92	1.94	1.96
	ft ins	$5.6\frac{3}{4}$	$5.7\frac{3}{4}$	$5.8\frac{1}{2}$	$5.9\frac{1}{4}$	5.10	$5.10\frac{3}{4}$	$5.11\frac{3}{4}$	$6.0\frac{1}{2}$	$6.1\frac{1}{4}$	6.2	$6.2\frac{3}{4}$	$6.3\frac{3}{4}$	$6.4\frac{1}{2}$	$6.5\frac{1}{4}$

4   Inflammatory bowel disease record form

A card containing essential information, filed at the front of the notes, is very helpful when managing patients with ulcerative colitis or Crohn's disease (p. 256). The following diagrammatic format, adapted from that used at the Central Middlesex Hospital, London, can be updated as necessary.

INFLAMMATORY BOWEL DISEASE RECORD FORM

Name: ....   Diagnosis: ....

Hospital No.: ....   Date of diagnosis: ....

Sheet No.: ....   Date of onset of symptoms: ....

Small bowel Radiology	Barium enema	Colonoscopy	Operation	Histology	Complications/ Special features
Date:	Date:	Date:			
Date:	Date:	Date:			
Date:	Date:	Date:			
Date:	Date:	Date:			

5   Diagnostic dilemmas

When the diagnosis is in doubt, or investigations contribute to rather than resolve the confusion, the following approach is recommended.

- Take a careful history again, paying attention to what the patient says
- Re-examine the patient, paying special attention to lymph nodes, external genitalia and rectal examination, because these areas are often overlooked on the initial examination
- List the investigations and results, in chronological order
- Seek advice if the way ahead remains unclear
- Do *not* order another test and hope that someone else sees the patient next time!

Index

Page numbers in *italic* refer to figures, those in **bold** refer to tables.

Index

Index

Index

Index